D0852463

Obesity
Etiology
Assessment
Treatment
and Prevention

Ross E. Andersen, PhD
Johns Hopkins School of Medicine

Editor

Human Kinetics

L.C.C. SOUTH CAMPUS LIBRARY

Library of Congress Cataloging-in-Publication Data

Obesity : etiology, assessment, treatment, and prevention / Ross E.
Andersen, editor.
    p. ; cm.
Includes bibliographical references and index.
 ISBN 0-7360-0328-2 (hard cover)
 1. Obesity.
 [DNLM: 1. Obesity--diagnosis. 2. Obesity--etiology. 3.
Obesity--therapy. 4. Risk Assessment. 5. Socioeconomic Factors. WD
210 O11215 2003] I. Andersen, Ross.
 RC628.O264 2003
 616.3'98--dc21   2002156665

ISBN: 0-7360-0328-2

Copyright © 2003 by Human Kinetics Publishers, Inc.

All rights reserved. Except for use in a review, the reproduction or utilization of this work in any form or by any electronic, mechanical, or other means, now known or hereafter invented, including xerography, photocopying, and recording, and in any information storage and retrieval system, is forbidden without the written permission of the publisher.

Acquisitions Editor: Michael S. Bahrke, PhD
Developmental Editor: D.K. Bihler
Assistant Editor: Kathleen D. Bernard
Copyeditor: Patsy Fortney
Proofreader: Pamela Johnson
Indexer: Susan Danzi Hernandez
Permission Manager: Dalene Reeder
Graphic Designer: Andrew Tietz
Graphic Artist: Yvonne Griffith
Photo Manager: Kareema McLendon
Cover Designer: Robert Reuther
Photographer (interior): Photo on p. 1 © Kim Karpeles; photo on p. 57 © DigitalVisionOnline; and photo on p. 139 © Raw Talent Photo
Art Manager: Kelly Hendren
Illustrator: Accurate Art
Printer: Sheridan Books

Printed in the United States of America   10 9 8 7 6 5 4 3 2 1

Human Kinetics
Web site: www.HumanKinetics.com

United States: Human Kinetics; P.O. Box 5076; Champaign, IL 61825-5076
800-747-4457
e-mail: humank@hkusa.com

Canada: Human Kinetics; 475 Devonshire Road Unit 100; Windsor, ON N8Y 2L5
800-465-7301 (in Canada only)
e-mail: orders@hkcanada.com

Europe: Human Kinetics; 107 Bradford Road; Stanningley; Leeds LS28 6AT, United Kingdom
+44 (0) 113 255 5665
e-mail: hk@hkeurope.com

Australia: Human Kinetics; 57A Price Avenue; Lower Mitcham, South Australia 5062
08 8277 1555
e-mail: liahka@senet.com.au

New Zealand: Human Kinetics; P.O. Box 105-231, Auckland Central
09-523-3462
e-mail: hkp@ihug.co.nz

RC
628
.O264
2003

JUN 1 7 2004

Contents

Foreword

Over the past 20 years, the prevalence of obesity has increased dramatically in North America and Europe, a trend that now appears to be spreading throughout the world. The seriousness of this problem was not fully appreciated until about five years ago. Prior to that time there was no scientific consensus as to how to classify individuals as overweight or obese. Consequently, research studies reporting prevalence data used several different cutoff points, so prevalence estimates varied considerably from study to study. In 1997, the World Health Organization convened a consultation of experts in the field of obesity to deal with issues related to this growing epidemic. Out of this consultation came a formal report, published in 1998 (World Health Organization 1998). Included in this report was a recommendation to classify overweight and obesity on the basis of body mass index (BMI), defined as the ratio of weight in kilograms to height in meters squared (kg/m^2). This recommendation was widely accepted, thus providing a rational basis for more objectively classifying people into the categories of underweight (BMI <18.5), normal weight (BMI 18.5-24.9), overweight (BMI 25.0-29.9), and obese (BMI ≥30.0).

With this new classification system in place, experts now estimate that more than 60% of U.S. men and women are overweight or obese (BMI ≥25.0). Further, between the data collection periods of 1976-1980 and 1999-2000 the prevalence of obesity (BMI ≥30.0) increased from 12.7 to 27.7% in men and from 17.0 to 34.0% in women (Flegal et al. 2002). The problem is much more significant in Mexican American men and women and black women.

Concern is not limited to adults, as similar trends have been reported in children and adolescents. Using the criteria of ≥95th percentile for body mass index, the prevalence of overweight in 6- to 11-year-old children increased from 6.5 to 15.3%, and in 12- to 19-year-old adolescents from 5.0 to 15.5%, between the data collection periods of 1976-1980 and 1999-2000. The largest increases were in blacks and Mexican Americans (Ogden et al.

2002). These figures point to a serious epidemic that has already manifested itself in an increase in hypertension and type 2 diabetes, and will likely increase the prevalence of coronary artery disease. In fact, type 2 diabetes, formerly known as adult-onset diabetes, is now being diagnosed in children and is appearing in adolescents at an alarming rate.

Public health, medical, nutrition, and exercise researchers and practitioners clearly must mobilize their resources to combat this epidemic by developing more effective strategies for treating people who are overweight and obese. Many have turned to pharmacological and surgical interventions out of frustration with the disappointing results from nutrition and exercise interventions. However, considering the magnitude of the problem, the economy will simply not be able to afford the costs associated with surgery and long-term drug use for everyone who is overweight or obese. Rather, researchers and practitioners will have to address the integration of behavioral, nutritional, and exercise interventions in a more focused and creative manner.

More important, however, is the need for health professionals to address prevention. Presently, the success rate in getting overweight and obese people to lose weight and maintain that weight loss for a five-year period or longer is not encouraging. Preventing undesirable weight gain, starting with children and continuing throughout life, should have a more positive outcome, although few data are available to support this. Clearly we need to emphasize healthy patterns of eating and physical activity. Yet it is difficult to compete with people's desire for supersized food portions, high intake of dietary fat, excessive watching of television and playing of video games, and other forces of modern society that work against maintaining a healthy weight.

This book, *Obesity: Etiology, Assessment, Treatment, and Prevention*, is an attempt by its editor, Dr. Ross Andersen from the Johns Hopkins School of Medicine, and some of the top scientists and practitioners in the world who specialize in the area of weight control, to provide clinicians and scientists with the most current information on the prevention and treatment of overweight and obesity. The book is divided into three sections. The first section addresses the etiology of obesity and considers the prevalence and psychosocial consequences of overweight and obesity. It also addresses the economic aspects of, and genetic influences on, obesity. The second section deals with assessment, including quality of life, body composition, clinical evaluation, diet, and physical activity. The third section concerns treatment and prevention, with chapters on aging, pediatric obesity, medical nutrition therapy, reducing physical inactivity, and increasing physical activity. This section ends with a chapter on medication for weight management and a chapter on future directions in the treatment of obesity.

This book has been written at a very critical time in the war against overweight and obesity. For those engaged in this battle, this book will be invaluable.

Jack H. Wilmore
Distinguished Professor, Department of Health and Kinesiology, Texas A&M University

References

Flegal, K.M., Carroll, M.D., Ogden, C.L., and Johnson, C.L. 2002. Prevalence and trends in obesity among U.S. adults, 1999-2000. *JAMA* 288: 1723-1727.

Ogden, C.L., Flegal, K.M., Carroll, M.D., and Johnson, C.L. 2002. Prevalence and trends in overweight among U.S. children and adolescents, 1999-2000. *JAMA* 288: 1728-1732.

World Health Organization. 1998. *Obesity: Preventing and managing the global epidemic*. Geneva: World Health Organization.

List of Contributors

Barbara E. Ainsworth, PhD, MPH
University of South Carolina at Columbia

David B. Allison, PhD
Clinical Nutrition Research Center, University of Alabama at Birmingham

Judith M. Ashley, PhD, MSPH, RD
University of Nevada School of Medicine

Susan J. Bartlett, PhD
Division of Rheumatology, Johns Hopkins School of Medicine

Adrian Bauman, MD, PhD
University of New South Wales, Sydney, Australia

Brock A. Beamer, MD
Johns Hopkins Geriatrics Center and Johns Hopkins School of Medicine

Vicki H. Bovee, MS, RD
University of Nevada School of Medicine

Dana M. Catanese, BA
Mid America Heart Institute and University of Missouri at Kansas City

Paul A. Cavazos, BA
Center for Eating and Weight Disorders, San Diego State University

David Crawford, PhD
Deakin University, Melbourne, Australia

Carlos J. Crespo, DrPH, MS, FACSM
University at Buffalo, State University of New York

Loretta DiPietro, PhD, MPH
Yale University School of Medicine

Samuel C. Durso, MD
Johns Hopkins School of Medicine

James Dziura, PhD, MPH
Yale University School of Medicine

Myles S. Faith, PhD
University of Pennsylvania School of Medicine

Kevin R. Fontaine, PhD
Division of Rheumatology, Johns Hopkins School of Medicine

John P. Foreyt, PhD
Baylor College of Medicine

Shawn C. Franckowiak, BS
Johns Hopkins School of Medicine

William Hartman, PhD
Weight Management Program of San Francisco

Helen Hayden-Wade, PhD
Children's Hospital, San Diego

Melissa L. Hyder, BA
Mid America Heart Institute and University of Missouri at Kansas City

John M. Jakicic, PhD
University of Pittsburgh

Michael J. LaMonte, PhD, MPH
University of Utah

Timothy G. Lohman, PhD
University of Arizona at Tucson

Patty E. Matz, PhD
Weill Medical College, Cornell University

Laurie Milliken, PhD
University of Massachusetts at Boston

Walker S. Carlos Poston, PhD, MPH
Mid America Heart Institute and University of Missouri at Kansas City

Nicolaas P. Pronk, PhD
HealthPartners Research Foundation

Brian E. Saelens, PhD
Cincinnati Children's Hospital Medical Center and the University of Cincinnati College of Medicine

Joan Saxton, MD
Weight Management Program of San Francisco and University of California at San Francisco

Ellen Smit, PhD, RD
University at Buffalo, State University of New York

Laure Sullivan, RD
Johns Hopkins School of Medicine

Marian Tanofsky-Kraff, MA
The National Institute of Child Health and Human Development, National Institutes of Health

Catrine Tudor-Locke, PhD
Arizona State University East

Denise E. Wilfley, PhD
Washington University School of Medicine, St. Louis

Jack H. Wilmore, PhD
Texas A&M University

Preface

Obesity is increasing in the United States and around the world at an alarming rate. It is well known that many adverse health outcomes are associated with being obese, and in many cases, weight reduction can result in dramatic improvements in health. Unfortunately, consumers are confused as to which approach to use to lose and ultimately manage their weight. Each day the public is bombarded with infomercials, magazines, and popular books that offer conflicting information.

Clinicians who work with overweight and obese patients come from many different backgrounds, including clinical nutrition, psychology, exercise science, and medicine. This book is written for any health professional who works with obese clients or patients. The purpose of this text is to offer the clinician working with overweight individuals a comprehensive reference manual so they will have a working knowledge of the many complex fields of study that are involved in treating overweight individuals. All of the authors who contributed chapters to this text have extensive experience in their respective areas.

This book is divided into three sections. The first consists of four chapters that describe the scope and gravity of the obesity epidemic. In chapter 1, Drs. Crespo and Smit report the current statistics related to the prevalence of obesity. In chapter 2, Dr. Faith and colleagues describe the psychosocial correlates that are associated with being obese; while in chapter 3, Dr. Pronk reports on the economic burden that obesity places on our society. Dr. Beamer reports on the importance of understanding the genetic influences of obesity in chapter 4.

The following section, Assessment of the Obese Patient, contains five chapters that offer clinicians tools for assessing the overweight patient. Specific details of assessing the patient's quality of life are offered in chapter 5, while Drs. Lohman and Milliken offer strategies and considerations for assessing body composition in obese individuals in chapter 6. In chapter 7, Dr. Durso explains how to provide a comprehensive clinical evaluation. Assessing dietary records and physical activity are covered in chapters 8 and 9.

The final section presents eight chapters with treatment strategies to help patients better manage their weight. Chapter 10 addresses the importance of weight maintenance, and chapter 12 presents strategies for helping patients make dietary changes, while the authors of chapters 13 and 14 describe innovative strategies for promoting physical activity. In chapter 15, Dr. Saelens offers strategies on how to help individuals reduce sedentary activity. Drs. Bauman and Crawford have described the environmental changes that can be implemented as a strategy for obesity prevention in chapter 16. This section of the book also includes a chapter on pediatric obesity, chapter 11, as well as a chapter on using medications for weight management, chapter 17. The final chapter by Dr. John Foreyt and colleagues offers insights into the future directions of obesity treatment.

Obesity is a complex medical problem. Health care professionals are no longer preaching a single approach to losing weight. It has become clear that treatment must integrate physical activity, nutrition, psychology, and medicine. This is a unique and timely text that should offer practitioners up-to-date strategies in each of these fields to help their obese and overweight patients better manage their weight.

Acknowledgments

I am grateful to all of the contributors, who took time out of their busy schedules to write chapters and share their knowledge in this text. In addition, thanks are due to Richard (Dick) Cotton, who served as a scientific reviewer of all chapters. I would also like to thank Mike Bahrke and D.K. Bihler from Human Kinetics, who have helped tremendously in moving this book through the lengthy production process. Finally, I would like to thank my wife, Susan, and my two daughters, Katie and Nicole, for their love and encouragement.

PART I

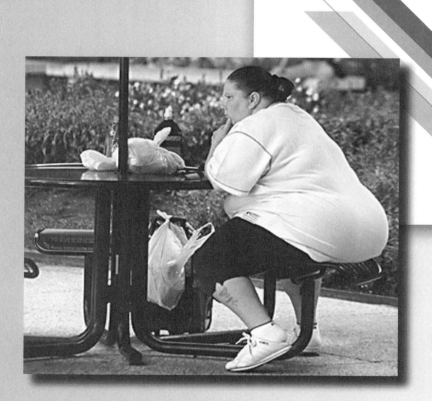

Etiology
of Obesity

Chapter 1

Prevalence of Overweight and Obesity in the United States

Carlos J. Crespo, DrPH, MS, FACSM
Ellen Smit, PhD, RD
Department of Social and Preventive Medicine, School of Medicine and Biomedical Sciences, University at Buffalo, State University of New York

Obesity is unquestionably a condition of public health significance in the United States. Pre-obesity (BMI 25-29.9) and obesity (BMI ≥30), as well as other conditions for which these serve as a major risk factor, are highly prevalent in all groups of the population (Allison and Saunders 2000; Pi-Sunyer 1999). It is therefore of interest to know which groups are affected, and to what extent this condition is disproportionately represented in certain segments of the U.S. population. In this chapter, we will examine how obesity occurs in various groups. For adults the prevalence of overweight (BMI ≥25) is consistently high, regardless of how the data were obtained (e.g., home interviews, telephone interviews, physical examination surveys, or surveillance systems). What the different data systems confirm is that U.S. adults are becoming more and more obese as time goes on. In fact, the number of adults who are morbidly obese (BMI ≥39) ranks in the millions (Blair and Nichaman 2002; Flegal et al. 1998; Kuczmarski 1993; Schoenborn, Adams, and Barnes 2002).

Prevalence of Obesity Among Adults

An estimated 97 million adults in the United States are overweight or obese, and with obesity comes a host of other preventable chronic diseases and conditions (Pi-Sunyer 1999). In addition to increasing mortality from all causes, obesity is closely linked to hypertension, type 2 diabetes mellitus, dyslipidemia, gallbladder disease, osteoarthritis, coronary heart disease, stroke, sleep apnea, and other respiratory problems. Other studies have found that obesity is a risk factor for endometrial, breast, prostate, and colon cancer, making this condition a substantial contributor to premature mortality (Bianchini, Kaaks, and Vainio 2002; Terry, Miller, and Rohan 2002).

Earlier data from the National Health Examination Survey (NHES) and the National Health and Nutrition Examination Survey (NHANES) used the 85th percentile of BMI for persons 20 to 29 years of age as a cutoff point to estimate the prevalence of overweight (Kuczmarski et al. 1994). Using these previous cutoff points, men with BMI ≥27.8 or women with BMI ≥27.3 were considered overweight. More recently, the World Health Organization and the U.S. National Institutes of Health (NIH) modified the excess body weight cutoff points to distinguish between overweight and obesity. The evidence-based report titled "Clinical Guidelines on the Identification, Evaluation, and Treatment of Overweight and Obesity in Adults" recommended that overweight be defined as a BMI between 25 and 29.9, and that obesity be defined as a BMI greater than or equal to 30 (Pi-Sunyer 2000). Table 1.1 shows the NIH's National Obesity Education Initiative proposed classification and the disease risk relative to normal weight and waist circumference.

This chapter includes some data that predate the recent WHO and NIH BMI cutoffs. Therefore, we will use the terms *excess body weight* to refer to the cutoff points for men with BMI ≥27.8 or women with BMI ≥27.3, *pre-obesity* to refer to cutoffs of BMI between 25 and 29.9, *overweight* for BMI ≥25, and *obesity* for BMI ≥30. Overweight and obesity are not necessarily mutually exclusive conditions since obese persons are also overweight (Arroyo et al. 2000; Flegal et al. 1998; Kuczmarski 1993; Pi-Sunyer 2000). More information on the value of BMI in the characterization of obesity will be discussed in later chapters.

The prevalence of obesity is a major public health concern throughout the United States (see figure 1.1 for the percent distribution of the

Table 1.1 — National Obesity Education Initiative Classification Table

	BMI (kg/m²)	Obesity class	Disease risk relative to normal weight and waist circumference	
			Men ≤102 cm (≤40 in.) Women ≤88 cm (≤35 in.)	>102 cm (>40 in.) >88 cm (>35 in.)
Underweight	<18.5			
Normal	18.5-24.9			
Overweight	25-29.9		Increased	High
Obese	30-34.9	I	High	Very high
	35-39.9	II	Very high	Very high
Extremely obese	≥40	III	Extremely high	Extremely high

Reprinted from Obesity Education Initiative Clinical Guidelines.

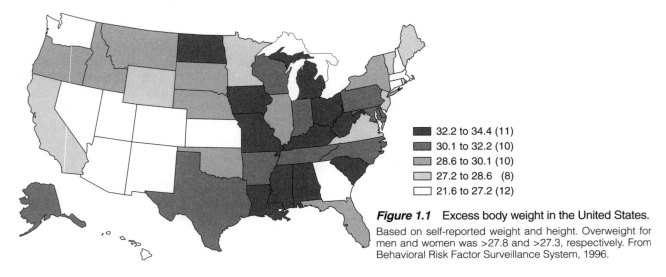

Figure 1.1 Excess body weight in the United States.
Based on self-reported weight and height. Overweight for men and women was >27.8 and >27.3, respectively. From Behavioral Risk Factor Surveillance System, 1996.

32.2 to 34.4 (11)
30.1 to 32.2 (10)
28.6 to 30.1 (10)
27.2 to 28.6 (8)
21.6 to 27.2 (12)

prevalence of adults with excess body weight), with higher prevalence mostly occurring in the middle to eastern part of the United States with the exception of Georgia and the New England states (Bolen et al. 2000). Data from the Third National Health and Nutrition Examination Survey (NHANES III), conducted between 1988 and 1994, revealed that overweight is a pervasive condition among non-Hispanic whites and blacks, and among Mexican Ameri-cans (Flegal 1999). Unfortunately, data on other minority groups have not been collected sys-tematically (Kuczmarski et al. 1994).

Surveys prior to NHANES III had an age limit of 74. During NHANES III, persons two months of age and older were eligible to participate in the study. Data from NHANES is unique, in that sampled persons went through a battery of an-thropometric measurements including weight and height measurements. Table 1.2 shows the

Table 1.2 — Body Weight Distribution Among U.S. Adults

	Sample size	Healthy weight (BMI = 18.5-24.9) %	Overweight (BMI ≥25) %	Obese (BMI ≥30) %
All	17,030	42.8	54.8	22.1
Men	7,953	39.6	59.1	19.4
Non-Hispanic white	3,271	39.2	59.5	19.5
Non-Hispanic black	2,094	40.8	56.8	20.7
Mexican American	2,233	32.2	66.6	22.4
Women	9,077	45.8	50.3	24.5
Non-Hispanic white	3,813	49.6	46.6	22.2
Non-Hispanic black	2,577	30.3	66.4	36.4
Mexican American	2,253	31.2	66.4	33.2
Education				
<12 years	7,016	38.9	58.0	25.8
12 years	5,106	40.1	57.8	24.4
13-15 years	2,696	44.9	52.3	20.7
16 or more years	2,087	50.6	46.5	14.5
Income				
<$10,000	2,638	40.8	55.1	27.0
$10,000-$19,999	4,347	39.5	57.8	25.9
$20,000-$34,999	3,695	41.1	56.1	22.4
$35,000-$49,999	2,109	44.9	53.2	20.4
$50,000+	3,792	46.2	51.2	19.0
Poverty				
Below poverty	3,617	37.9	58.7	27.6
1-1.85 above poverty	3,756	40.5	56.4	25.8
1.85+ above poverty	9,657	44.2	53.2	20.4

age-adjusted prevalence (per 100) of persons of normal weight (BMI 18.5-24.9), overweight (BMI ≥25), and obese (BMI ≥30) in U.S. adults 20 years and older. Overweight was higher among men (59.1%, 95th confidence interval (CI): 57.4-61.4) than among women (50.3%, 95th CI: 48.6-52.8), yet more women (24.5%, 95th CI: 22.7-26.6) were obese than men (19.4%, 95th CI: 18.1-20.9). These results indicate that more men have a BMI greater than or equal to 25, but more women have a BMI greater than or equal to 30.

The prevalence of overweight (BMI ≥25) is highest among Mexican American men, as shown in figure 1.2, and it peaks between the ages of 50 and 59. The prevalence is lowest among persons between the ages of 20 and 29 and among those 70 and older. There may be several explanations for the differences in the age distribution of overweight. First, the prevalence observed among those 20 to 29

years may not change in subsequent years, thus producing a "cohort effect." Similarly, the cohort of men with the highest prevalence of overweight, those 50 to 59 years old, may still be the most overweight cohort 30 years from now, when they are 80 years old and older. Another explanation for the lower prevalence of overweight among persons 70 and older may be that those who were overweight died before age 70 and were not available to be randomly selected for the study, producing a "survivor effect." Thus, those persons with healthier body weight tend to live longer, and obese individuals are less likely to survive past age 60.

As shown in figure 1.3, the prevalence of overweight among minority women is greater than among non-Hispanic white women before age 70. As observed in Mexican American men, Mexican American women consistently

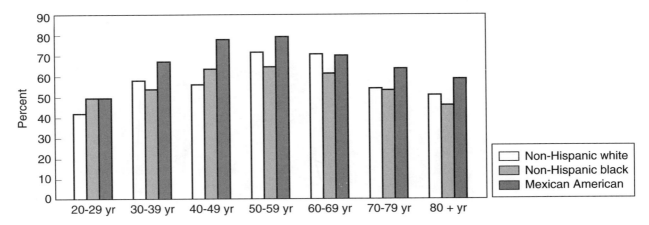

Figure 1.2 Prevalence of overweight in U.S. men.
From NHANES III, 1988-1994.

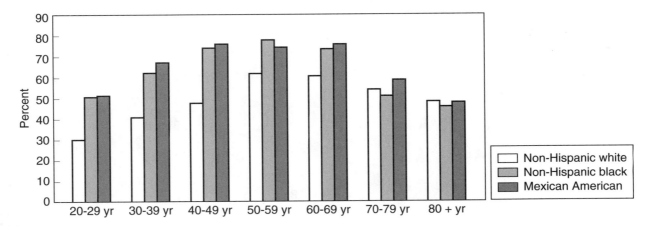

Figure 1.3 Prevalence of overweight in U.S. women.
From NHANES III, 1988-1994.

have a higher prevalence of overweight than any other group of non-Hispanic whites and across all age groups. Non-Hispanic black women also experience a higher prevalence of overweight and obesity between ages 20 and 69, whereas in the older age groups the prevalence is similar to non-Hispanic whites. As with men, overweight peaks for non-Hispanic black women at ages 50 to 59 and for Mexican American women at ages 60 to 69. These estimates of overweight are concomitant with the excess burden of other chronic diseases such as type 2 diabetes, heart disease, hypertension, breast cancer, and other conditions that occur during this period of life for both men and women (Kopelman 2000; Martorell et al. 2000; Ostir et al. 2000). To what extent overweight and obesity are causative or predisposing factors will be discussed later in this book.

Overweight (BMI ≥25), which also includes obese persons (BMI ≥30), peaks during the ages of 40 to 69, as illustrated in figures 1.2 and 1.3. To distinguish between overweight and obesity, we show the prevalence of obesity (BMI ≥30) in figures 1.4 and 1.5. Among men (see figure 1.4), the prevalence of obesity was lowest among those 80 years and older. This may again be due to a survivor effect. Non-Hispanic black men between the ages of 20 and 29 had a higher prevalence of obesity than their non-Hispanic white and Mexican American counterparts in the same age group. Between the ages of 40 and 59, Mexican American men had the highest prevalence of obesity, yet the lowest prevalence of obesity was observed among Mexican American men age 80 or older.

Obesity was more prevalent among non-Hispanic black and Mexican American women

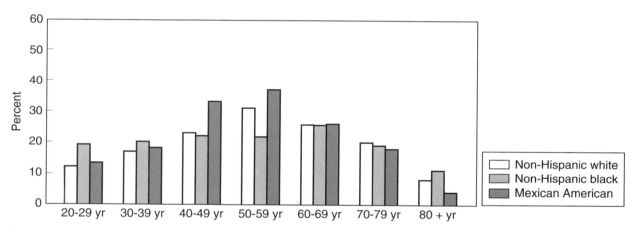

Figure 1.4   Prevalence of obesity in U.S. men.
From NHANES III, 1988-1994.

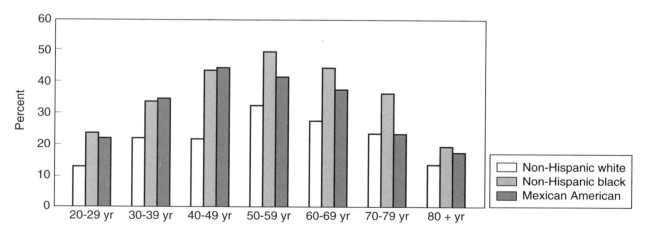

Figure 1.5   Prevalence of obesity in U.S. women.
From NHANES III, 1988-1994.

than among non-Hispanic white women in every age group. Among women ages 70 to 79, black women had the highest prevalence of obesity when compared to their non-Hispanic white and Mexican American counterparts in the same age group. Almost half of all black women between the ages of 50 and 59 were obese, and consistently over 40% of all black women between the ages of 40 and 69 were obese (see figure 1.5).

Prevalence of Obesity Among College Students

More female college students think of themselves as being overweight than do their male counterparts; however, the percent of college males and females who were overweight, according to their BMI, was not drastically different. It is interesting to note that only among male black college students was the percent of persons with excess body weight greater than the percent that thought that they were overweight. In every other group, more persons considered themselves overweight than actually were. These results revealed that not only may gender differences play a role in who considers themselves overweight, but cultural differences may also play an important role (Bolen et al. 2000; Debate, Topping, and Sargent 2001; Kumanyika 1993).

Gregg and Narayan (1998) studied 2,205 black and white girls aged 9 and 10 and reported racial variation in the relationship between self-esteem and adiposity, with the magnitude of the effect somewhat less in black girls. Whether this racial difference extends to college students needs to be further studied (Gregg and Narayan 1998). Several investigators (Faith et al. 2001; Epstein 1996; Epstein et al. 2000; Jeffery 1991) have suggested that obesity in minority groups in the United States is best understood as a variation on a larger cultural theme—the creation of an environment in which highly palatable foods are accessible to all at low cost and physical activity is not required. A cultural acceptance toward higher body weight among blacks and Hispanics may also explain why minorities may be at higher risk for overweight, but this remains to be studied further (Gregg and Narayan 1998).

Prevalence of Obesity Among Children

Adults have been classified as obese based on a variety of studies, reference population criteria, and more recently, data relating morbidity as well as mortality to weight status (Pi-Sunyer 1999). In the absence of outcome-based criteria for children, a statistical approach is the most practical choice for classification (Bellizzi and Dietz 1999; Cole et al. 2000; Guillaume 1999; Malina and Katzmarzyk 1999). Overweight or obesity will therefore be defined relative to a selected sex- and age-specific percentile of a reference population. In this chapter, we will define overweight and obesity as the 85th and 95th percentiles, respectively, based on sex- and age-specific groups of children examined during two national representative health examination surveys: NHES II (1963-1965) and NHES III (1966-1970) (Troiano and Flegal 1999). A recent workshop on childhood obesity concluded that although body mass index is not a perfect measure in children because it covaries with height, it has been validated against measurements of body density (Dietz and Bellizzi 1999). Obese children (95th percentile) do tend to become overweight adults and therefore may have a better positive predictive value than overweight children (85th percentile) (Guo and Chumlea 1999; Malina and Katzmarzyk 1999).

Overweight and obesity in children ages 8 to 16 has increased dramatically in the United States. Data from NHANES III conducted from 1988 to 1994 showed that approximately 25% of children ages 8 to 16 were overweight, and 12% were obese. Preliminary data from the NHANES of 1999 showed continued increments in obesity prevalence among both boys and girls (National Center for Health Statistics 2002). Overweight and obesity were not drastically different between boys and girls, although more girls tried to lose weight than did boys (Bolen et al. 2000; Bowen, Tomoyasu, and Cauce 1991).

Both Mexican American boys and girls, and non-Hispanic black girls, aged 8 to 16 have some of the highest prevalence of obesity in the United States, ranging from 15.5 to 17.1% (see table 1.3). It is unclear what cultural, lifestyle, genetic, or environmental factors may explain these differences (Bowen et al. 1991;

Table 1.3   *Overweight and Obesity in U.S. Children*

	N	Overweight		Obese	
		Prevalence (SE)	95% CI	Prevalence (SE)	95% CI
Total	4,113	27.2 (1.3)	24.4, 30.0	12.4 (0.9)	10.5, 14.4
Boys	2,021	29.0 (1.6)	25.8, 32.3	13.8 (1.5)	10.7, 16.8
8-10 years	809	31.4 (2.5)	26.3, 36.4	17.3 (2.7)	11.9, 22.8
11-13 years	660	28.3 (2.3)	23.6, 33.0	11.9 (2.0)	8.0, 15.9
14-16 years	552	27.4 (3.8)	19.8, 35.0	12.0 (2.8)	6.4, 17.5
Girls	2,092	25.3 (1.7)	21.7, 28.8	11.1 (1.1)	8.8, 13.4
8-10 years	759	24.5 (2.5)	19.5, 29.4	11.8 (1.7)	8.3, 15.3
11-13 years	711	25.8(2.9)	19.9, 31.6	11.4 (1.8)	7.8, 15.0
14-16 years	622	25.7 (3.0)	19.6, 31.7	10.0 (1.7)	6.6, 13.5
Race/ethnicity:					
Non-Hispanic whites	1,071	26.4 (1.9)	22.7, 30.2	11.9 (1.3)	9.3, 14.5
Boys	513	29.1 (2.2)	24.7, 33.5	12.8 (1.9)	9.0, 16.6
Girls	558	23.6 (2.3)	18.9, 28.2	10.9 (1.5)	7.8, 13.9
Non-Hispanic blacks	1,450	29.3 (1.2)	27.0, 31.6	15.5 (1.1)	12.9, 17.2
Boys	722	28.9 (1.7)	22.6, 29.2	14.4 (1.3)	11.8, 17.0
Girls	728	32.8 (1.9)	29.0, 36.5	15.7 (1.6)	12.5, 19.0
Mexican Americans	1,406	33.7 (2.6)	28.4, 38.9	16.3 (2.0)	12.2, 20.4
Boys	695	35.1 (2.3)	30.5, 39.7	17.1 (2.1)	12.9, 21.4
Girls	711	32.2 (3.6)	24.9, 39.5	15.5 (2.9)	9.6, 21.4

Prevalence (per 100) of U.S. children aged 8 to 16 who were overweight (using age- and gender-specific 85th percentile of BMI from NHES 1963-1970) and obese (using age- and gender-specific 95th percentile of BMI from NHES 1963-1970) by age and race and ethnicity, 1988-1994. SE=standard error; CI=confidence interval

Cole et al. 2000; Jeffery 1991; Roberts 2000). Public health officials have tried to identify modifiable risk factors to implement policies that will have an impact on obesity prevalence in minority populations.

We have found that television watching is positively related to adiposity (Andersen et al. 1998) and that obesity also increases with more television viewing (Crespo et al. 2001; Gortmaker et al. 1996). *Healthy People 2010* has also identified television viewing as an important public health target to reduce the percent of children who watch television for two or more hours a day (U.S. Department of Health and Human Services 2000). Figure 1.6 shows the prevalence of obesity increasing with the number of hours watched. The lowest prevalence was observed among those who watch one hour of television or less per day. Although television watching is not the only cause of physical inactivity, it does serve as a good estimate of the number of hours that children spend being inactive (Andersen et al. 1998).

Ogden and colleagues (1997), in their examination of the prevalence of obesity in preschool children, observed notable increases among children 4 and 5 years of age between NHANES II (1976-1980) and NHANES III (1988-1994), but not in younger children. The prevalence of obesity was twice as high for Mexican American boys and girls than it was for non-Hispanic white boys and girls ages 1 and 2. Non-Hispanic black girls also exhibited a higher prevalence of obesity than did non-Hispanic white girls younger than 2 years of age (Dennison, Erb, and Jenkins 2002; Ogden et al. 1997). It is therefore not surprising to observe a greater prevalence of obesity among minority adolescents and adults.

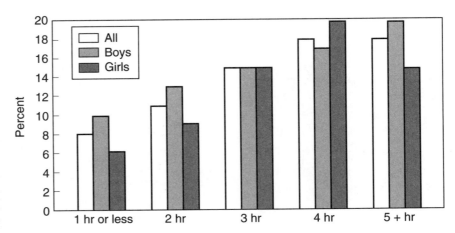

Figure 1.6 Prevalence of obesity by hours of television watching in children 8 to 16 years of age.

Reprinted, by permission, from C.J. Crespo et al. 2001, "Television watching, energy intake, and obesity in U.S. children," *Archives of Pediatric Adolescence Medicine* 155: 360-365.

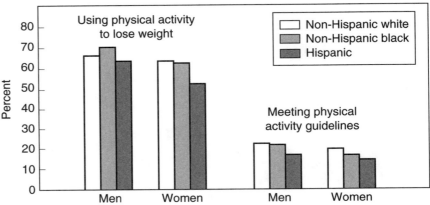

Figure 1.7 Physical activity among overweight adults.

From MMWR, April 21 2000 Vol 47, 326-330.

Prevalence of Obesity and Physical Activity

Lack of physical activity and excess caloric consumption are some of the reasons epidemiologists suggest for the increase of obesity in the last 20 years (Allred 1995; Andersen et al. 1998; Crespo et al. 2001; Gortmaker et al. 1999; Roberts, Lucas, and Hirsch 2000). A panel of experts met at the 1999 American College of Sports Medicine to more clearly understand the role of exercise in the prevention and treatment of obesity (Blair and Brodney 1999). The evidence reviewed suggested that exercise is beneficial in the prevention of weight gain and is also an important adjunct therapeutic modality in the treatment of obesity. In the general population, however, barely 24% of the population engages in physical activity for

30 minutes a day, five or more days a week as recommended by the U.S. surgeon general. It is unclear whether overweight persons accurately report their exercise habits, and whether those who report exercising do so at the recommended frequency, intensity, and duration.

Figure 1.7 presents the percent of overweight adults who reported using physical activity as a way to lose weight. Although two out of three (67% for men and 62% for women) of the overweight adults reported using physical activity as a strategy to lose weight, only one out of five (22% of men and 20% of women) met the recommended physical activity guidelines of being physically active for 30 minutes most days of the week. Given that between 22 and 25% of the general population report meeting the recommended amount of moderate-intensity physical activity (30 minutes a day, most days of the week), the findings from this study show that overweight adults are no more active than the general population. The authors reported that, for both sexes, using physical activity to lose weight was inversely related to age and BMI and directly related to education levels. Additionally, the prevalence of using physical activity to lose weight was highest among black men and lowest among Hispanics of both sexes. The southern states had the lowest percent of people who reported using physical activity as a strategy to lose weight (Gordon et al. 2000).

Prevalence of Obesity and Social Class

Some researchers have suggested that the prevalence of obesity is related to social class (Cole et al. 2000; Gortmaker et al. 1993; Messina and Barnes 1991; Stern et al. 1995). Three social class indicators (education, income, and poverty) were used to describe the prevalence of normal weight, overweight, and obesity. Table 1.2 on page 5 shows that overweight and obesity were highest in the least educated and in those living in households earning less than $10,000 a year. Poverty Index Ratio is calculated by the federal government and combines the number of persons in the household and household income, and also takes into account some regional differences. Those living 185% above the poverty line had the lowest prevalence of overweight and obesity.

In an attempt to better understand how education and income are related to obesity, figures 1.8 and 1.9 show the prevalence of obesity by different strata of social class using nine mutually exclusive categories of education and income. In men (see figure 1.8), the highest prevalence of obesity was observed among those with less than a high school education, but living in a household with earnings of $35,000 or more a year. Among those earning less than $20,000 a year, the prevalence of obesity was highest among those who completed 12 years of school (high school). The prevalence of obesity among those with more than 12 years of education (more than high school) was highest among those earning between $20,000 and $35,000.

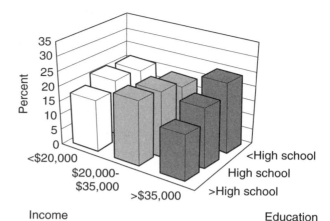

Figure 1.8 Social class and its relation to obesity in men 20 years and older.
From NHANES III, 1988-1994.

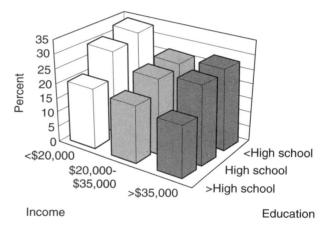

Figure 1.9 Social class and its relation to obesity in women 20 years and older.
From NHANES III, 1988-1994.

Among women, the prevalence of obesity was consistently highest among those with less than 12 years of education (less than high school), and lowest among those with more than 12 years of education (greater than high school) in every income category (see figure 1.9). These results are different from those observed in men, where the most educated men did not always have the lowest prevalence of obesity. In both men and women, the most educated and those with the highest income had the lowest prevalence of obesity.

Gender, poverty, and race are three major risk factors of weight-related problems that are often ignored in the literature on weight management (Bowen et al. 1991; Crawford et al. 2001; Livingstone 2000). Kumanyika and Golden (1991) established that poverty and lower educational attainment are associated with obesity, independent of ethnicity, and therefore affect a relatively higher percent of persons in minority populations than in white populations. Thus, minorities may be at higher risk for obesity because of their increased poverty rate and lower educational attainment.

Our understanding of how and why obesity develops requires the integration of social, behavioral, cultural, physiological, metabolic, and genetic factors. Obesity affects millions of U.S. adults and children, representing one of the most challenging public health problems. Labor-saving devices, overconsumption of calories, and the percent of persons who engage in little or no leisure time physical activity may partially explain the current prevalence of obesity.

body mass index does not change significantly over time. Weight and height are among the most valid and reliable biological measurements commonly available.

More than 60% of white men and black women were overweight between 1988 and 1994. Although overweight (BMI ≥25) estimates were highest in white men, the prevalence of obesity (BMI ≥30) was higher among white women than men (see figures 1.10 and 1.11). The prevalence of obesity was highest among black women. Alarming increases in the prevalence of obesity have been observed in children as illustrated in figure 1.12. The prevalence of obesity in 1999 revealed an alarming increase in the percent of obese persons when compared to previous reference points on data collected between 1960 and 1980 (Schoenborn et al. 2002). Ruling out measurement error, other changes must have

Trends in Prevalence

Since 1960 the National Center for Health Statistics has been tracking weight and height data on adults as well as children. Some of these data produced the growth charts used by every pediatrician to track the weight and height of children in the United States and throughout the world. More recently, these charts were updated using data from a national representative sample of children two months and older from NHANES III, and other pertinent data from infant birth records (Kuczmarski et al. 2002). Data collected on adults has yielded fairly accurate information to track the percent of adults who are overweight and obese. Contrary to other health indicators, the accuracy of calculating

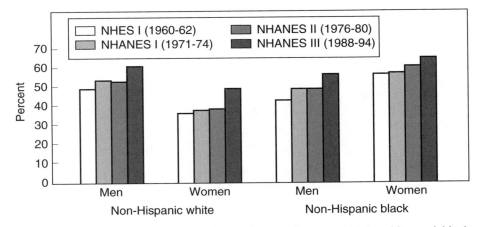

Figure 1.10 Trends in age-adjusted prevalence of overweight in white and black adults, age 20 to 74.

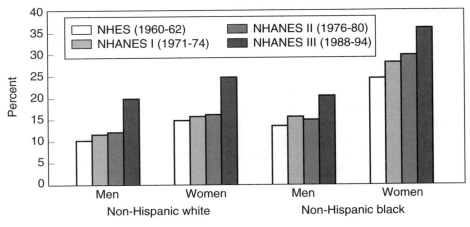

Figure 1.11 Trends in age-adjusted prevalence of obesity in white and black adults, age 20 to 74.

occurred during the 1980s to account for the observed increases in obesity. It is unlikely that the genetic pool could have been responsible for this increase in such a short period of time. (A discussion of the genetic influence on obesity can be found in chapter 4.)

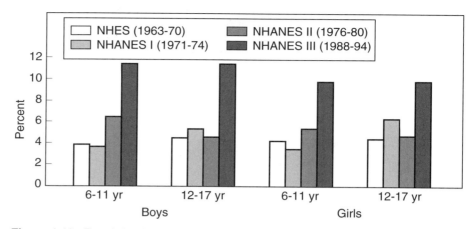

Figure 1.12 Trends in obesity among U.S. children.
From *Healthy People 2000*, Progress Review, CDC/NCHS 1999.

Some have suggested that the increase in overweight and obesity may in part be due to the increase in smoking cessation, although it probably does not explain most of the increase (Flegal et al. 1995). Others have suggested that the recent trend in overemphasizing low-fat foods and underemphasizing total caloric intake may have contributed to increased consumption and thus increased caloric intake (Cummings, Parham, and Strain 2002; Lee et al. 2001).

Decreases in physical activity may also account for some of the increase in overweight and obesity (Blair and Brodney 1999; Prentice and Jebb 1995). Participation in physical activity, either occupational or recreational, has not been tracked in a systematic way until recently (1985), when the National Health Interview Survey obtained baseline data for the *Healthy People 1990* survey. In that survey, roughly 24% of the population reported participating in no leisure time physical activity. Data collected from phase I (1988-1991) of the NHANES III confirmed that less than a quarter of the population engaged in no leisure time physical activity (Crespo et al. 1996). Other updates using NHANES III and other surveys confirmed that the percent of sedentary adults and children has either increased or not changed (Crespo et al. 1999; Kimm et al. 2002; Pate et al. 2002).

Summary

Obesity is highly prevalent and rising in the United States. Contributing factors may include reduction in all types of physical activities (e.g., leisure time, occupational, and transportation) and increases in caloric intake and smoking cessation, among others. The data presented in this chapter show that from 1976 to 1980 and 1988 to 1994, the percent increase in obesity was substantially greater than the increases observed from 1960 to 1976. These dramatic increases were observed in both adults and children. Racial and ethnic minorities, especially non-Hispanic blacks and Mexican Americans, also experienced obesity increases that were greater than those observed among non-Hispanic whites. More research is needed to understand the interaction among genetic, social, cultural, and environmental factors that may have influenced the dramatic increases in obesity in this nation.

References

Allison, D.B., and Saunders, S.E. 2000. Obesity in North America. An overview. *Med. Clin. North Am.* 84: 305-332.

Allred, J.B. 1995. Too much of a good thing? An overemphasis on eating low-fat foods may be contributing to the alarming increase in overweight among U.S. adults. *J. Am. Diet. Assoc.* 95: 417-418.

Andersen, R.E., Crespo, C.J., Bartlett, S.J., Cheskin, L.J., and Pratt, M. 1998. Relationship of physical activity and television watching with body weight and level of fatness among children: Results from the Third National Health and Nutrition Examination Survey. *JAMA* 279: 938-942.

Arroyo, P., Loria, A., Fernandez, V., Flegal, K.M., Kuri-Morales, P., Olaiz, G., and Tapia-Conyer, R. 2000. Prevalence of pre-obesity and obesity in urban adult Mexicans in comparison with other large surveys. *Obes. Res.* 8: 179-185.

Bellizzi, M.C., and Dietz, W.H. 1999. Workshop on childhood obesity: Summary of the discussion. *Am. J. Clin. Nutr.* 70: 173S-175S.

Bianchini, F., Kaaks, R., and Vainio, H. 2002. Overweight, obesity, and cancer risk. *Lancet Oncol.* 3: 565.

Blair, S.N., and Brodney, S. 1999. Effects of physical inactivity and obesity on morbidity and mortality: Current evidence and research issues. *Med. Sci. Sports Exerc.* 31: S646-S662.

Blair, S.N., and Nichaman, M.S. 2002. The public health problem of increasing prevalence rates of obesity and what should be done about it. *Mayo Clin. Proc.* 77: 109-113.

Bolen, J.C., Rhodes, L., Powell-Griner, E.E., Bland, S.D., and Holtzman, D. 2000. State-specific prevalence of selected health behaviors, by race and ethnicity—Behavioral Risk Factor Surveillance System, 1997. *Mor. Mortal. Wkly. Rep. CDC Surveill. Summ.* 49: 1-60.

Bowen, D.J., Tomoyasu, N., and Cauce, A.M. 1991. The triple threat: A discussion of gender, class, and race differences in weight. *Women Health* 17: 123-143.

Cole, T.J., Bellizzi, M.C., Flegal, K.M., and Dietz, W.H. 2000. Establishing a standard definition for child overweight and obesity worldwide: International survey. *BMJ* 320: 1240-1243.

Crawford, P.B., Story, M., Wang, M.C., Ritchie, L.D., and Sabry, Z.I. 2001. Ethnic issues in the epidemiology of childhood obesity. *Pediatr. Clin. North Am.* 48: 855-878.

Crespo, C.J., Ainsworth, B.E., Keteyian, S.E., Heath, G.W., and Smit, E. 1999. Prevalence of physical inactivity and its relation to social class in U.S. adults: Results from the Third National Health and Nutrition Examination Survey, 1988-1994. *Med. Sci. Sports Exerc.* 31: 1821-1827.

Crespo, C.J., Keteyian, S.J., Heath, G.W., and Sempos, C.T. 1996. Leisure-time physical activity among U.S. adults. Results from the Third National Health and Nutrition Examination Survey. *Arch. Intern. Med.* 156: 93-98.

Crespo, C.J., Smit, E., Troiano, R.P., Bartlett, S.J., Macera, C.A., and Andersen, R.E. 2001. Television watching, energy intake, and obesity in U.S. children: Results from the Third National Health and Nutrition Examination Survey, 1988-1994. *Arch. Pediatr. Adolesc. Med.* 155: 360-365.

Cummings, S., Parham, E.S., and Strain, G.W. 2002. Position of the American Dietetic Association: Weight management. *J. Am. Diet. Assoc.* 102: 1145-1155.

Debate, R.D., Topping, M., and Sargent, R.G. 2001. Racial and gender differences in weight status and dietary practices among college students. *Adolescence* 36: 819-833.

Dennison, B.A., Erb, T.A., and Jenkins, P.L. 2002. Television viewing and television in bedroom associated with overweight risk among low-income preschool children. *Pediatrics* 109: 1028-1035.

Dietz, W.H., and Bellizzi, M.C. 1999. Introduction: The use of body mass index to assess obesity in children. *Am. J. Clin. Nutr.* 70: 123S-125S.

Epstein, L.H. 1996. Family-based behavioural intervention for obese children. *Int. J. Obes. Relat. Metab. Disord.* 20 (Suppl. 1): S14-S21.

Epstein, L.H., Paluch, R.A., Gordy, C.C., and Dorn, J. 2000. Decreasing sedentary behaviors in treating pediatric obesity. *Arch. Pediatr. Adolesc. Med.* 154: 220-226.

Faith, M.S., Berman, N., Heo, M., Pietrobelli, A., Gallagher, D., Epstein, L.H., Eiden, M.T., and Allison, D.B. 2001. Effects of contingent television on physical activity and television viewing in obese children. *Pediatrics* 107: 1043-1048.

Flegal, K.M. 1999. The obesity epidemic in children and adults: Current evidence and research issues. *Med. Sci. Sports Exerc.* 31: S509-S514.

Flegal, K.M., Carroll, M.D., Kuczmarski, R.D., and Johnson, C.L. 1998. Overweight and obesity in the United States: Prevalence and trends, 1960-1994. *Int. J. Obes. Relat. Metab. Disord.* 22: 39-47.

Flegal, K.M., Troiano, R.P., Pamuk, E.R., Kuczmarski, R.J., and Campbell, S.M. 1995. The influence of smoking cessation on the prevalence of overweight in the United States. *N. Engl. J. Med.* 333: 1165-1170.

Gordon, P.M., Heath, G.W., Holmes, A., and Christy, D. 2000. The quantity and quality of physical activity among those trying to lose weight. *Am. J. Prev. Med.* 18: 83-86.

Gortmaker, S.L., Must, A., Perrin, J.M., Sobol, A.M., and Dietz, W.H. 1993. Social and economic consequences of overweight in adolescence and young adulthood. *N. Engl. J. Med.* 329: 1008-1012.

Gortmaker, S.L., Must, A., Sobol, A.M., Peterson, K., Colditz, G.A., and Dietz, W.H. 1996. Television viewing as a cause of increasing obesity among children in the United States, 1986-1990. *Arch. Pediatr. Adolesc. Med.* 150: 356-362.

Gortmaker, S.L., Peterson, K., Wiecha, J., Sobol, A.M., Dixit, S., Fox, M.K., and Laird, N. 1999. Reducing obesity via a school-based interdisciplinary intervention among youth: Planet Health. *Arch. Pediatr. Adolesc. Med.* 153: 409-418.

Gregg, E.W., and Narayan, KM. 1998. Culturally appropriate lifestyle interventions in minority populations. More than meets the eye? *Diabetes Care* 21: 875-877.

Guillaume, M. 1999. Defining obesity in childhood: Current practice. *Am. J. Clin. Nutr.* 70: 126S-130S.

Guo, S.S., and Chumlea, W.C. 1999. Tracking of body mass index in children in relation to overweight in adulthood. *Am. J. Clin. Nutr.* 70: 145S-148S.

Jeffery, R.W. 1991. Population perspectives on the prevention and treatment of obesity in minority populations. *Am. J. Clin. Nutr.* 53: 1621S-1624S.

Kimm, S.Y., Glynn, N.W., Kriska, A.M., Barton, B.A., Kronsberg, S.S., Daniels, S.R., Crawford, P.B., Sabry, Z.I., and Liu, K. 2002. Decline in physical activity in black girls and white girls during adolescence. *N. Engl. J. Med.* 347: 709-715.

Kopelman, P.G. 2000. Obesity as a medical problem. *Nature* 404: 635-643.

Kuczmarski, R.J. 1993. Trends in body composition for infants and children in the U.S. *Crit. Rev. Food Sci. Nutr.* 33: 375-387.

Kuczmarski, R.J., Flegal, K.M., Campbell, S.M., and Johnson, C.L. 1994. Increasing prevalence of overweight among US adults. The National Health and Nutrition Examination Surveys, 1960 to 1991. *JAMA* 272: 205-211.

Kuczmarski, R.J., Ogden, C.L., Guo, S.S., Grummer-Strawn, L.M., Flegal, K.M., Mei, Z., Wei, R., Curtin, L.R., Roche, A.F., and Johnson, C.L. 2002. 2000 CDC Growth Charts for the United States: Methods and development. *Vital Health Stat.* 11: 1-190.

Kumanyika, S.K. 1993. Special issues regarding obesity in minority populations. *Ann. Intern. Med.* 119: 650-654.

Kumanyika, S.K., and Golden, P.M. 1991. Cross-sectional differences in health status in U.S. racial/ethnic minority groups: Potential influence of temporal changes, disease, and life-style transitions. *Ethn. Dis.* 1: 50-59.

Lee, I.M., Blair, S.N., Allison, D.B., Folsom, A.R., Harris, T.B., Manson, J.E., and Wing, R.R. 2001. Epidemiologic data on the relationships of caloric intake, energy balance, and weight gain over the life span with longevity and morbidity. *J. Gerontol Biol. Sci. Med. Sci.* 56 (Spec. no. 1): 7-19.

Livingstone, B. 2000. Epidemiology of childhood obesity in Europe. *Eur. J. Pediatr.* 159 (Suppl. 1): S14-S34.

Malina, R.M., and Katzmarzyk, P.T. 1999. Validity of the body mass index as an indicator of the risk and presence of overweight in adolescents. *Am. J. Clin. Nutr.* 70: 131S-136S.

Martorell, R., Kettel, K.L., Hughes, M.L., and Grummer-Strawn, L.M. 2000. Overweight and obesity in preschool children from developing countries. *Int. J. Obes. Relat. Metab. Disord.* 24: 959-967.

Messina, M., and Barnes, S. 1991. The role of soy products in reducing risk of cancer. *J. Natl. Cancer Inst.* 83: 541-546.

National Center for Health Statistics. 2002. Overweight among U.S. children and adolescents. NHANES Data Briefs, 1-2.

Ogden, C.L., Troiano, R.P., Briefel, R.R., Kuczmarski, R.J., Flegal, K.M., and Johnson, C.L. 1997. Prevalence of overweight among preschool children in the United States, 1971 through 1994. *Pediatrics* 99: E1.

Ostir, G.V., Markides, K.S., Freeman, Jr., D.H., and Goodwin, J.S. 2000. Obesity and health conditions in elderly Mexican Americans: The Hispanic EPESE. Established Population for Epidemiologic Studies of the Elderly. *Ethn. Dis.* 10: 31-38.

Pate, R.R., Freedson, P.S., Sallis, Taylor, W.C., Sirard, J., Trost, S.G., and Dowda, M. 2002. Compliance with physical activity guidelines: Prevalence in a population of children and youth. *Ann. Epidemiol.* 12: 303-308.

Pi-Sunyer, F.X. 1999. Comorbidities of overweight and obesity: Current evidence and research issues. *Med. Sci. Sports Exerc.* 31: S602-S608.

Pi-Sunyer, F.X. 2000. Obesity: Criteria and classification. *Proc. Nutr. Soc.* 59: 505-509.

Prentice, A.M., and Jebb, S.A. 1995. Obesity in Britain: Gluttony or sloth? *BMJ* 311: 437-439.

Roberts, S.B., Lucas, A., and Hirsch, J. 2000. Low energy expenditure as a contributor to infant obesity. *Am. J. Clin. Nutr.* 71: 154-56.

Roberts, S.O. 2000. The role of physical activity in the prevention and treatment of childhood obesity. *Pediatr. Nurs.* 26: 33-41.

Schoenborn, C., Adams, P., and Barnes, P.M. Body weight status of adults: United States, 1997-98. Advance Data 330, 1-16. 9-6-2002. National Center for Health Statistics, Department of Health and Human Services, Centers for Disease Control and Prevention. Ref Type: Generic

Stern, J.S., Hirsch, J., Blair, S.N., Foreyt, J.P., Frank, A., Kumanyika, S.K., Madans, J.H., Marlatt, G.A., St Jeor, S.T., and Stunkard, A.J. 1995. Weighing the options: Criteria for evaluating weight-management programs. The Committee to Develop Criteria for Evaluating the Outcomes of Approaches to Prevent and Treat Obesity. *Obes. Res.* 3: 591-604.

Terry, P.D., Miller, A.B., and Rohan, T.E. 2002. Obesity and colorectal cancer risk in women. *Gut* 51: 191-194.

Troiano, R.P., and Flegal, K.M. 1999. Overweight prevalence among youth in the United States: Why so many different numbers? *Int. J. Obes. Relat. Metab. Disord.* 23 (Suppl. 2): S22-S27.

U.S. Department of Health and Human Services. 2000. *Healthy People 2010.* 2nd ed. With Understanding and Improving Health and Objectives for Improving Health. 2 vols. 11-1-2000. Washington, DC: U.S. Government Printing Office.

Chapter 2

Psychosocial Correlates and Consequences of Obesity

Myles S. Faith, PhD

Weight and Eating Disorders Program, University of Pennsylvania School of Medicine

Patty E. Matz, PhD

Weill Medical College, Cornell University

David B. Allison, PhD

Department of Biostatistics, Section on Statistical Genetics, Clinical Nutrition Research Center, University of Alabama at Birmingham

The medical complications of obesity have been well cataloged (Pi-Sunyer 1993) and justify weight loss recommendations for many individuals. Equally pernicious for obese individuals, however, may be the psychological tolls of obesity in Western culture. Antiobese attitudes are common in society and often translate into discriminatory practices in multiple settings (Yuker and Allison 1994). Obesity-related stigma and discrimination can detrimentally affect body image appraisal, self-esteem, and other psychological characteristics in obese individuals of all ages.

This chapter reviews the psychological correlates and consequences of obesity. We begin with an overview of the psychological correlates of obesity from general population studies, as well as studies examining subgroups of obese persons that may be more prone to psychological disorders. Following this we summarize data on obesity-related prejudices and discrimination. Studies suggest that such prejudices affect obese individuals of all ages,

can have economic consequences, can be found among healthcare professionals, and may be moderated by attribution style. Next, we explore the notion that antifat biases and discriminatory behaviors may perpetuate obesity-promoting behaviors such as overeating and reduced physical activity in some individuals. Finally, we review interventions designed to foster self-acceptance, which may confer psychological benefits independent of weight loss (Wilson 1997). At the same time, enhancing self-acceptance and related coping skills might also promote changes in eating behavior and physical activity that are consistent with better weight control.

Throughout this chapter, we primarily speak of associations rather than causal pathways, as much of the literature has relied on correlational research designs. When analyzing relationships between obesity and psychological traits, one often faces the "chicken-and-egg" problem that cannot be easily resolved. Studies using experimental, longitudinal, or genetically sensitive designs may provide greater clarity into causal pathways.

Psychological Correlates of Obesity in the General Population

Population-level studies are critical for understanding whether obesity is associated with psychological disorders or conditions. Clinical studies that recruit obese patients may be prone to sampling biases since obese individuals seeking weight loss treatment have greater psychopathology than obese individuals not seeking treatment (Fitzgibbon, Stolley, and Kirschenbaum 1993; Prather and Williamson 1988). Moreover, clinical studies have often relied on unreliable outcome measures or unvalidated assessment strategies (Smoller, Wadden, and Stunkard 1987). Hence, the advantages of population-based studies with validated measures cannot be overstated.

Several investigators have qualitatively reviewed population-based sampling studies comparing obese to nonobese individuals on various psychological indexes (Faith and Allison 1996; O'Neil and Jarrell 1992; Striegel-Moore and Rodin 1986; Wadden and Stunkard 1985). Most conclude that, on average, obese and nonobese individuals are psychologically comparable. Perhaps in part for these reasons, obesity per se is not considered a mental disorder and by itself is not included in the *Diagnostic and Statistical Manual of Mental Disorders* (*DSM-IV*; American Psychiatric Association 1994). On the other hand, it may be premature to simply conclude that obesity has no psychological correlates or that psychological conditions cannot promote weight gain. Because studies of the obesity–psychopathology association have had methodological limitations, clear conclusions remain elusive (Friedman and Brownell 1995). The obese population appears to be psychologically heterogeneous, and certain subgroups may be more prone to psychological problems than others are.

Moreover, recent studies using superior sampling methods and clinical assessment challenge the null findings from previous studies.

Friedman and Brownell (1995) quantitatively reviewed the association between body mass index (BMI: kg/m^2) and various psychiatric/psychological symptoms. Figure 2.1 summarizes these associations, expressed as Pearson's correlation coefficients. Depression is one of the most common psychological disorders in the general population. Its association with obesity status has been evaluated in several community-based studies and is relatively small in magnitude ($r = -0.03$). Thus, there seems to be little association between obesity and depression. However, this relationship may depend on gender. An analysis of the National Health and Nutrition Examination Survey (NHANES I) (Istvan, Zavela, and Weidner 1992) indicated a positive association between BMI and depression among women, but not men. A recent study that used nationally representative sampling and a structured clinical interview reached similar conclusions.

Carpenter and colleagues (2000) tested the probability of DSM-IV Past-Year Major Depressive Disorder as a function of obesity status in Caucasian and African American men and women. They found that the relationship between BMI and depression was gender dependent. Being obese rather than average weight was associated with an *increased* risk of depression for women (odds ratio, OR, = 1.37) but a *decreased* risk of depression for men (OR = 0.63). Associations were comparable for Caucasians and African Americans. These results suggest that being obese may be

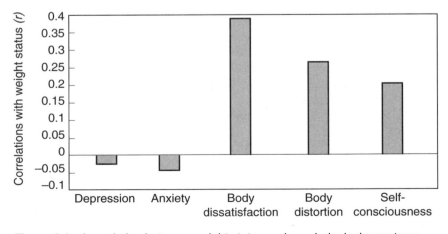

Figure 2.1 Association between weight status and psychological symptoms.

more psychologically disturbing for women than it is for men. Clinical experience suggests that, for many men, being too thin or nonmuscular is more bothersome than being somewhat overweight. This does not appear to be the case clinically among women. As an overweight female indicated, "I wish I were more like my husband in terms of how he sees his body. He'd much rather be a bit heavy and muscular than thin and scrawny. Being too thin is not something I worry much about."

Body image disparagement, or body dissatisfaction, may be the most common psychological complication of obesity. As figure 2.1 illustrates, a sizable association exists between BMI and body image disparagement such that heavier individuals tend to see their bodies in a more negative light. This finding probably relates to the increasingly slender "ideal" body type celebrated in Western culture in conjunction with obesity-related prejudices (Yuker and Allison 1994). Individuals who are more likely to compare themselves to peers or others in the media also tend to have greater body image disparagement (Faith, Leone, and Allison 1997; Heinberg and

Thompson 1995). Body image disparagement may be especially problematic for obese individuals who binge eat. Results from a national body image survey found that, among obese men and women, self-identified binge eaters reported poorer evaluations of their overall bodies and specific body parts, greater "fat-anxiety," and a greater value and emphasis placed on their physical appearance (Cash 1991). Obese adults who were also obese during adolescence tend to have greater body image disparagement compared to those who were not obese during adolescence (Stunkard and Burt 1967).

Because obese individuals do not fit a distinct profile (Faith, Allison, and Geleibter 1997), researchers are attempting to identify subgroups of obese individuals with greater psychological difficulties. Obese binge eaters have been studied extensively and consistently demonstrate greater psychopathology than non-binge-eating obese individuals or normal weight controls. Table 2.1 summarizes DSM-IV diagnostic criteria for binge eating disorder (BED). Clinically, one of the most common experiences of the obese binge eater

Table 2.1 — DSM-IV Diagnostic Criteria for Binge Eating Disorder

A. Recurrent episodes of binge eating*. An episode of binge eating is characterized by both of the following:

- Eating, in a discrete period of time (e.g., within any two-hour period), an amount of food that is definitely larger than most people would eat in a similar period of time under similar circumstances.

- A sense of a lack of control over eating during the episode (e.g., a feeling that one cannot stop eating or control what or how much one is eating).

B. The binge eating episodes are associated with three (or more) of the following:

- Eating much more rapidly than normal
- Eating until feeling uncomfortably full
- Eating large amounts of food when not feeling physically hungry
- Eating alone because of being embarrassed by how much one is eating
- Feeling disgusted with oneself, depressed, or very guilty after overeating

C. Marked distress regarding binge eating is present.

D. The binge eating occurs, on average, at least two days a week for six months.

Note: The method of determining frequency differs from that used for bulimia nervosa; future research should address whether the preferred method of setting a frequency threshold is counting the number of days on which binges occur or counting the number of episodes of binge eating.

*The binge eating is not associated with the regular use of inappropriate compensatory behaviors (e.g., purging, fasting, or excessive exercise) and does not occur exclusively during the course of anorexia nervosa or bulimia nervosa.

is to feel "out of control" when eating. As an obese BED patient expressed, "It's as if there is an uncontrollable force in me that cannot be stopped. Even if I need to go out of the way in the middle of the evening to get foods to eat, I will do so when these feelings are awake."

Compared to non-binge-eating obese individuals, obese individuals with BED are more likely to experience anxiety, depression, obsessive-compulsive disorder, paranoid ideation, psychoticism, and borderline personality disorder. BED patients also displayed greater somatization, hostility, and interpersonal sensitivity (Marcus, Wing, and Hopkins 1988). Table 2.2 summarizes results from Yanovski and colleagues' (1993) comparison of obese individuals with and without BED. The table shows the relative risk of having been diagnosed with various axis I and axis II disorders as a function of having BED (as opposed to

not having BED); the results demonstrate that BED patients are more likely to have psychiatric diagnoses.

Increased psychopathology might be common among people in other obese subgroups as well. Weight fluctuation is also associated with increased psychological disorders in some studies (Brownell and Rodin 1994). On the other hand, weight cycling is not necessarily associated with psychology. Foster, Sarwer, and Wadden (1997) reviewed the literature on the relationship between weight cycling and various psychological outcome measures. Table 2.3 summarizes their findings and demonstrates that, across the studies reviewed, weight cycling seemed to have little relation to depression, psychopathology, cognitive style, general well-being, or stress. Clinical experience supports these data, as many obese individuals who lose and regain weight are nonetheless psychologically healthy. As a patient indicated, "It is a struggle for me to maintain my weight loss. I lose it and then regain, and on and on. But I've learned to get back on the horse when I fall off. I know that, if I regain weight, it's not forever and I'll get it back off again—hopefully for good." Thus, repeated bouts of weight loss and regain among obese patients should not necessarily be interpreted as symptomatic or causative of underlying psychological distress.

In sum, population-based studies have yielded mixed results. Greater body image disparagement among obese individuals seems to be one of the most robust findings in the literature. Also, recent studies suggest that obesity is associated with elevated depression in African American and Caucasian women, but not men. Elevated psychopathology may be unique to subgroups of the obese population, although the studies that suggest this provide

Table 2.2   *Relative Risks of DSM Psychiatric Disorders (Lifetime) Associated With BED Among Obese Patients*

Disorder	Relative risk
Axis I	
Major depression	6.4
Dysthymia	2.2
Obsessive-compulsive disorder	0.7
Social phobia	4.1
Panic disorder	8.6
Agoraphobia	4.1
Drug abuse	1.5
Alcohol abuse	1.6
Any substance abuse	1.5
Any Axis I diagnosis	3.0
Axis II	
Borderline personality disorder	13.6
Obsessive-compulsive personality disorder	1.0
Self-defeating personality disorder	4.3
Any Axis II diagnosis	2.7

Data from Yanovski et al. 1993.

Table 2.3   *Association of Weight Cycling With Psychological Constructs in Obese Persons*

Construct	N studies	Resulting effect	
		Not statistically significant	Not clinically significant or mixed
Depression	7	86%	14%
Psychopathology	2	0%	100%
Cognitive style	3	75%	25%
General well-being and health	3	33%	67%
Stress	2	50%	50%

Data from Foster, Sarwer, and Wadden 1997.

limited insight into causal mechanisms. That many obese individuals do not experience psychological problems is arguably impressive, given the stigma of obesity in our culture. A discussion of this literature proceeds in the following section.

Antiobese Attitudes and Discrimination

Obesity-related prejudices and discrimination are widespread in Western culture. Personal characteristics often thought to be associated with obesity include laziness, gluttony, and self-indulgence. As Wadden and Stunkard (1985, p. 164) noted, "In virtually every aspect of their lives, the overweight are reminded that they live in a society that hates fat."

Prejudices Across the Age Span

Antiobese attitudes start early in life (Cramer and Steinwert 1998). Obese children are often perceived as "lazy," "stupid," "dirty," and "immature" (Sherman 1981). In a study of nine-year-old girls and boys who rated silhouettes varying in body size, the overweight silhouette was associated with poor social functioning, impaired academic success, and poor perceived health (Hill and Silver 1995). When ranking a drawing of the same child portrayed as being physically healthy and then with five different "physical disabili-

ties," the obese figure received the poorest ratings (Richardson et al. 1961). Phillips and Hill (1998) found that self-esteem related to physical appearance and athletic competence was compromised in obese children and adolescents, although measures of global self-esteem were not affected. However, different findings come from Strauss (2000), who tested changes in global self-esteem over a four-year period among 9- to 10-year-old children from the National Longitudinal Study of Youth. Compared with nonobese Hispanic and Caucasian girls, obese Hispanic and Caucasian girls showed significant reductions in self-esteem over time. Compared to nonobese boys, obese boys in all ethnic groups showed mild reductions in self-esteem. Decreasing levels of self-esteem in obese children were associated with increased sadness, loneliness, and nervousness.

Adults are also the recipients of the antifat stigma. Falkner and associates (1999) examined perceived mistreatment related to weight and the sources of this mistreatment in a nonclinical sample enrolled in a weight gain prevention program. Twenty-two percent of the women and 17 percent of the men reported weight-related mistreatment, most frequently at the hands of strangers and spouses or loved ones. Reported mistreatment was ten times higher among persons above the highest quartile of BMI relative to below the lowest BMI quartile. Other studies confirm that greater exposure to weight-related mistreatment is directly associated with psychological distress (Myers and Rosen 1999). The "scars" of these negative attitudes can be found among formerly obese adults as well. In one study, formerly morbidly obese persons unanimously preferred deafness, dyslexia, acne, or heart disease to resumed obesity (Rand and MacGregor 1991).

Attribution Style and Obesity Prejudice

People who attribute obesity to "uncontrollable" factors (e.g., genetics) tend to have fewer negative attitudes than those who attribute obesity to "controllable" factors (e.g., poor willpower or a weak constitution) (Allison, Basile, and Yuker 1991; Crandall and Martinez 1996; Crandall and Moriarty 1995). These same findings hold for obese individuals themselves. In a sample of 9- to 11-year-old overweight children, self-esteem was more compromised among those children who perceived themselves as being responsible for their weight or who believed that being overweight impaired their social relations (Pierce and Wardle 1997). These data are reflected in the following comments of an obese adult patient who recognized her family history of obesity, "Why should I drive myself crazy and make myself miserable about my body size? My parents were both heavy, and so were their parents. It's not my fault, so I'll just do my best to exercise and try to maintain my weight."

Research by Crandall and others indicates that antiobese attitudes are part of a larger constellation of authoritarian attitudes (Crandall and Biernat 1990; Morrison and O'Connor 1999). Individuals holding more negative attitudes toward obese persons tend to be politically conservative, more racist, in favor of capital punishment, less supportive of nontraditional marriages, and less tolerant of sexuality among handicapped, homosexual, and elderly persons (Crandall and Biernat 1990).

Weight Teasing

Weight-related teasing can be particularly stigmatizing for children, adolescents (Neumark-Sztainer, Story, and Fabisch 1998), and adults (Falkner et al. 1999; Myers and Rosen 1999; Rothblum et al. 1989). Retrospective reports by college students (Cash 1995; Rieves and Cash 1996; Thompson and Psaltis 1988) and obese adults seeking weight loss treatment (Grillo et al. 1994) indicate that weight teasing during childhood is associated with poorer body image during adulthood. Weight teasing can come from family members and friends (Rieves and Cash 1996), although teasing from family members may be more detrimental to body image (Wardle and Collins 1998). Thompson and associates (1995) conducted a three-year longitudinal study that examined the prospective relationships among weight status, teasing, and the development of body image dissatisfaction. They found that teasing mediated the relationship between weight status and body image dissatisfaction, such that the negative effects on body image of being overweight were dependent on weight teasing history.

Weight teasing psychologically affects not only sedentary children and adults, but professional athletes as well. Take the case of baseball pitcher David Wells, whose weight was discussed in a feature article published in *Sports Illustrated*. Concerning this article, Wells stated, "It's an honor to be on the cover, but the story is a total joke. It's terrible. . . . All it talks about is me being fat. . . . It's stupid." (Pearlman 2000).

Economic, Employment, and Interpersonal Relations

The consequences of obesity also pertain to overt acts of discrimination in interpersonal relationships, housing opportunities, educational level, job attainment, and income. Compared to nonobese individuals, obese persons are discriminated against in job interviews (Klesges et al. 1990), receive lower salaries (Frieze, Olson, and Good 1990), are less likely to receive financial support for college from their parents (Crandall 1991), are less likely to be offered jobs (Klesges et al. 1990), and are less likely to be rented apartments (Karris 1977). Analyses of the National Longitudinal Study of Youth (Gortmaker et al. 1993) provide some of the strongest data on this issue.

Longitudinal analyses followed up and compared young adults who were either overweight or not overweight during adolescence. Results are summarized in table 2.4

Table 2.4   *Adolescent Weight Status and Social and Economic Characteristics*

Adult outcome	Adolescent weight status			
	Females		Males	
	Overweight	Nonoverweight	Overweight	Nonoverweight
Married (%)	28	56	40	48
Household income ($)	18,372	30,586	26,008	31,462
Education (yr)	12.1	13	12.4	13.1
Completed college (%)	9	33.6	10	23

Adapted from Gortmaker et al. 1993.

and indicate that the consequences of obesity are especially detrimental for females. Females who were overweight as adolescents had completed fewer years of school, had a lower household income and higher rates of household poverty, and were less likely to be married as young adults. Other studies confirm that obese women may be discriminated against more than obese men. Relative to overweight men and average weight men and women, overweight women dated less frequently, had less mate satisfaction, and received more criticism (Stake and Lauer 1987).

Prejudices From Health Care Professionals

Antifat attitudes can come from health care professionals as well (Garner and Nicol 1998; Maiman et al. 1979). Wadden and Stunkard (1985) noted that weight loss professionals often blame overweight persons for weight regain, with comments such as, "I guess he didn't really want be thin" (p. 174). Prejudicial beliefs about overweight persons have been documented among rehabilitation counselors (Kaplan 1984), physicians (Najman, Klein, and Munro 1982; Price et al. 1987), nurses (Garner and Nicol 1998), and mental health professionals (Young and Powell 1985).

Physicians often view obesity as a psychologically based problem (Liese 1986) and underemphasize genetic and metabolic factors. Harris, Hamaday, and Mochan (1999) surveyed 210 osteopathic family physicians regarding the impact of motivational, lifestyle, and biological factors on obesity etiology. Results indicated that 38.5% perceived lack of willpower, 56.4% perceived physical inactivity, and 68% perceived poor diet as the most significant contributors to obesity. In contrast, genetic factors (12.8%) and metabolic processes (2%) were perceived to be less important factors.

Physicians' prejudices may discourage some obese individuals from seeking medical services (Olsen, Schumaker, and Yawn 1994). Many health care professionals acknowledge their reluctance to perform preventive health care examinations on obese individuals (Adams et al. 1993). Analyzing data from the 1992 National Health Interview survey, Fontaine and colleagues (1998) tested the association between BMI and the use of preventive medical care services in a nationally representative sample of women. They investigated whether the time intervals since the most recent mammography, clinical breast examination, gynecological examination, and Papanicolaou smear were greater for heavier individuals. Results supported this hypothesis, even after adjusting for various sociodemographic variables such as age, race, income, and smoking status. Compared to nonobese women, obese women were 26% more likely to have delayed breast examinations, 39% more likely to have delayed gynecological examinations, and 29% more likely to have delayed Papanicolaou examinations for at least three years.

In sum, ample evidence shows that obese individuals are discriminated against across a range of life domains. Prejudices and discrimination are not limited to strangers, but occur from friends, family members, and health care professionals as well. An issue that has received less attention is whether such prejudices and discrimination might affect health behaviors that are related to weight regulation. We discuss this issue in the next section.

Antiobese Attitudes and Obesity-Promoting Behaviors

Several recent studies have addressed whether obesity prejudices and stigmatizing behaviors are associated with eating behavior and physical activity. These data await more rigorous evaluation, as existent studies have relied on correlational designs that do not allow for causal inference. However, addressing these issues may be clinically informative. To the extent that stigmatizing behaviors influence eating or physical activity among individuals who are obese or at risk for obesity, these issues might be relevant for obesity treatment and prevention efforts.

Weight Stigma, Eating Behavior, and Body Weight

To what extent might social pressures to be thin or to lose weight promote eating behaviors that are conducive to weight gain? Several studies have tested the hypothesis that increased dietary restraint promotes greater-than-average weight gain or obesity onset over time, with dietary restraint defined as a person's tendency to try to eat less than he or she desires (Gorman and Allison 1995). Several studies in adults found that dieting practices predicted increased weight gain over time (Klesges, Isbell, and Klesges 1992; Klesges, Klem, and Bene 1989), although other studies did not (Heatherton, Polivy, and Herman 1991).

Stice and colleagues addressed this question in a community study of over six hundred female adolescents from three California high schools (Stice 1998; Stice et al. 1998). Recently, Stice and colleagues (1999) conducted a four-year longitudinal analysis to determine whether baseline measures of dietary restraint and self-labeled dieting predicted subsequent obesity onset. Cox proportion hazard analyses indicated that baseline dietary restraint and self-labeled dieting had risk ratios of 2.92 and 3.24, respectively. That is, a one-unit increase on each of these measures was associated

with a 192% and 324% increase, respectively, in the hazard for obesity onset. Separate analyses of this same sample indicated that dieting predicted binge eating onset, which in turn predicted greater relative body weight (Stice 1998).

Stice's findings jibe with controlled laboratory studies by Birch, Johnson, and colleagues that carefully measured *ad libitum* child eating and self-reported maternal feeding practices. They found that greater maternal control during feeding was associated with poorer caloric regulation by the child (Fisher and Birch 1999) and increased child body fat (Johnson and Birch 1994). Finally, Wertheim and colleagues (1997) examined the specific reasons adolescent females diet or watch their weight using a structured interview with 10-year-old girls. Approximately 17% of the respondents indicated that peer teasing about their bodies was a factor. Muir, Wertheim, and Paxton (1999) also reported that body image dissatisfaction, social comparison, and teasing history were the most commonly reported triggers of dieting in a sample of adolescent females. Teasing history significantly discriminated dieters from nondieters in a sample of approximately 400 Swedish students, 10 to 16 years olds (Edlund et al. 1999).

Clinical experience suggests that, for some obese adults, overly restrictive dieting practices can be counterproductive and result in overeating at subsequent meals. One obese adult noted, "I can only cut back so much on what I take in before I lose control and need to eat more food. It's too uncomfortable otherwise, although I know it doesn't help my weight problem."

Additional studies are needed to test whether food restriction "causes" obesity. As Stice and colleagues (1999) acknowledged, reported dietary restraint may actually be a marker for obesity propensity. Indeed, dietary restraint and other eating disorders symptoms appear to have a genetic component (Wade et al. 1999), suggesting the potential utility of genetically sensitive designs for addressing such questions (Faith, Johnson, and Allison 1997). Korkeila and colleagues (1999) conducted a pertinent study to address this question; they tested the effects of weight loss attempts on future weight gains of 10 kg (22 lb) or greater in the Finnish Twin Cohort. This behavior-genetic study allowed the authors to test whether weight loss attempts predict future weight gain even after controlling for concomitant genetic influences on weight change. Results indicated a significant genetic contribution to weight change, although weight loss attempts still had a significant effect. For example, among middle-aged women, those who had attempted to lose weight were 2.43 times more likely to have gained at least 10 kg (22 lb) over a six-year period.

Weight Stigma, Physical Activity, and Body Weight

Might social factors similarly operate to discourage physical activity in certain individuals? Faith and colleagues (2002) tested whether weight teasing during physical activity was associated with attitudes toward physical activity and reported physical activity levels in a sample of fifth- to eighth-grade children. Moreover, they tested whether an ability to cope with weight teasing moderated these associations. In general, BMI was positively correlated with weight teasing during physical activity. Regression analyses consistently indicated that weight teasing during physical activity was associated with poorer attitudes toward sports and reduced mild-intensity physical activity. Moreover, coping skills for teasing moderated these associations. Thus, these relationships were less pronounced among children better able to cope with weight teasing. However, this study could not address the causal mechanisms underlying these associations.

In another correlational study, Pierce and Wardle (1997) examined the associations among self-esteem, teasing history, peer relations, and sport and game participation in clinically obese 9- to 11-year-old children. Overweight children commonly reported being "embarrassed doing physical activity and playing sports" (p. 649). Seventy-two percent of the subjects indicated that they were excluded from games and sports because of their body size. Ninety percent of the students thought the teasing would stop if they lost weight, and 72% of the students thought their sports and game performance would improve if they lost weight. Together, these data seem consistent with certain clinical reports of exercise treatments with obese adults. As Lyons

and Miller (1999) argued, overweight persons encounter powerful social disincentives to exercise. The hardships that overweight individuals encounter during exercise can impede the perceived psychological benefits of exercise as well.

These data are consistent with the notion that the social stigma of overweight could discourage participation in physical activity and, theoretically, perpetuate the obese condition. However, studies using more rigorous research designs are needed. Weight teasing may be secondary to the obesity or physical ineptness and may not have a unique causal influence on sport participation or body weight. Experimental or longitudinal designs would be particularly informative, as would behavior-genetic designs that could control for putative genetic influences on body size, physical performance, or both (Faith, Johnson, and Allison 1997).

Enhancing Size Acceptance and Self-Esteem for Obese Individuals

Given the stigma of obesity, increasing attention is being paid to treatment methods to enhance self-acceptance and psychological well-being among obese individuals (Brown 1997; Faith et al. 2000; Wooley 1995). In these treatments, weight loss is usually considered a secondary goal of intervention. Treatment often uses cognitive and behavioral methods to discourage patients from evaluating self-worth based on their body size (Lyons and Miller 1999), conceptualizing enhanced quality of life as a legitimate treatment outcome. Several investigations have examined the effects of self-acceptance treatment among obese individuals. This section reviews these studies, after which we conduct a brief and informal meta-analysis to quantitatively estimate the effects of intervention on self-esteem. We only review studies that partially or exclusively focused on obese patients.

Roughan, Seddon, and Vernon-Roberts (1990) studied 87 obese women for two years after these women received a 10-week "psychologically based group therapy programme, which aims at changing disordered eating behaviour and promoting a more positive body image and self-image" (p. 136). No control group was included. Data were available for between 47 and 56 subjects at follow-up. Results showed that, in general, treatment was associated with statistically significant improvements in psychological variables and a statistically significant decrease of one BMI unit.

Ciliska (1990) conducted a 12-week clinical trial of a nondieting program for modestly obese women. The purpose of this intervention was to "re-establish normal eating, improve self-esteem, and learn to deal with . . . negative messages about our body shape in order to be more accepting of ourselves" (p. 49). Ciliska's program resulted in significant improvements in self-esteem, self-reported eating behavior, body satisfaction, mood, and social functioning. However, improvements in certain variables were only partially maintained at follow-up. There was no statistically significant weight change among the groups.

Polivy and Herman (1992) provided the same "undieting" program to 18 obese women over 10 sessions. At the end of treatment, the women demonstrated significant improvements in a number of psychological measures including self-esteem and reductions in bulimia symptoms and restrained eating. Other measures did not improve. Of concern is that the subjects gained approximately 5.5 kg (12 lb) on average. Although the difference was not significant, five individuals (or 28% of the sample) had no weights reported at posttreatment; this raises concern about nonresponse biases influencing the final results. No control group was included.

Rosen (1996) and colleagues (Rosen, Orosan, and Reiter 1995) developed an intervention that specifically targets negative body image among obese women. In a randomized clinical trial, 51 obese women were assigned to either a no-treatment control group or a multifaceted cognitive-behavioral program, which met for 8 two-hour sessions. This program was inspired by previous work by Cash (1991) and included the following components: (1) exploration of the social consequences of obesity; (2) exploration of the variables causing and maintaining negative body image; (3) teaching clients to tolerate distress surrounding physical appearance; (4) cognitive restructuring regarding assumptions about physical appearance; and (5) behavioral assignments

in which subjects gradually allowed greater body exposure in social situations (e.g., wearing tight-fitting as opposed to loose clothes).

A variety of measures were taken before and two weeks after treatment for both groups, and at a four-and-a-half-month follow-up for the treatment group only. The investigators found significant improvements in body image, general psychological functioning, and self-esteem. Moreover, treatment was not associated with weight change, attendance was excellent, and 88% of the participants who completed treatment said that that they would recommend the program.

Lewis, Blair, and Booth (1992) conducted a group therapy program for 24 practitioner- or self-referred women, a proportion of whom were obese. Over the course of eight weekly sessions, subjects were provided information on dieting behavior, nutrition, and cognitive strategies for coping with negative emotions associated with dieting, emotional eating, methods to increase personal effectiveness, and assertiveness against social pressures. Treatment was associated with significant improvement in a number of variables including self-esteem, weight loss self-efficacy, food- and weight-related assertiveness, and desired and actual emotional eating. These effects were maintained at six-month follow-up. BMI significantly decreased between pretest and posttest, as well as pretest and follow-up, although the magnitude of change was relatively small (e.g., the mean BMI decreased from 30.8 at pretest to 29.8 at six-month follow-up).

Robinson and Bacon (1996) developed the "If Only I Were Thin . . . " program, a multifaceted intervention consisting of two assessment, nine group, and two individual sessions. Program components included information on the social transmission of negative body attitudes, reducing blame, examining eating patterns through diaries, redefining beauty, decreasing restricted activities, and increasing social action and assertion. Using a pretest/posttest design, Robinson and Bacon tested the effects of their intervention on various psychological measures among 58 nonobese and obese women. Treatment was associated with significant reductions in "fat phobia" and depression. Self-esteem and self-reported physical activity also increased.

Tanco, Linden, and Earle (1998) examined the efficacy of a cognitive group treatment for morbidly obese women that included a nondieting approach, regular exercise, and the use of coping skills. The program consisted of eight weekly meetings and focused on "fostering insight into maladaptive behaviors, enhancing emotional well-being, and promoting regular physical exercise and nondisordered eating in the absence of any attempt at weight reduction" (p. 329). Fifty obese women were randomly assigned to cognitive treatment (CT), a standard behavioral weight loss treatment (BT), or a wait list control group. The main outcome measures were regular exercise, weight loss, nonchaotic eating, and psychological well-being. Only the CT group showed significant decreases in depression, anxiety, and eating-related psychopathology, along with an increase in perception of self-control. Regular exercise increased among the CT and BT groups. BMI significantly decreased in the CT and BT groups relative to the control group, among whom a nonsignificant increase in BMI was observed. Six-month follow-up data revealed that treatment benefits were maintained in both the CT and BT groups.

Table 2.5 presents a meta-analysis of a subset of these studies with respect to the effects of treatment on self-esteem. Because each study provided pre- and postintervention data on self-esteem, effect sizes represent *change* in self-esteem associated with treatment. Results indicated a surprisingly large effect size, with a weighted mean d value of 1.57 (standard error, SE, = 0.11). That is, on average, self-esteem increased by approximately 1.5 standard deviation units. To put these data into perspective, Abelson (1995) examined distributions of effect sizes from three meta-analyses published in the *Psychological Bulletin* and concluded that it was "unusual" for d to be as large as 1.0, "quite rare" for it to be 1.4, and "extraordinary" for it to be 2.0 (p. 89). This encouraging finding should be tempered for methodological reasons. The lack of control groups in most studies does not allow one to rule out the alternative explanations such as spontaneous recovery, regression to the mean, or factors associated with the mere passage of time. Effects may be due in part to demand characteristics such that patients gave the "right" or socially desirable answers on reported outcome measures (Faith, Wong, and Allison 1998). Studies testing the efficacy of self-acceptance treatments should include control groups, long-term follow-up, and measures shown to be resistant to socially desirable measures.

Table 2.5   Studies on Self-Esteem and Obesity

Study	Control group?	Exclusively obese subjects?	Total sessions	Follow-up duration	d^* (improvements in self-esteem)
Polivy & Herman 1992	No	No ("almost all")	10	6 months	1.16
Robinson & Bacon 1996	No	No	13-14	None	1.08
Roughan et al. 1990	No	No	10	6 months, 1 year, 2 year	3.79
Ciliska 1990	Yes	Yes	12	6 months, 1 year	0.67
Lewis et al. 1992	No	No	8	6 months	1.49
Rosen et al. 1995	Yes	Yes	8	4 months	1.05

*d values were computed using Hedges and Olkin's (1985) adjustment on Cohen's g, where g is defined as the preintervention mean minus the postintervention mean, divided by the pooled standard deviation. Hedges and Olkin's d adjusts for g, which overestimates the population parameter when sample size is small. For Lewis et al. (1992), d was calculated from the t-value (repeated-measured) provided by the authors. Calculations were performed on the D-STAT software (Johnson 1989).

M.S. Faith et al. *Behavior Modification* 24: 459-493, © 2000 by Sage Publications, Inc. Reprinted by permission of Sage Publications, Inc.

Clinically, it is our experience that few obese patients will come to fully accept their weight and give up the hope of one day being thin. Nonetheless, the treatments described herein can be very valuable for many obese individuals, especially with respect to encouraging obese individuals to live active and interpersonally rich lives despite their weight. Obese individuals can still join social organizations, attend singles events, take courses, and attempt to make new friends. As one obese individual stated, "I learned to be a bit more comfortable going out in public places, how to dress better given my body size, and to try one new social event each month to be around more people. That won't make me thin, but may make me a little bit happier."

Summary

Obese individuals cannot be depicted by a single psychological profile. Nonetheless, a substantial literature documents pervasive psychosocial prejudices against obese individuals. Treatments are currently being developed to enhance the psychological well-being and self-acceptance among obese persons. An important question remains as to whether social stigma, discriminatory comments and behaviors, and related phenomena can promote overeating or avoidance of physical activity. Stronger research designs will be needed to address these questions. Enthusiasm for interventions targeting self-acceptance is expected to increase if they are shown to promote behavior changes that are consistent with better weight control.

References

Abelson R.P. 1995. *Statistics as principled argument.* Hillsdale, NJ: Erlbaum.

Adams, C.H., Smith, N.J., Wilbur, D.C., and Grady, K.E. 1993. The relationship of obesity to the frequency of pelvic examinations: Do physician and patient attitudes make a difference? *Women and Health* 20: 45-57.

Allison, D.B., Basile, V.C., and Yuker, H.E. 1991. The measurement of attitudes toward and beliefs about obese persons. *International Journal of Eating Disorders* 10: 599-807.

American Psychiatric Association. 1994. *Diagnostic and statistical manual of mental disorders, 4th edition.* Washington, DC: American Psychiatric Association.

Brown, D.K. 1997. Childhood and adolescent weight management. In *Overweight and weight management: The health professional's guide to understanding and practice,* ed. S. Dalton, 497-525. Gaithersburg, MD: Aspen.

Brownell, K.D., and Rodin, J. 1994. Medical, metabolic, and psychological effects of weight cycling. *Archives of Internal Medicine* 154: 1325-1330.

Carpenter, K.M., Hasin, D.S., Allison, D.B., and Faith, M.S. 2000. Relationships between obesity and DSM-IV Major Depressive Disorder, suicide ideation, and suicide attempts: Results from a general population study. *American Journal of Public Health* 90: 251-257.

Cash, T.F. 1991. Binge eating and body images among the obese: A further evaluation. *Journal of Social Behavior Personality* 6: 367-376.

Cash, T.F. 1995. Developmental teasing about physical appearance: Retrospective descriptions and relationships with body image. *Journal of Social Behavior Personality* 23: 123-130.

Ciliska, D. 1990. *Beyond dieting: Psychoeducational interventions for chronically obese women: A nondieting approach.* New York: Brunner/Mazel.

Cramer, P., and Steinwert, T. 1998. Thin is good, fat is bad: How early does it begin? *Journal of Applied Developmental Psychology* 19: 429-451.

Crandall, C., and Martinez, R. 1996. Culture, ideology, and antifat attitudes. *Personality and Social Psychology Bulletin* 22: 1165-1176.

Crandall, C.S. 1991. Do heavy weight students have more difficulty paying for college? *Personality and Social Psychology Bulletin* 17: 606-611.

Crandall, C.S., and Biernat, M. 1990. The ideology of anti-fat attitudes. *Journal of Applied Social Psychology* 20: 227-243.

Crandall, C.S., and Moriarty, D. 1995. Physical illness stigma and social rejection. *British Journal of Social Psychology* 34: 67-83.

Edlund, B., Halvarsson, K., Gebre-Medhin, M., and Sjoeden, P-O. 1999. Psychological correlates of dieting in Swedish adolescents: A cross-sectional study. *European Eating Disorders Journal* 7: 47-61.

Faith, M.S., and Allison, D.B. 1996. Assessment of psychological status in obese persons. In *Body image, eating disorders, and obesity: A practical guide for assessment and treatment,* ed. J.K. Thompson, 365-387. Washington, DC: American Psychological Association.

Faith, M.S., Allison, D.B., and Geleibter, A. 1997. Emotional eating and obesity: Theoretical considerations and practical recommendations. In *Obesity and weight control: The health professional's guide to understanding and treatment,* ed. S. Dalton, 439-465. Gaithersburg, MD: Aspen.

Faith, M.S., Fontaine, K.R., Cheskin, L.J., and Allison, D.B. 2000. Behavioral approaches to the problems of obesity. *Behavior Modification* 24: 459-493.

Faith, M.S., Johnson, S.L., and Allison, D.B. 1997. Putting the "behavior" into the behavior genetics of obesity research. *Behavior Genetics* 27: 423-439.

Faith, M.S., Leone, M., and Allison, D.B. 1997. The effects of self-generated comparison targets, BMI, and social comparison tendencies on body image appraisal. *Eating Disorders: Journal of Treatment Prevention* 5: 34-46.

Faith, M.S., Leone, M., Ayers, T.S., Heo, M., and Pietrobelli, A. 2002. Weight-criticism during physical activity, coping skills, and reported physical activity in children. *Pediatrics* 110: e23.

Faith, M.S., Wong, F.Y., and Allison, D.B. 1998. Demand characteristics of the research setting can influence indexes of negative affect-induced eating in obese individuals. *Obesity Research* 6: 134-136.

Falkner, N.H., French, S.A., Jeffery, R.W., Neumark-Sztainer, D., Sherwood, N.E., and Morton, N. 1999. Mistreatment due to weight: Prevalence and sources of perceived mistreatment in women and men. *Obesity Research* 7: 572-576.

Fisher, J.O., and Birch, L.L. 1999. Restricting access to foods and children's eating. *Appetite* 32: 405-419.

Fitzgibbon, M.L., Stolley, M.R., and Kirschenbaum, D.S. 1993. Obese people who seek treatment have different characteristics than those who do not seek treatment. *Health Psychology* 12: 342-345.

Fontaine, K.R., Faith, M.S., Allison, D.B., and Cheskin, L.J. 1998. Body weight and health care among women in the general population. *Archives of Family Medicine* 7: 381-384.

Foster, G.D., Sarwer, D.B., and Wadden, T.A. 1997. Psychological effects of weight cycling in obese persons: A review of research agenda. *Obesity Research* 5: 474-488.

Friedman, M.A., and Brownell, K.D. 1995. Psychological correlates of obesity: Moving to the next research generation. *Psychological Bulletin* 117: 3-20.

Frieze, I.H., Olson, J.E., and Good, D.C. 1990. Perceived and actual discrimination in the salaries of male and female managers. *Journal of Applied Social Psychology* 20: 46-67.

Garner, C.M., and Nicol, G.T. 1998. Comparison of male and female nurses' attitudes toward obesity. *Perceptual and Motor Skills* 86: 1442.

Gorman, B.S., and Allison, D.B. 1995. Measures of restrained eating. In *Handbook of assessment methods for eating behaviors and weight-related problems*, ed. D.B. Allison, 149-184. Thousand Oaks, CA: Sage.

Gortmaker, S.L., Must, A., Perrin, J.M., Sobol, A.M., and Dietz, W.H. 1993. Social and economic consequences of overweight in adolescence and young adulthood. *New England Journal of Medicine* 329: 1008-1012.

Grillo, C.M., Wilfley, D.E., Brownell, K.D., and Rodin, J. 1994. Teasing, body image and self-esteem in a clinical sample of obese women. *Addictive Behaviors* 19: 443-450.

Harris, J.E., Hamaday, V., and Mochan, E. 1999. Osteopathic family physicians' attitudes, knowledge, and self-reported practices regarding obesity. *Journal of the American Dietetic Association* 99: 358-365.

Heatherton, T.F., Polivy, J., and Herman, C.P. 1991. Restraint, weight loss, and variability of body weight. *Journal of Abnormal Psychology* 100: 78-83.

Heinberg, L.J., and Thompson, J.K. 1995. Body image and televised images of thinness and attractiveness: A controlled laboratory investigation. *Journal of Social and Clinical Psychology* 7: 335-344.

Hill, A.J., and Silver, E.K. 1995. Fat, friendless, and unhealthy: 9-year-old children's perception of body shape stereotypes. *International Journal of Obesity* 19: 423-430.

Istvan, J., Zavela, K., and Weidner, G. 1992. Body weight and psychological distress in NHANES I. *International Journal of Obesity* 16: 999-1003.

Johnson, S.L., and Birch, L.L. 1994. Parents' and children's adiposity and eating style. *Pediatrics* 94: 653-661.

Kaplan, S.P. 1984. Rehabilitation counseling students' perceptions of obese male and female clients. *Rehabilitation Counseling Bulletin* 27: 172-181.

Karris, L. 1977. Prejudice against obese renters. *Journal of Social Psychology* 101: 159-160.

Klesges, R.C., Isbell, T.R., and Klesges, L.M. 1992. Relationship between dietary restraint, energy intake, physical activity, and body weight: A prospective analysis. *Journal of Abnormal Psychology* 101: 668-674.

Klesges, R.C., Klem, M., and Bene, C. 1989. Effects of dietary restraint, obesity, and gender on holiday eating behavior and weight gain. *Journal of Abnormal Psychology* 98: 499-503.

Klesges, R.C., Klem, M.L., Hanson, C.L., Eck, L.H., Ernst, J., O'Laughlin, D., Garrott, A., and Rife, R. 1990. The effects of applicant's health status and qualifications on simulated hiring decisions. *International Journal of Obesity* 14: 525-535.

Korkeila, M., Rissanen, A., Kaprio, J., Sorensen, T.I., and Koskenvuo, M. 1999. Weight-loss attempts and risk of major weight gain: A prospective study in Finnish adults. *American Journal of Clinical Nutrition* 70: 965-975.

Lewis, V.J., Blair, A.J., and Booth, D.A. 1992. Outcome of group therapy for body-image emotionality and weight-control self-efficacy. *Behavioral Psychotherapy* 20: 155-165.

Liese, B.S. 1986. Physicians' perceptions of the role of psychology in medicine. *Professional Psychology: Research and Practice* 17: 276-277.

Lyons, P., and Miller, W.C. 1999. Effective health promotion and clinical care for large people. *Medicine and Science in Sports and Exercise* 31: 1141-1146.

Maiman, L.A., Wang, V.L., Becker, M.H., Finlay, J., and Simonson, M. 1979. Attitudes toward obesity and the obese among professionals. *Journal of the American Dietetic Association* 74: 331-336.

Marcus, M.D., Wing, R.R., and Hopkins, J. 1988. Obese binge eaters: Affect, cognitions, and response to behavioral weight control. *Journal of Consulting and Clinical Psychology* 56: 433-439.

Morrison, T.G., and O'Connor, W.E. 1999. Psychometric properties of a scale measuring negative attitudes toward overweight individuals. *Journal of Social Psychology* 139: 436-445.

Muir, S., Wertheim, E.H., and Paxton, S.J. 1999. Adolescent girls' first diets: Triggers and the role of multiple dimensions of self-concept. *Eating Disorders: Journal of Treatment and Prevention* 7: 259-270.

Myers, A., and Rosen, J.C. 1999. Obesity stigmatization and coping: Relation to mental health symptoms, body image, and self-esteem. *International Journal of Obesity* 23: 221-230.

Najman, J.M., Klein, D., and Munro, C. 1982. Patient characteristics negatively stereotyped by doctors. *Social Science Medicine* 16: 1781-1789.

Neumark-Sztainer, D., Story, M., and Fabisch, L. 1998. Perceived stigmatization among overweight African American and Caucasian adolescent girls. *Journal of Adolescent Health* 23: 264-270.

Olsen, C.H., Schumaker, H., and Yawn, B. 1994. Overweight women delay medical care. *Archives of Family Medicine* 3: 888-892.

O'Neil, P.M., and Jarrell, M.P. 1992. Psychological aspects of obesity and very-low-calorie diets. *American Journal of Clinical Nutrition* 56: 185S-189S.

Pearlman, J. The David Wells Diet: Chips, Beer, and American League Batters. *Sports Illustrated,* 6 July 2000.

Phillips, R.G., and Hill, A.J. 1998. Fat, plain, but not friendless: Self-esteem and peer acceptance of obese pre-adolescent girls. *International Journal of Obesity* 22: 287-293.

Pierce, J.W., and Wardle, J. 1997. Cause and effect beliefs and self-esteem of overweight children. *Journal of Child Psychology and Psychiatry* 6: 645-650.

Pi-Sunyer, F.X. 1993. Medical hazards of obesity. *Annals of Internal Medicine* 119: 655-660.

Polivy, J., and Herman, C.P. 1992. Undieting: A program to help people stop dieting. *International Journal of Eating Disorders* 11: 261-268.

Prather, R.C., and Williamson, D.A. 1988. Psychopathology associated with bulimia, binge eating, and obesity. *International Journal of Eating Disorders* 7: 177-184.

Price, J.H., Desmond, S.M., Krol, R.A., Snyder, F.F., and O'Connel, J.K. 1987. Family practice physicians' beliefs, attitudes, and practices regarding obesity. *American Journal of Preventive Medicine* 3: 339-345.

Rand, C.S.W., and MacGregor, A.M.C. 1991. Successful weight loss following obesity surgery and the perceived liability of morbid obesity. *International Journal of Obesity* 15: 577-579.

Richardson, S.A., Hastorf, A.H., Goodman, N., and Dornbusch, S.M. 1961. Cultural uniformity in reaction to physical disabilities. *American Sociological Review* 26: 241-247.

Rieves, L., and Cash, T.F. 1996. Social developmental factors and women's body image attitudes. *Journal of Social Behavior and Personality* 11: 63-78.

Robinson, B.E., and Bacon, J.G. 1996. The "If Only I Were Thin . . . " treatment program: Decreasing the stigmatizing effects of fatness. *Professional Psychology: Research and Practice* 27: 175-183.

Rosen, J.C. 1996. Improving body image in obesity. In *Body image, eating disorders, and obesity*, ed. J.K. Thompson, 425-440. Washington, DC: American Psychological Association.

Rosen, J.C., Orosan, P., and Reiter, J. 1995. Cognitive behavior therapy for negative body image in obese women. *Behavior Therapy* 26: 25-42.

Rothblum, E.D., Brand, P., Miller, C., and Oetjen, H. 1989. Results of the NAAFA survey on employment discrimination: Part II. *NAAFA Newsletter* 17: 4-6.

Roughan, P., Seddon, E., and Vernon-Roberts, J. 1990. Long-term effects of a psychologically based group programme for women preoccupied with body weight and eating behaviour. *International Journal of Obesity* 14: 135-147.

Sherman, A.A. 1981. *Obesity and sexism: Parental child preferences and attitudes toward obesity.* Unpublished master's thesis, University of Cincinnati.

Smoller, J.W., Wadden, T.A., and Stunkard, A.J. 1987. Dieting and depression: A critical review. *Journal of Psychosomatic Research* 31: 429-440.

Stake, J., and Lauer, M.L. 1987. The consequences of being overweight: A controlled study of gender differences. *Sex Roles* 17: 31-47.

Stice, E. 1998. Prospective relation of dieting behaviors to weight change in a community sample of adolescents. *Behavior Therapy* 29: 277-279.

Stice, E., Cameron, R.P., Killen, J.D., Hayward, C., and Taylor, C.B. 1999. Naturalistic weight-reduction efforts prospectively predict growth in relative weight and onset of obesity among female adolescents. *Journal of Consulting and Clinical Psychology* 67: 967-974.

Stice, E., Killen, J.D., Hayward, C., and Taylor, C.B. 1998. Age of onset for binge eating and purging during adolescence: A four-year survival analysis. *Journal of Abnormal Psychology* 107: 671-675.

Strauss, R.S. 2000. Childhood obesity and self-esteem. *Pediatrics* 105: e15.

Striegel-Moore, R., and Rodin, J. 1986. The influence of psychological variables in obesity. In *Handbook of eating disorder: Physiology, psychology, and treatment of obesity, anorexia, and bulimia*, eds. K.D. Brownell and J.P. Foreyt, 99-121. New York: Basic Books.

Stunkard, A.J., and Burt, V. 1967. Obesity and body images: II. Age at onset of disturbances in the body image. *American Journal of Psychiatry* 123: 1443-1447.

Tanco, S., Linden, W., and Earle, T. 1998. Well-being and morbid obesity in women: A controlled therapy evaluation. *International Journal of Eating Disorders* 23: 325-339.

Thompson, J.K., Covert, M.D., Richards, K.J., Johnson, S., and Catering, J. 1995. Development of body image, eating disturbance, and general psychological functioning in female adolescents: Covariance structure modeling and longitudinal investigations. *International Journal of Eating Disorders* 18: 221-236.

Thompson, J.K., and Psaltis, K. 1988. Multiple aspects and correlates of body figure ratings: A replication and extension of Fallon and Rosin (1985). *International Journal of Eating Disorders* 7: 813-818.

Wadden, T.A., and Stunkard, A.J. 1985. Psychopathology and obesity. *Annals of the New York Academy of Sciences* 499: 55-65.

Wade, T., Martin, N.G., Neale, M.C., Tiggermann, M., Treloar, S.A., Bucholz, K.K., Madden, P.A., and Heath, A.C. 1999. The structure of genetic and environmental risk factors for three measures of disordered eating. *Psychological Medicine* 29: 925-934.

Wardle, J., and Collins, E. 1998. Body dissatisfaction—Social and emotional influences in adolescent girls. Unpublished manuscript, University College, London, England.

Wertheim, E.H., Paxton, S.J., Schutz, H.K., and Muir, S.L. 1997. Why do adolescent girls watch their weight? An interview study examining sociocultural pressures to be thin. *Journal of Psychosomatic Research* 42: 345-355.

Wilson, G.T. 1997. Acceptance and change in the treatment of eating disorders and obesity. *Behavior Therapy* 27: 417-439.

Wooley, S.C. 1995. Is self-acceptance a reasonable goal? In *Obesity treatment: Establishing goals, improving outcomes, and reviewing the research agenda*, eds D.B. Allison, and F.X. Pi-Sunyer, 75-78. New York: Plenum Press.

Yanovski, S.Z., Nelson, J.E., Bubbert, B.K., and Spitzer, R.L. 1993. Association of binge eating disorder and psychiatric comorbidity in obese subjects. *American Journal of Psychiatry* 150: 1472-1479.

Young, L.M., and Powell, B. 1985. The effects of obesity on the clinical judgments of mental health professionals. *Journal of Health and Social Behavior* 26: 233-246.

Yuker, H.E., and Allison, D.B. 1994. Obesity: Sociocultural perspectives. In *Understanding eating disorders: Anorexia nervosa, bulimia nervosa, and obesity*, eds. L.A. Alexander-Mott, and D.B. Lumsden, 243-270. Philadelphia: Taylor & Francis.

Chapter 3

Economic Aspects of Obesity: A Managed Care Perspective

Nicolaas P. Pronk, PhD

HealthPartners, Center for Health Promotion
and HealthPartners Research Foundation,
Minneapolis, Minnesota

This chapter presents an overview of economic aspects related to overweight and obesity. The prevalence of overweight and obesity in the United States has risen steadily over the past couple of decades. Since the relationship between increased adiposity and morbidity is well documented, it is not surprising that the burden of illness is accompanied by a concomitant increase in the cost of illness. However, the *total* cost of illness is the result of direct medical expense as well as the increased indirect costs associated with lost productivity and premature death.

From a public health perspective, it is important to understand the overall impact of overweight and obesity on costs. From a managed care perspective, however, it may be more meaningful to consider the excess costs associated with individual-level overweight and obesity profiles in relation to the prevalence of the defined population that receives coverage. The difference is that the former applies to the public at large and presents a general overview of the issue, whereas the latter represents the scope of the issue at the local level and would allow for individual follow-up. In formulating clinical policy and deciding how to apply scarce health care resources, managed care organizations (MCOs) are interested in how these issues apply to their populations, preferably in the short term.

Given the priority to address the rapid increase in overweight and obesity and its associated economic impact, health plans or payers may wish to invest in interventions that effectively modify this adverse health risk. From a clinical perspective, how could MCOs support caregivers and providers in this effort? A coordinated effort that involves multiple settings, multiple teams, and multiple technologies holds much potential. Such an approach, termed a *systems approach* to obesity prevention and treatment (Pronk and Labat 1999; Pronk and O'Connor 1997), can bring multiple treatment options to those ready to take action at the most opportune time. The reach into the population of interest is critical and, when done well, has a considerable potential to address the economic burden of overweight and obesity.

Prevalence of Obesity

Despite persistent efforts to lose weight (Serdula et al. 1994), the U.S. population has experienced a dramatic and rapid rise in the prevalence of overweight and obesity over the past several decades (Flegal et al. 1998). Data based on the National Health and Nutrition Examination Surveys (NHANES) indicate that the proportion of the U.S. population considered obese (as defined by a body mass index (BMI) of ≥ 30 kg/m^2) has increased from 14.5% between 1976 and 1980 to 22.5% between 1988 and 1994 up to 30.5% in 1999 and 2000 (Flegal et al. 1998; Mokdad et al. 1999; Mokdad et al. 2001; Popkin and Drewnowski 1997; Flegal et al. 2002). When overweight is considered as well (as defined by a BMI of ≥ 25 kg/m^2), prevalence estimates suggest that 64.5% of adults in the United States today meet this criteria (Flegal et al. 2002). Furthermore, this dramatic increase has occurred across multiple racial and ethnic groups and both sexes (Flegal et al. 2002; Flegal et al. 1998; Mokdad et al. 1999; Mokdad et al. 2001).

The increase in prevalence of overweight and obesity has not been limited to specific areas of the United States. Recent data have profiled the spread of the "obesity epidemic" in terms of adult obesity prevalence statistics at the state level from 1991 to 1998 (Mokdad et al. 2001). Using data obtained from the Behavioral Risk Factor Surveillance System (BRFSS), the prevalence of obesity increased from 12% in 1991 to 17.9% in 1998 (Mokdad et al. 2001). The magnitude of the increased prevalence varied by region and by state. In 1991, states with prevalence statistics of >15% were an exception—by 1998, they had become the rule.

Obesity and the Burden of Disease

Excess weight is strongly associated with a burden of disease. Overweight and obesity cluster with cardiovascular disease, type 2 diabetes mellitus (DM), hypertension, stroke, dyslipidemia, osteoarthritis, depression, and some cancers (Burton et al. 1985). Recently, Must and colleagues (1999) described the relationship between weight status and the prevalence of health conditions in relation to severity of overweight and obesity. This analysis, based on NHANES III data, documented prevalence ratios for DM, gallbladder disease, coronary heart disease, high blood cholesterol, and hypertension by age and sex across weight status categories. With normal weight individuals as the reference (BMI range 18.5-

24.9 kg/m^2), a strong statistically significant trend emerged for an increasing prevalence of comorbid conditions for all diseases except coronary heart disease and high blood cholesterol in older men and women. As compared to normal-weight individuals, among those younger than 55 years and having class III obesity (BMI >40 kg/m^2), prevalence ratios were highest for DM (prevalence ratio of 18.1 for men and 12.9 for women) and gallbladder disease (prevalence ratios of 21.1 for men and 5.2 for women). Prevalence ratios tended to be greater in younger than in older adults, and the prevalence of having two or more health conditions increased across weight status categories regardless of race or ethnicity.

In a study conducted in a managed care setting, Quesenberry, Caan, and Jacobsen (1998) also reported an association between increasing BMI and a higher incidence of comorbid chronic conditions. The study was conducted on 17,118 members of a large MCO in northern California. Table 3.1 outlines this relationship by presenting the proportion of patients who have a chronic condition and fall into one of four BMI categories.

Obesity and the Total Cost of Illness

The total cost of illness includes more than just the costs associated with medical treatment. Broadly defined, costs may be measured in terms of direct or indirect expenditures. Direct costs would include the expenses associated with patient care ranging from physician visits, clinic services, medications, hospitalization, and others. Indirect costs would include the costs associated with a quantification of the value of lost productivity and premature death. This component is especially difficult to measure since it requires putting a price tag on concepts such as lost opportunity costs (e.g., forgone sales due to illness of the salesperson) and nonmedical payouts related to replacement staff and increased time spent on training, extra administration, and so on. Therefore, the total cost of obesity may be represented as the combination of direct and indirect costs associated with overweight and obesity.

However, as discussed previously, overweight and obesity cluster with many chronic

Table 3.1   *Relationship Between Body Mass Index and Chronic Disease*

Chronic condition	Percent of patients with chronic disease by BMI category			
	20-24.9 kg/m²	25-29.9 kg/m²	30-34.9 kg/m²	≥35 kg/m²
Diabetes	4	7	12	15
Hypertension	18	29	37	39
High cholesterol	13	19	20	14
Heart disease	10	15	17	17
Depression	13	14	16	22
Musculoskeletal	21	24	28	31

Data from Quesenberry, Caan, and Jacobsen 1998.

conditions that also have medical care costs. The costs associated with the medical treatment for obese individuals are therefore partly related to DM care, heart disease care, gallbladder care, depression care, and so forth. Overweight and obesity independent of associated disease also account for excess costs. To better understand the fraction of costs associated with obesity, analyses will need to control, at least to some degree, for chronic conditions. No doubt, most of the medical treatment cost for obese patients is related to chronic comorbidities—but not all. Excess weight and adiposity will create health concerns that need to be addressed even in the absence of chronic diseases. Furthermore, the indirect cost may well be much larger than the independent contribution of obesity to the medical treatment costs. For example, absenteeism and decrements in workplace performance have been related to overweight and obesity (Burton et al. 1998; Narbro et al. 1996; Tucker and Friedman 1998).

Measuring Costs

The measurement of medical care costs is not trivial and has many inherent challenges and limitations. First, the collection of cost data imposes many challenges on researchers and evaluators. Often, several databases are used to track medical charges, that is, the amount billed for services rendered. Medical care claims databases may be completely separate from pharmacy databases, and the two may

not be relational. Not being able to directly relate charges incurred at the individual member level poses challenges to the analyses.

Next, MCOs may have different contracts and payment arrangements with multiple providers, and therefore, one procedure may have differential pricing depending on who provides the service. As a result, actual utilization may be most appropriately modeled from a cost perspective by measuring the incurred charges as opposed to the amount paid.

In assessing the costs associated with, for example, obesity for a defined population, a proportion of the members will likely not have accessed the medical care delivery system over the study period and thus will have zero costs. Dealing with zero charges is a statistical challenge. Medical cost data tend to be severely skewed and therefore need to be transformed prior to statistical manipulation in order to meet normality assumptions—zero charges present a problem for transformation approaches. In addition, once the statistical computations have been made, the coefficients are not meaningful in terms of dollars since they were transformed. Hence, a retransformation that recreates the variable in its original form (i.e., dollars) needs to be applied. When this is done, the results only apply to that segment of the population that had positive, nonzero, charges. It is therefore paramount that the analytical approach deal appropriately with zero charges.

The skewness of medical cost data also affects the upper end of the distribution—the high-cost cases. Typically, a very small

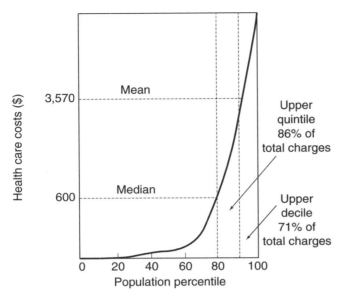

Figure 3.1 Obesity and cost distribution.
Data from Pronk et al. 1999, *Journal of American Medical Association* 282: 2235-2239.

proportion of the population studied incurs the majority of the expenses. For example, in an attempt to examine the relationship of modifiable health risks to subsequent health care charges, Pronk and colleagues (1999) studied 5,689 adult MCO members aged 40 and older. Resource use was measured by billed health care charges over an 18-month period. The distribution of the charges was such that the upper quintile of subjects accounted for 86% of the total charges, and the upper decile accounted for 71% of total charges. The median annual charge in the study population was $600 (interquartile range, $151-$2,080) compared with a mean (± SD) of $3,570 ± $12,823. Also, over this relatively short follow-up period, 15% of the study subjects had no medical encounter that generated a medical claim. This distribution is depicted in figure 3.1.

Societal Perspective

From a societal perspective, the cost associated with overweight and obesity may be calculated based on prevalence estimates. Analyses conducted in this area have provided important insight into the relationship between obesity and its economic burden. The data used in these types of analyses are limited to mostly secondary sources, including large prospective studies that analyzed the propor-

tion of certain diseases attributable to obesity or literature reviews that generate average (mean) data. Total direct cost estimates may then be developed for the disorders associated with obesity, and subsequent total cost statistics can be generated.

A study by Wolf and Colditz (1998) used a prevalence-based approach to quantifying the total cost of illness attributable to obesity in 1995 dollars. Direct costs were presented in the context of obesity-related diseases, while indirect costs were calculated following an analysis of excess physician visits, work-lost days, restricted activity, and bed days attributable to obesity and obtained from the 1988 and 1994 National Health Interview Survey (NHIS). The total cost attributable to obesity amounted to $99.2 billion in 1995. Approximately $51.6 billion was related to direct medical care costs. The direct costs of obesity represented 5.7% of the 1995 national health expenditure in the United States. This amount is approximately 1.25 times the cost of coronary heart disease and 2.7 times the cost of hypertension in the United States. Colditz (1999) presented updates to these data using prevalences from NHANES III. Overall, the direct costs of obesity were approximately $70 billion, accounting for approximately 7% of the total health care cost. Table 3.2 shows a summary of the direct costs in both of these studies.

The economic burden of overweight and obesity on society is clearly substantial. Moreover, since the direct cost of obesity expresses itself through morbidity-related medical care delivery system interactions, the burden of illness associated with obesity is also overwhelmingly high. In fact, it may be considered greater than that of heart disease or hypertension.

Individual-Level and Defined Population Perspectives

The sum of the health of all individuals within a defined population may be considered equal to that of the population (Evans and Stoddart 1994). In a defined population, such as the membership of a MCO, individual-level data on the cost of medical care may be tracked. In such cases, the association between overweight and obesity (expressed using BMI) and health services use and costs may be quantified and directly related to policy and resource allocation decisions at the local level of the MCO.

Table 3.2   *Costs of Diseases Attributed to Obesity*

Condition	Direct costs ($ billions)*	Direct costs ($ billions) **
Type 2 diabetes	32.40	36.6
Coronary heart disease	6.99	16.2
Osteoarthritis	4.30	3.6
Hypertension	3.23	7.6
Gallbladder disease	2.59	4.3
Breast cancer	0.84	0.53
Endometrial cancer	0.286	0.23
Colon cancer	1.01	0.89
Total	51.64	70

* Data from Wolf and Colditz 1998.
** Data from Colditz 1999.

Table 3.3   *Health Care Utilization Rates and Costs by BMI Categories*

Variable	BMI categories			
	25-29.9 kg/m^2	30-34.9 kg/m^2	≥35 kg/m^2	*p*
Inpatient services	0.83	1.33	1.70	<0.001
Inpatient cost	0.83	1.33	1.70	<0.001
Pharmacy cost	1.23	1.60	1.78	<0.001
Laboratory cost	0.97	1.24	1.85	<0.001
Outpatient visits	1.02	1.14	1.25	<0.001
Outpatient cost	0.99	1.21	1.37	0.003
Total cost of care	0.95	1.25	1.44	<0.001

Rate ratio reference group is BMI 20-24.9 kg/m^2. Data from Quesenberry et al. 1998.

Obesity and Health Care Utilization

Quesenberry, Caan, and Jacobsen (1998), as discussed earlier, studied the health care utilization and direct annual cost of 17,118 Kaiser Permanente Medical Care Program members. The type of health care utilization was expressed according to BMI ranges, and costs collected included all hospitalizations, laboratory services, outpatient visits, outpatient pharmacy, radiology services, and the direct costs of providing these services during 1993.

The researchers found a strong association between BMI and these services. Relative to a BMI of 20 to 24.9 kg/m^2, mean annual total costs were 25% greater among those with BMI of 30 to 34.9 kg/m^2 and 44% greater among those with BMI of ≥35 kg/m^2. The direct cost of care associated with obesity amounted to approximately 6% of total health plan health care expenditure for 1997. Table 3.3 describes the increasing rates (expressed as rate ratios) between health care utilization and direct costs.

Body Mass Index and Short-Term Excess Health Care Charges

Defining the financial feasibility of care improvement and prevention investments should not only consider cost-effectiveness and cost-benefit, but also the high cost of inaction, that is, the cost of not preventing or not improving. In the context of a defined population, the cost of inaction becomes very meaningful since financial risk may be related back to specific individuals who are, by definition, included in the population.

Pronk and colleagues (1999) studied the relationship between modifiable health risks and short-term health care charges in a sample of HealthPartners health plan members in the upper midwestern United States. A stratified random sample of health plan members age 40 and older was selected from the MCO in Minnesota. This sample was stratified according to the presence of none, one, or two or more chronic conditions including diabetes, hypertension, heart disease, and dyslipidemia ($N = 7,535$). A total of 5,689 subjects (75.5% response rate) completed surveys. Resource use was measured by billed health care charges during the following 18 months. After adjustment for age, sex, race, and chronic disease status, each BMI unit was prospectively related to 1.9% higher charges. That is, for each incremental unit of BMI, health care costs increased by 1.9%. Furthermore, as overweight was combined with other modifiable health risks, such as physical inactivity and tobacco use, risk-specific profiles (low- and high-risk profiles) indicated significantly higher excess costs incurred due to the presence of high modifiable risks by as much as 49% per year. The characteristics of the low-risk profile were a BMI of 25 kg/m², never smoked, and did physical activity three days per week; the characteristics of the high-risk profile were a BMI of 27.5 kg/m², currently smoking, and engaging in zero days of phyiscal activity per week. Both the low- and high-risk profiles were controlled for age, heart disease, and diabetes. These results are depicted in figure 3.2.

Direct Cost of Obesity in Employed Population

Pronk, Tan, and O'Connor (1999) studied the association between obesity and cost in a multi-employer data set. As part of ongoing health improvement initiatives, they obtained health risk information from 8,822 employed health plan members. The population for this study was defined as all employees who were associated with a worksite health promotion program implemented at 298 companies ($N = 24,720$). Therefore, the response rate was 35.7%. Unlike other non-population-based studies, however, the researchers were able to compare responders to nonresponders regarding their health care expenditures since all employees received their medical care benefits from the same health plan. Nonresponders included more males, were older, and had significantly more clinic visits and higher charges, a conclusion supporting the notion that all relationships found among respondents should be regarded as conservative findings.

Control was exerted for age, sex, asthma, breast cancer, other cancer, diabetes, heart disease, hypercholesterolemia, hypertension, back pain, lung disease, emotional function, and physical function. Obesity-related risk levels were assigned according to the level of BMI. A BMI <27.8 kg/m² for men and <27.3 kg/m² for women was considered low risk, and all levels above those were considered high risk. Charges

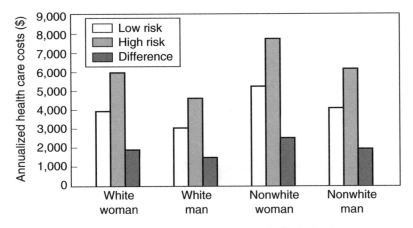

Figure 3.2 Excess annual cost impact of modifiable behaviors.

Data from Pronk et al. 1999, *Journal of American Medical Association* 282: 2235-2239.

were collected retrospectively for an average of 33 months and subsequently annualized.

Multivariate analyses indicated a significant relationship between obesity and annualized health care costs. Relative to low-risk individuals, the mean medical costs for high-risk individuals were 8% per year higher. This 8% translated to an excess cost of $135 per high-risk individual per year.

Willingness to Communicate

In order to present a compelling argument for the need for investments in health improvement programs that effectively address weight-related concerns, we must know whether an "audience" exists that is willing to engage in a two-way communication around issues of health and weight management. O'Connor and coworkers conducted a survey of all adults attending two health maintenance organization clinics and asked them about their willingness to communicate regarding processes and programs designed to help them improve their health (O'Connor et al. 1996). The survey was conducted by telephone and completed by 3,826 members (82% response rate); 86% of the respondents were willing to engage in a two-way communication with health professionals.

These study results indicate that, in general, adults appear to be interested in a two-way communication around health issues. In a subsequent study, we hypothesized and demonstrated that this willingness to communicate would also be related to higher health care cost (Pronk, Tan, and O'Connor 1999). The hypothesis was based on the premise that those interested in knowing their options for health improvement already realized the presence of modifiable health risk factors in their lives. Using similar control variables and adding BMI and predicted fitness, willingness to communicate remained an independent predictor for excess annualized costs. This variable was associated with 22% higher annualized costs as compare to individuals not willing to communicate, or $358 per year. In other words, individuals interested in learning more about options available to them to improve their health are more likely to also have higher annual health care costs. This finding supports strategic efforts to reach out proactively to individuals who are willing to learn of their options for health improvement and invite them to join programs.

Interventions for Defined Populations

Whereas cross-sectional analyses describe associations of overweight and obesity with health care expenditures, there is a need to consider specific interventions designed to support achievement of healthy weight in the context of program costs and benefits incurred. It is important to consider the need for information that is based on the study of clearly defined populations and interventions that may be considered scalable and sustainable. Hence, issues related to the feasibility of program implementation and the overall logic framework used for program justification is quite important for program administrators.

Economic Feasibility

The studies presented in this chapter provide strong evidence of significant excess medical expenses associated with overweight and obesity. The total excess costs incurred by health plans and payers for the entire populations of interest are clearly substantial. This amount is directly related to the prevalence of overweight and obesity and the amount of change that is achieved in the context of the cost of the intervention.

Unfortunately, not much information is available in the area of return on investment (ROI) for weight management programs in which program benefits are considered against program costs. Several studies that present individual-level data for defined populations have outlined the fraction of excess charges that may be reversed (Pronk et al. 1999; Pronk, Tan, and O'Connor 1999; Quesenberry, Caan, and Jacobsen 1998). However, in these analyses the cost of the intervention is not addressed. Hence, implementation of programs is hindered by the absence of studies that outline return on investment for these programs. Nevertheless, studies have emerged in the literature that address the issue of ROI for health improvement programs (Goetzel, Juday, and Ozminkowski 1999; Ozminkowski et al. 1999; Pelletier 1997). Despite the fact that weight management programs are not analyzed separately, the overall trend for health improvement programs is in a favorable direction for cost-related outcome (Aldana 2001; Goetzel, Juday, and Ozminkowski 1999).

Furthermore, skepticism exists regarding the efficacy and effectiveness of interventions designed to manage weight from the perspective of populations. When considering specific programs, managed care organizations can calculate total implementation costs. Regardless of the costs, however, if the returns are unknown, organizations may have difficulty investing unless they do so for reasons other than economic

benefit. A continued need exists for effectiveness studies of weight management programs that document long-term success.

Economic Logic Model

Evans and Stoddart (1994, p. 55) state: "A society that spends so much on health care that it cannot or will not spend adequately on other health enhancing activities may actually be reducing the health of its population." The studies presented here indicate that the cost of inaction, that is, the costs associated with maintaining a status quo regarding the issues of overweight and obesity, may be unacceptably high. There is an apparent need for a logic that would describe a closed-loop rationale linking economic justification of investing in health improvement programs

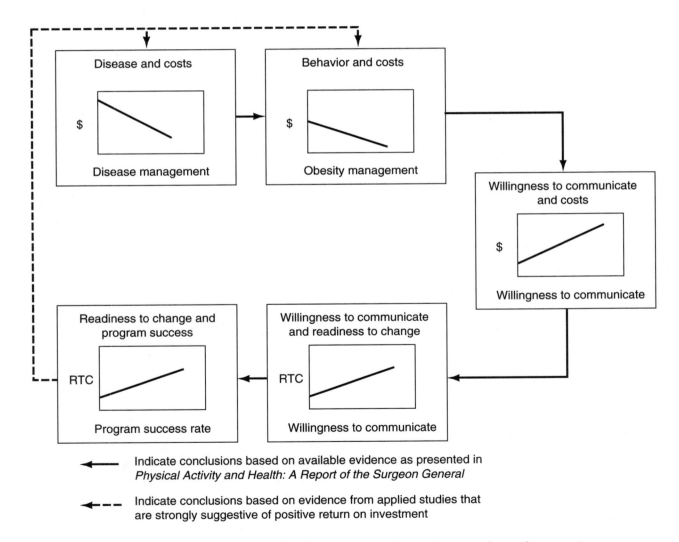

Figure 3.3 Closed-loop logic for economic rationale for investment in obesity prevention and treatment.

designed to manage disease and weight, reaching a sufficiently large audience, getting good participation, and relating outcomes back to the programs that were implemented. In such a model, logic needs to flow from one question to the next, linking disease to behavior to reach a defined target population and showing program success. Pronk, O'Connor, and Martinson (2002) proposed such a model in the area of physical activity and economic impact. This model was derived from population-based studies on the relationship between health care charges and disease or lifestyle. Furthermore, this model is consistent with a systems approach to health improvement for defined populations, which calls for cost-related outcomes as one of its performance measures (Pronk and O'Connor 1997).

Considering that an audience needs to be available to hear the messages and act on opportunities, the concept of "willingness to communicate" must be quantified in terms of the size of the audience and the economic impact (O'Connor et al. 1996; Pronk, Tan, and O'Connor 1999). Furthermore, among health plan members, readiness to make changes related to diet and physical activity appears significantly greater in those who have one or more chronic conditions than in their healthier counterparts (Boyle et al. 1998). Hence, based on the notion that readiness to change is directly related to successful behavior change (Prochaska and Velicher 1997), outreach programs that proactively invite individuals who are willing to communicate, at higher stages of readiness to make changes, and overweight or obese appear to be a worthwhile economic consideration. Figure 3.3 outlines this rationale in closed-loop logic.

Summary

Overweight and obesity are strong predictors of excess direct and indirect health care costs. The economic burden of not changing the prevalence of overweight and obesity presents us with an opportunity to act. Since the short-term cost of overweight is tremendous, effective weight management programs may be a good investment. This may be especially true since overweight and obesity are strongly related to a variety of diseases and disorders that also create an unacceptably high burden of illness. A closed-loop logic may be helpful in supporting strategic decision making and resource allocation criteria for key stakeholders in this process.

References

Aldana, S.G. 2001. Financial impact of health promotion programs: A comprehensive review of the literature. *American Journal of Health Promotion* 15: 296-320.

Boyle, R.G., O'Connor, P.J., Pronk, N.P., and Tan, A. 1998. Stages of change for physical activity, diet, and smoking among HMO members with chronic conditions. *American Journal of Health Promotion* 12: 170-175.

Burton, B.T., Foster, W.R., Hirsch, J., and VanItallie, T.B. 1985. Health implications of obesity: NIH consensus development conference. *International Journal of Obesity* 9: 155-169.

Burton, W.N., Chen, C-Y., Schultz, A.B., and Edington, D.W. 1998. The economic costs associated with body mass index in a workplace. *Journal of Occupational and Environmental Medicine* 40: 786-792.

Colditz, G.A. 1999. Economic costs of obesity and inactivity. *Medicine and Science in Sports and Exercise* 31: S663-S667.

Evans, R.G, and Stoddart, G.L. 1994. Producing health, consuming health care. In *Why are some people healthy and others not?* eds. R.G. Evans, M.L. Barer, and T.R. Marmor, 27-66. New York: Aldine de Gruyter.

Flegal, K.M., Carrol, M.D., Kuczmarski, R.J., and Johnson, C.L. 1998. Overweight and obesity trends in the United States: Prevalence and trends, 1960-1994. *International Journal of Obesity* 22: 39-47.

Flegal, K.M., Carrol, M.D., Ogden, C.L., and Johnson, C.L. 2002. Prevalence and trends in obesity among U.S. adults, 1999-2000. *Journal of the American Medical Association* 288: 1723-1727.

Goetzel, R.Z., Juday, T.R., and Ozminkowski, R.J. 1999. What's the ROI? A systematic review of return-on-investment studies of corporate health and productivity management initiatives. *AWHP's Worksite Health* summer: 12-21.

Mokdad, A.H., Bowman, B.A., Ford, E.S., Vinicor, F., Marks, J.S., and Koplan, J.P. 2001. The continuing epidemics of obesity and diabetes in the United States. *Journal of the American Medical Association* 286: 1195-1200.

Mokdad, A.H., Serdula, M.K., Dietz, W.H., Bowman, B.A., Marks, J.S., and Koplan, J.P. 1999. The spread of the obesity epidemic in the United States, 1991-1998. *Journal of the American Medical Association* 282: 1519-1522.

Must, A., Spadano, J., Coakley, E.H., Field, A.E., Colditz, G., and Dietz, W.H. 1999. The disease burden associated with overweight and obesity. *Journal of the American Medical Association* 282: 1523-1529.

Narbro, K., Jonsson, E., Larsson, B., Waaler, H., Wedel, H., and Sjostrom, L. 1996. Economic consequences of sick-leave and early retirement in obese Swedish women. *International Journal of Obesity* 20: 895-903.

O'Connor, P.J., Rush, W.A., Rardin, K.A., et al. 1996. Are HMO members willing to engage in two-way communications to improve health? *HMO Practice* 10: 17-19.

Ozminkowski, R.J., Dunn, R.L., Goetzel, R.Z., Cantor, R.I., Murnane, J., Harrison, M. 1999. A return on investment evaluation of the Citibank, N.A., health management program. *American Journal of Health Promotion* 14: 31-43.

Pelletier, K. 1997. Clinical and cost outcomes of multifactorial, cardiovascular risk management interventions in worksites: A comprehensive review and analysis. *Journal of Occupational and Environmental Medicine* 39: 1154-1169.

Popkin, B.M., and Drewnowski, A. 1997. Dietary fats and the nutrition transition: New trends in the global diet. *Nutrition Reviews* 55: 31-33.

Prochaska, J.O., and Velicher, W.F. 1997. The transtheoretical model of health behavior change. *American Journal of Health Promotion* 12: 38-48.

Pronk, N.P., Goodman, M., O'Connor, P.J., and Martinson, B.C. 1999. Relationship between modifiable health risks and short-term health care charges. *Journal of the American Medical Association* 282: 2235-2239.

Pronk, N.P., and Labat, J. 1999. Systems approach to childhood and adolescent obesity prevention and treatment in a managed care organization. *International Journal of Obesity* 23: S38-S42.

Pronk, N.P., and O'Connor, P.J. 1997. Systems approach to population health improvement. *Journal of Ambulatory Care Management* 20: 24-31.

Pronk, N.P., O'Connor, P.J., and Martinson, B.C. 2002. Population health and active living: Economic potential of physical activity promotion. *American Journal of Medicine and Sports* 4: 51-57.

Pronk, N.P., Tan, A., and O'Connor, P.J. 1999. Obesity, fitness, willingness to communicate and health care costs. *Medicine and Science in Sports and Exercise* 31: 1535-1543.

Quesenberry, C.P., Caan, B., and Jacobsen, A. 1998. Obesity, health services use, and health care costs among members of a health maintenance organization. *Archives of Internal Medicine* 158: 466-472.

Serdula, M.K., Williamson, D.F., Anda, R.F., Levy, A., Heaton, A., and Byers, T. 1994. Weight control practices in adults. *American Journal of Public Health* 84: 1821-1824.

Tucker, L.A., and Friedman, G.M. 1998. Obesity and absenteeism: An epidemiologic study of 10,825 employed adults. *American Journal of Health Promotion* 12: 202-207.

Wolf, A.M., and Colditz, G.A. 1998. Current estimates of the economic cost of obesity in the United States. *Obesity Research* 6: 97-106.

Chapter 4

Genetic Influences on Obesity

Brock A. Beamer, MD
Johns Hopkins Geriatrics Center
and Johns Hopkins School of Medicine

"You are what you eat." Well, not quite. You are what you eat *after* what you eat has been altered quite a bit. The instructions for that alteration are contained in your genes, which hold the recipes for the proteins that form the structure and machinery of the human food-processing factory. These genes direct an incredible process by which a single cell uses food to develop into an incredibly organized multitude of unique cells, each with different properties, and each in just the right place.

Having many very similar genes makes different collections of cells develop very similarly. Hence all mammals are warm-blooded, four-limbed, furry creatures that bear live offspring. Having somewhat different genes is what makes an elephant big and a mouse small, even if they are both mammals and even if they both eat the same food (albeit in different quantities). Having the same basic genes makes all dogs a single species, but having some variation in those genes is what makes a Great Dane great and a Miniature Poodle miniature.

Of course, there is not nearly as much variety in the bodies of various humans as there is in the bodies of various dogs. This suggests that the genes controlling human body shape and size are more uniform throughout the population. (Indeed, it is estimated that 99.9% of our genome is identical between persons.) There are relatively narrow absolute ranges of heights and weights (and shapes) of human bodies ["absolute" in that no adults are <2 or >10 ft tall (<0.5 or >3 m), nor weigh <10 or >2,000 lb (<5 or >1,000 kg)]. There is an even narrower range of "normal" within which most humans fall. But certainly we are not all *exactly* the same. Some are tall and some are short. Some are thin and some are obese. How much of that variety is due to differences in our genes and how much is due to other differences among us (our behaviors, environments, and so on) is not entirely clear yet. Estimates range as low as 30%, but it is more probable that 50 to 70% of that variation is due to genetic differences. In any case, it does seem increasingly clear that a considerable portion of the variation seen in the size of human bodies can be explained by genetic variation.

The purpose of this chapter is to discuss genetic influences on obesity. Because the rapid pace of discovery will make a detailed review obsolete by press time, we refer only briefly to specific gene variants known thus far to influence obesity. Instead of comprehensively reviewing a relatively new field, we will try to prepare readers to understand basic concepts that will help in following this field as it develops further ("Give a man a fish and he eats for a day. Teach a man to fish and he eats for a lifetime.") We will begin by considering genetic influences on obesity in historical and social contexts, then discuss how obesity is a complex disease with special concerns regarding genetic analysis. Finally, we will discuss how we are approaching this analysis and how a reader can evaluate our progress. Readers are encouraged to write or e-mail if any issues are not addressed adequately for their particular purposes. The basic goals of this chapter are to enable readers (1) to understand the importance of looking for genetic influences on obesity, (2) to follow the search for those influences, and (3) to appreciate why we will need to be patient and thoughtful in that search.

Historical Context

In some ways, it is surprising that not long ago experts disagreed about whether obesity is genetically influenced. Selective breeding of livestock, particularly swine, has long been very successful at increasing total body fat (and more recently, at reducing it again). In humans, historical and literary references abound with accounts of obese parents having obese offspring (although many often added "slovenly," "lazy," or "greedy" to the inherited traits). Over the past few decades, classical, or Mendelian, geneticists have tried to identify a pattern of inheritance for obesity. While a very few pedigrees do suggest an autosomal dominant or recessive mode of inheritance, most suggest that obesity "tends to run in families" but without a clear pattern of inheritance. Exceptions include heritable syndromes in which obesity is one of several features, such as Prader-Willi disease. Also, it has been known for some time that Down's syndrome is caused by the dramatic genetic abnormality of an extra chromosome, and that it carries an increased risk of obesity.

While a primary genetic basis appears to underlie the tendency for typical obesity to run in families, there are other plausible explanations. It may be simply that children learn to eat in excess from parents who do likewise (as they learn to smoke or to be racist). Certainly many familial and cultural traits are "inherited" in a nongenetic fashion, and dietary habits are prominent examples. Chinese cuisine has few sweets, and Chinese people tend to be thinner than those from cultures that prize desserts. The opposite extreme is seen in some North African cultures, where plumpness remains a prominent sign of prosperity, and it is customary to force-feed young daughters.

That the generally accepted (and well-documented) tendency for obesity to run in families is not due solely to social or postnatal environmental influences was elegantly demonstrated even before modern molecular genetics could identify specific mutations as causal. For instance, the body habitus of adoptees was shown to more closely resemble that of their birth parents than of their adoptive parents (Stunkard et al. 1986). Similarly, the bodies of monozygotic twins resemble each other more so than do those of dizygotic twins (Stunkard, Foch, and Hrubec 1986). While these studies cannot exclude prenatal environmental effects, they are suggestive enough to have warranted considerable research into genetic factors underlying obesity. Certainly they suggest that not all the factors influencing the development of obesity are behavioral or volitional.

Social Context

From a social perspective, the recognition that obesity has strong genetic influences may be of greater importance than is the similar recognition for many other common (and most uncommon) diseases. We are all familiar with the great potential that molecular biology and genetics hold for improved diagnosis or treatment of diseases such as cystic fibrosis or coronary artery disease. Obesity, however, is not "just another medical disease." Obese people often face condemnation rather than compassion, and discrimination rather than accommodation. Obese people are often viewed not as sick, but rather as lazy, and even ugly, dumb, slovenly, or disgusting. These sentiments are well documented to lead to a lack of appropriate employment opportunities and a dearth of fashionable clothes. Unfortunately, these sentiments are also evident in the indifference if not antagonism expressed at all levels of the health care community. Most tragically, they are evident in the psyche of obese persons who believe that all the terrible things our society says about them are true.

Not only may understanding the molecular bases of obesity lead to improved means of preventing its adverse effects on health, but it may also begin to address some of its social, emotional, and, for some people, ethical ramifications. Indeed, one may argue that the greatest impact of improved understanding of the etiology of disorders such as leprosy, schizophrenia, and epilepsy has not been the development of effective medical therapies, but the alteration in the way others viewed people suffering from them, and the way those suffering from them viewed themselves. No longer do we believe people with these disorders to be cursed, sinful, or possessed by demons—we view them as unfortunate sufferers of an inevitable biological process. Current knowledge supports such a change in attitude for obesity as well. It is increasingly clear that genetic influences contribute to most, if not all, cases of typical obesity, and to all cases of profound obesity. Translating this information to effective therapies may take some time, but using it to remove stigma and to bolster self-esteem should be well under way already.

Biological Context

At first glance, obesity seems to be a very simple disorder: If you eat too much, you become obese. It's not quite so simple since if you exercise a lot, you won't get quite as obese. But isn't it true that two different people can eat and exercise the same amount, and one will become obese but the other won't? Could it be because they have different genes? But isn't it also true that identical twins never weigh *exactly* the same? It must not be *all* genes.

Obesity As a Complex, Polygenic Disease

Typical obesity is a complex disorder with multiple genetic and nongenetic influences. Mathematical models and statistical analyses help prove this. But proof or not, at some level we all know it to be true because we see it in action every day. McDonald's wouldn't spend millions of dollars on advertising if it didn't make people want to eat more; Jenny Craig wouldn't be getting rich if people could lose weight just because they wanted to; people in the same family wouldn't look so very similar if genes didn't play a large role. We all know that the development of obesity is complex because we all see it every day, every place we look. It really is that simple.

While "simple," when referring to a disease, may seem to refer to how simple the disease is to figure out, more specifically it refers to the number of factors that contribute to the etiology of the disease. If a disease has one necessary and sufficient cause, it is simple. If it has dozens of possible interacting causes, it is complex. Generally, traumatic injuries and infections are simple, as are single gene disorders with absolute penetrance (i.e., everyone with the mutation has the disease). Coronary artery disease and childhood asthma are complex, with probable contributions from multiple genetic and environmental influences (and others, such as personality and infectious influences).

One could debate whether a clear dichotomy of simple versus complex exists when diseases are scrutinized carefully. For instance, the flu seems pretty simple: The influenza virus makes you sick. On the one hand, this is true—no virus, no disease. On the other hand, the virus can be quite variable. Some people with the same virus feel lousy for a few days then recover while others get horribly sick and die. Surely factors other than simple exposure to the virus determine the outcome of a case of the flu (perhaps even a genetic abnormality in the patient's immune system). More germane to a discussion of genetics is the most widely recognized simple genetic disorder. Why do some people with sickle cell disease live fairly normal lives while others with the same mutation in the same gene have frequent painful attacks and disabling sequelae? Interactions with the environment, and with variation in other genes, certainly affect the outcome of even simple disorders.

This issue of semantics, however, should not detract from the utility of this conceptual construct. In genetics (as in most of medicine, as in most of science, as in most of life!) nothing is as simple as we once believed. Nonetheless, from a pragmatic standpoint the concept of simple versus complex can be quite useful, particularly when studying genetic traits and diseases. When trying to establish whether a genetic variation is influencing a particular trait, we must be mindful of other influences that may confound the characterization of an individual as positive versus negative for that trait. If one does not account for differences in environmental and behavioral factors (or other nongenetic factors), then one may mistakenly attribute some differences between people to genetic factors, or mistakenly dismiss genetic influences in people who appear similar.

For example, John is very obese and has a variation in gene X. Jim is very lean and has the normal gene X. It may appear that the gene X variant makes John obese, but this assessment may change when one realizes that John eats nothing but chicken-fried steak and never exercises, while Jim is a vegetarian who runs marathons. Conversely, what if John and Jim weighed exactly the same? It may appear that the gene variant has no effect at all, until those very different diet and exercise habits are considered.

Even if all nongenetic issues could be ignored, great complexity occurs when more than one genetic variant can lead to the same trait. Physiological systems generally have a multitude of proteins that work together to perform a given function. Each of these proteins is encoded by a gene that is subject to mutation. It is easy to imagine, then, that a mutation in any of these different genes may result in the same disease or physical trait. Further, the system may be able to compensate for a mutation in any one of these genes, but combinations of multiple mutations may not be adequately compensated and thus may result in the disease or abnormal trait.

Most complicated are diseases or traits that involve several physiological systems that can compensate for one another. The disease or trait may then be present only when multiple mutations impede the function of multiple systems (and perhaps then only if certain nongenetic factors are also present). These situations are very difficult to study, and most cases of obesity appear to be situations like this. Maintaining a stable body weight requires the balance of energy intake and energy expenditure. As illustrated in figure 4.1, however, even if these remain equal and weight does remain stable, differences in how our bodies use the energy determine whether

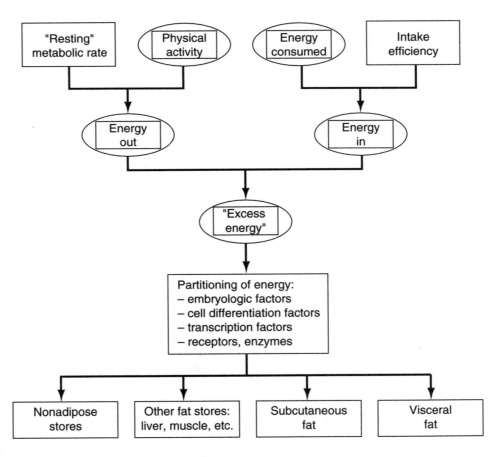

Figure 4.1 Partitioning of energy.

a weight stable person has a lot of muscles, a beer belly, or an extra seat cushion. The boxes in figure 4.1 indicate that the factor is largely influenced by genetic variation, and the ovals indicate that the factor is largely influenced by nongenetic factors. Both a box and an oval signify that genetic and nongenetic factors likely contribute to variation.

Of course, most people are not weight stable throughout adulthood, but rather take in more energy than they expend. Figures 4.2 (energy intake) and 4.3 (energy expended) illustrate only some of the many factors that contribute to this phenomenon. When one considers all the different physiological systems involved in each side of that "simple" equation, and all the different genetic and nongenetic factors that can influence those systems, it is easy to appreciate why there is such a wide range of adiposity in humans. In figures 4.2 and 4.3, boxes indicate the factor is likely largely influenced by genetic variation, and ovals indicate the factor is likely largely influenced by nongenetic factors. Both a box and an oval indicate that both likely contribute to variation. With so many factors on each side, in fact, it is remarkable how weight stable most people are.

Obesity As a Simple, Monogenic Disorder

Most cases of "typical obesity" likely are complex with multiple genetic and nongenetic influences. However, recently researchers have identified some very rare cases of "simple" obesity due to mutations in single genes. For the most part, these are so rare and so recently discovered that it is not yet known whether they are transmitted in classical Mendelian fashion, but it appears that they should be. That is, if we could observe enough families that have these mutations, we should be able to predict which individuals carried the mutation and which did not just by knowing who was very obese.

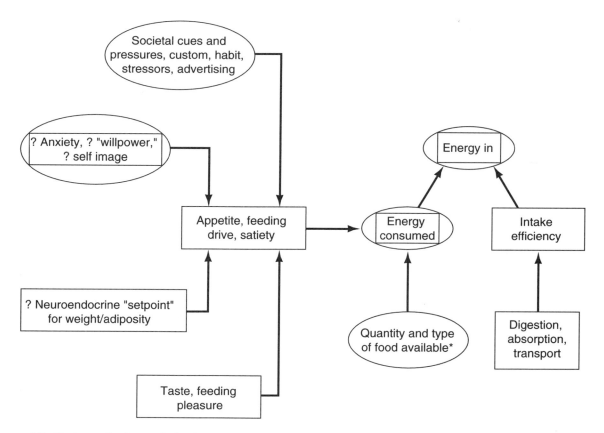

Figure 4.2 Factors affecting variation in energy intake.
*Note that until recently in human history, this factor kept most people "dieting" regardless of all the rest.

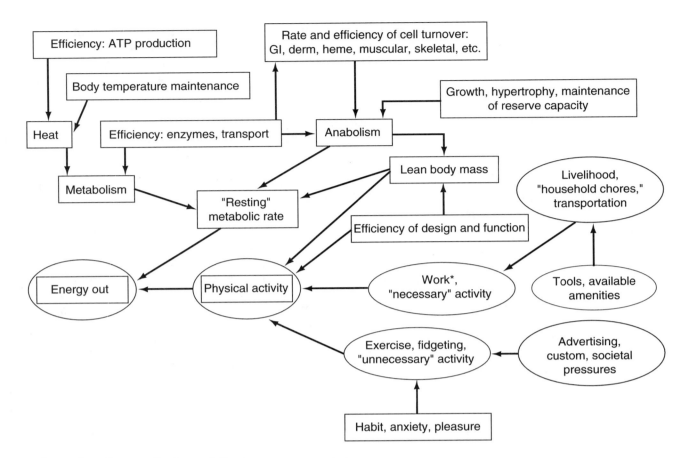

Figure 4.3 Factors affecting variation in energy expended.

*Note that until very recently in history, most people required this factor to be very high just for survival.

Most compelling is a mutation in the gene encoding the hormone leptin. Leptin was discovered as the factor involved in two of the most widely used rodent models of obesity, the diabetic and obese mice (now commonly referred to by their respective mutation, the db/db and ob/ob mice). Leptin is secreted by adipose tissue in amounts proportional to fat stores, and forms a feedback to the hypothalamus (the brain region most important in appetite regulation) to decrease appetite and increase energy expenditure. While this system appears very potent in rodents, a variety of evidence suggests it is less potent in most humans (for instance, obese people may have very high levels of leptin, yet be very hungry and continue to gain weight).

Confirmation that leptin is indeed an important regulator of appetite in humans (at least at lower levels) came not from the laboratory, but from the clinic. A girl was born who appeared normal except for an extremely ravenous appetite leading to incredible adiposity at a young age. She was found to be homozygous for a mutation in the leptin gene that resulted in no circulating leptin molecules (Montague et al. 1997). When she was treated with leptin injections, her appetite subsided and she began to lose weight (Farooqi et al. 1999). It appears quite clear that her severe obesity was due to variation in a single gene, and that environmental or other nongenetic factors played virtually no role (granted, diet restriction may have halted weight gain, but when attempted, she became extremely uncomfortable—as if starving).

The leptin gene (and leptin receptor gene) have been screened for mutation in hundreds if not thousands of other obese people, with very few, very rare mutations identified to cause significant obesity. Other genes that appear to be good candidates for influencing obesity have also been screened, and a few more very rare mutations have been found

Table 4.1   *Effects of Gene Variants Attributed to Obesity*

Gene	Potential/presumed mechanism	Gene effect* Minor	Gene effect* Major
Leptin (Ob or Lep)	Appetite; energy expenditure	Maybe	Yes
Leptin receptor (Ob-R or Lep-R)	Appetite; energy expenditure	Maybe	?
β-2 adrenergic receptor	Energy expenditure	Probably	No
β-3 adrenergic receptor	Energy expenditure	Yes	No
Uncoupling protein-1 (UCP-1)	Energy expenditure	Yes	No
Pro-opiomelanocortin (POMC)	Appetite	Maybe	Yes
Melanocortin 4-receptor (MC4-R)	Appetite	Maybe	Yes
PPAR-γ (γ1 and γ2)	Adipocyte differentiation; insulin sensitivity	Yes	Yes
Hormone-sensitive lipase	Lipid traffic/metabolism	Yes	No
Low-density lipoprotein receptor (LDL-R)	Lipid traffic/metabolism	Yes	No

* Identified in a few genes are some very rare mutations that have such a major effect as to cause obesity regardless of the remainder of an individual's genetic makeup, or even their environment (i.e., "monogenic obesity"). We believe the vast majority of "typical" obesity cases to be due to interactions of environment and behavior and combinations of multiple less severe mutations, each with a more minor effect in itself. Note that all genes that have very rare mutations with a major effect also have other more common variants that may or may not have minor effects.

that seem to be the primary cause of severe obesity in a small minority of people (see table 4.1).

Unlike genetic syndromes that include obesity among other more prominent traits (such as mental retardation in Prader-Willi disease), the most striking features of these individuals are obesity and its sequelae. While these monogenic forms account for a very small fraction of the number of cases of obesity, they are important for at least two reasons. First, they confirm that indeed obesity can be strongly influenced by genetic factors. Second, and more importantly, they provide insight into the pivotal role of those specific genes and physiological systems in the control of body weight. This helps focus research on potential therapies targeted at those systems (for use in any obese person) and on other genes in those systems that may harbor more common mutations that affect many more people.

Do all people with obesity have a single mutation that has a major effect on their body weight? This appears to be unlikely.

The obesity associated with these "major effect" mutations has high penetrance (i.e., no thin people have been found with the same genotype that causes obesity). Thus, families with such mutations (whether dominant or recessive) should demonstrate clear patterns of inheritance. The number of families that do is far too small to account for all the obese persons in the world. Furthermore, the increasing prevalence of obesity in recent years (as excess food has become more available) suggests that most cases are due to less dramatic genetic influences that become evident only in a calorie-rich environment.

Other factors also suggest that most people have multiple influences on how and why they gain weight. We see great variety in the degree of obesity, the age of onset of obesity, the ease of management (i.e., the effectiveness of weight loss regimens), the distribution of fat depots, and the associated features or sequelae of obesity. All of these factors provide circumstantial evidence of multiple genetic and nongenetic factors influencing body weight. This has been demonstrated in animal models. Most rodents show considerably variable responses to high-fat diets and exercise, and genetic studies suggest that at least 12 different genetic loci influence obesity in rodents.

Although the variation in weight of rodents can be influenced by several factors (e.g., high-fat versus low-fat diet), there are some rodent strains in which single mutations in specific genes have profound effects that overshadow differences in other factors ("obese," "diabetic," "mahogany," "tubby"). Most famous are the "obese mouse" and "diabetic mouse" models, both of which are quite prone to obesity and subsequent diabetes, and both of which display an autosomal recessive mode of inheritance. Although the extent of these traits can be manipulated, these mutations (labeled "ob" and "db" respectively) cause homozygous (ob/ob or db/db) mice to be markedly different from mice without the mutation (Ob/Ob or Db/Db) even under extreme dietary conditions or when bred into different strains of mice. Such mutations are often referred to as "major effect" genes/mutations, since other "effectors" (factors) can influence the severity but do not entirely negate their effect on a given trait (i.e., these lead to cases of a simple disorder of obesity). These are to be contrasted with "minor effect" genes/mutations, which may influence obesity to a lesser extent and/or only when other specific factors are present (i.e., in the more common complex disorder of obesity).

In the laboratory, there are lots of ob/ob and db/db mice (because we have bred them, fed them, and protected them from predators). In the real world, there appear to be very few human equivalents (presumably because it is neither healthy nor advantageous in evolutionary terms). There are a lot of obese people, to be sure, but the vast majority has no major effect obesity mutations, but rather multiple minor effect obesity mutations.

Research Context

Obesity is a complex, multifactorial, and polygenic disease. This should not be surprising to us. Most diseases are more complex than we used to think. (Does everyone exposed to viruses get sick to the same degree?) But obesity is even more so. The complexity extends to factors far beyond the individual who is struggling to maintain a slim figure, with powerful external influences intended to alter behavior that might limit weight gain (advertising for restaurants and junk food, suburbs designed to favor the automobile over walking, "modern conveniences" that eliminate household work). More relevant to this chapter, complexity arises from the numerous physiological systems that influence energy balance (see table 4.2). As suggested, a serious flaw in any one of these may contribute to the development of obesity, but obesity arises much more commonly from an interaction among them.

Screening for Mutations That Cause Obesity

Unlike sickle cell disease or Tay-Sachs disease, no single gene has a major defect in every case of obesity. While many other factors may influence its severity (including mutations in other genes), *everyone* with sickle cell disease does have a serious mutation in the hemoglobin gene. While rare individuals (or families) have defects in single genes that appear to play a dominant role in the development of obesity, the consensus opinion is that most obese people have multiple genes that are abnormal to varying degrees. This was suggested by the lack of a clear pattern of inheritance, and further confirmed by linkage analyses.

Linkage analysis is a powerful method combining classical genetics with molecular biology to see if transmission of a particular trait across generations corresponds with (is *linked* to) transmission of a specific chromosomal region. If one or very few genes account for all the variability in the obesity phenotype, this method should localize them readily. Such has not been the case. Several large well-designed studies have indeed found a few chromosomal regions that are somewhat linked to obesity in some populations, but none that account for a large portion of the variability we see in degree of obesity. That is, genes in those regions do influence obesity, but none is *the* obesity gene; for most individuals there is no single gene, but rather a cluster of genes with an aggregate effect that leads to a higher tendency to obesity in

Table 4.2   *Traits or Systems That Can Influence Obesity*

Resting metabolic rate	Physical activity	Energy storage
Lean body mass	Lean body mass	Mobilization efficiency
▫ Muscle/organ/bone ratio	▫ Muscle/organ/bone ratio	Adipose differentiation
Basal temperature	Nervousness	Adipose function
ATP generation efficiency	Fidget frequency	Partitioning
ATP utilization efficiency	Willpower	▫ Subcutaneous abdomen
Protein synthesis efficiency	Pleasure from work or exercise	▫ Visceral
Protein stability/turnover	Pain threshold	▫ Subcutaneous limb
Cell turnover rate	Self-image	▫ Liver
▫ Blood	Personality	▫ Bone marrow
▫ Gastrointestinal	Muscle work efficiency	▫ Intramuscular
▫ Skin	Body mechanical efficiency	▫ Other fat stores
▫ Other tissues	Glycogen storage efficiency	Other energy stores
Sebaceous function	Glycogen storage quantity	▫ Glycogen
Hair/nail growth	Lipolysis efficiency	▫ Protein
Thyroid function		▫ ATP
Adrenergic activity		

the setting of a permissive environment (e.g., lots of food with little exercise). Identification of some of those many genes (perhaps those with the greatest population effect, or perhaps those with the most consistent, albeit modest, effect) will likely come from the genome-wide scans (i.e., linkage analyses).

Further gene variants or mutations will be identified by a different, although complementary, approach called the candidate gene approach. This requires an educated guess as to which genes might be involved in the regulation of weight and adiposity and a detailed search for mutations in such genes (note that one of the best clues for such a guess is linkage from a genome-wide scan).

Table 4.1 lists some of the genes that have been screened for mutation based on their presumed importance in energy metabolism or storage. For most of these genes, several different variations were identified, yet further study suggests that very few of them have any major effect mutations (and those are present in very few people). Most of the mutations in these genes that are generally accepted to

contribute to obesity do so only slightly, and perhaps only in certain settings (i.e., effects are seen in some ethnic cohorts but not in others). Combining both linkage and candidate gene approaches has resulted in identification of mutations in the POMC gene. Using only functional clues, the candidate gene approach has also identified human major effect (e.g., leptin and PPAR-γ) and minor effect (e.g., β3-AR and a different PPAR-γ) mutations.

As suggested by this discussion, much of the work in the genetic influences on obesity has focused on adipose tissue itself. This has certainly yielded some promising results. Less easy to study, however, are some of the many other systems involved in energy homeostasis. Caloric intake is surely influenced by numerous genes expressed in the brain, oropharynx, gastrointestinal tract, and perhaps other tissues. These control how much energy is consumed in each meal and of what composition (e.g., fat versus carbohydrate), how efficiently this energy is absorbed, and how frequently meals will take place. Our understanding of these factors is quite rudimentary, relative to other physiological processes, and methods to detect variation between people are not well enough established to allow studies on how genetic differences may affect even appetite or satiety, much less absorption efficiency. We can measure how much people eat (at least when in controlled environments such as a laboratory) and how much weight they gain, but we have difficulty determining why they eat what they eat.

We are better prepared to study some components of energy expenditure, in part because we understand the chemical processes involved in the metabolism of fat, protein, and carbohydrate. Strong correlations exist between the energy used and the amount of oxygen consumed or the amount of water and carbon dioxide formed as by-products. Even here, though, we are not able to discern well where the energy is used or why. We can estimate whether the energy is used for "work" (exercise), as part of the basal or resting metabolic rate, or even as part of the energy expended to digest a meal, but for the most part these remain estimates. Even then, we know relatively little about what specific molecules contribute to each component. How much of the variation in resting metabolic rate is due to differences in mitochondrial function? How much to differences in efficiency in using ATP? How much for making new skin cells or for blinking one's eyes? We now know that fidgeting can significantly increase energy expenditure and lead to lower body weight, but what controls how much we fidget?

Clearly, many of the factors that contribute to energy balance are themselves quite complex. Isolating these factors in a way that permits measurement of the variation among individuals will be difficult. Therefore, identifying minor effect mutations that act through one of these systems will be difficult until we understand more about the physiology of specific systems and until we can measure these factors in large study populations. However, major effect mutations may still be detectable since they will associate significantly with morbid obesity, which is easy to measure.

So far the best-characterized component (and thus most amenable to detection of minor effect mutations) is the most obvious tissue involved in obesity, adipose tissue itself. For many years, this tissue was completely ignored by most physiologists. More recently, however, it has been studied extensively for its roles in obesity, diabetes, and dyslipidemia. As such, we are gaining considerable knowledge about its development and metabolism, and which genes are important for each.

Identifying Candidate Genes

It is beyond the scope of this chapter to perform a comprehensive review of how candidate genes can be identified in each obesity-relevant physiological system. The figures and tables give some general suggestion of where we need to look, and this section will briefly review how one of these systems (adipose tissue) has been approached.

The basic approach is to first identify a tissue or system that seems likely to contribute to obesity, then determine precisely by what mechanism it may do so, and then find some molecules important to that mechanism. Until recently, it was difficult to take the next steps of finding, characterizing, and screening the gene that encodes one of these molecules. However, technological advances and the Human Genome Project have made this much easier. The real challenge is gaining sufficient knowledge of which genes are important in the various physiological systems that can influence body weight or composition. The most productive approach to this—as in much of human physiology—has been to perform extensive laboratory work in more easily accessible and manipulable nonhuman systems and then confirm the importance of a finding in relatively simple human experiments.

Much of our most basic knowledge has come from the 3T3-L1 and similar mouse cell lines, which have been developed to survive long periods in culture (unlike most mammalian cells). This allows the study of fat cell differentiation (e.g., what molecules are important in the transition from precursor cells to fat cells) and metabolism (e.g., how cells handle sugar and lipid). Valuable "whole animal" experimental models include various means of overfeeding regular mice, and of course the obese and diabetic mouse strains mentioned earlier. Other obese mouse (and other rodent) strains have been studied to a lesser extent, and more recently researchers have developed transgenic mice lacking fat tissue (lipoatrophic mice). Less common are studies in larger mammals, but important work has been done with monkeys on restrictive diets. Any of these animals can be compared to controls in studies of energy expenditure, appetite, expression of molecules in the brain or fat tissue, response to drugs, and the like.

Recent developments in molecular biology have provided another powerful tool in the study of candidate genes—transgenic mice. We now are able to "knock out" normal genes and "knock in" a gene of interest (e.g., a mutated mouse gene or even a human gene) with increasing ease and precision. The inserted gene can be altered such that it is expressed only in certain tissues (e.g., "cre-lox" systems) or only in the presence or absence of an exogenous chemical (e.g., "tet-on" and "tet-off" systems). While these techniques are not yet perfect, they can help us estimate the importance and function of a specific gene or a specific mutation. We can detect response to altering a given gene in terms of which other genes are expressed in greater or lesser amounts, how nutrients are transported and stored differently, how responses to hormones or drugs are altered, and so on. One caveat to remember when interpreting these studies is that some of the traits seen in such mice may reflect unpredictable effects of the genetic manipulation (affecting embryogenesis, for instance), and not simply the effect of the gene we are studying. We study these mice for clues as to which molecules are important and why, not as definitive answers as to the role of a given gene. As long we remember this, they are powerful models indeed.

Once animal or in vitro models suggest that a gene could be involved in the development of obesity, it needs to be studied in humans. While it would be ideal to characterize the role of a given molecule in human physiology first, it is now easier and cheaper to go straight to screening for mutations. In the recent past, this has commonly been performed with SSCP (single-strand conformation polymorphism) analysis. This technique uses the fact that while DNA in its typical double-strand helix is very uniform in shape, it can be separated into single strands that fold into individualized shapes. Even slight variation in DNA sequence can alter this folding and change how that piece of DNA travels in an electrophoresis gel. If the gel pattern of an individual's single-stranded DNA differs from everyone else's, then there likely is a change somewhere in that gene's sequence. Determining where that change is then requires sequencing.

The SSCP technique appears to be very specific and sensitive when done correctly, but it is cumbersome and slow and requires some level of expertise. Thus, researchers have attempted to simplify this technique, or develop rival techniques to screen large numbers of persons quickly for the presence of genetic variation. Increasingly, screening for genetic variation has used direct sequencing, which eliminates the first layer of screening for people who may have a variant gene before sequencing the DNA of those relatively few persons. Automated sequencing machines have become faster, cheaper, and more reliable at detecting subtle changes (especially heterozygous changes, which are difficult), making it possible to sequence the genes of dozens (or hundreds) of people with less effort and time than other methods (such as SSCP). As technology continues to advance, screening very large numbers of persons for mutations in multiple genes at once will likely become commonplace. Given the number of gene variants that have been identified with the slower methods, we anticipate a flood of new variants to be unleashed.

Estimating the Significance of a Gene Variant

With so many variants detected, how do we decide which variants merit further study? If a gene is well characterized, it should be possible to estimate what the molecular effect of a given variant might be. For instance, if the change in DNA sequence is such that it might change an amino acid in a very important region of the protein, then that variant should be studied. Much more common, however, are variants in regions of the gene that have no known function in the expression of the gene or the function of the protein it encodes. These are generally much less interesting or important.

The next steps are to determine if the variant does indeed change the effectiveness of the protein and the functioning of the system involved. This determination has two aspects, which should be performed in conjunction with each other (although negative results on either may dampen enthusiasm to perform the other). The first aspect involves in vitro (or in vivo transgenic mouse) studies of the function of the mutated protein or the gene itself, such as the ability to bind other molecules normally or to alter expression levels appropriately to stimuli. The more the function is altered in vitro, the more likely the function will be to be altered in humans who carry that mutation. However, in vitro studies may be insensitive to subtle changes in function, in vitro and in vivo activity are not always similar, and there may be many levels of compensation for a given alteration (within the particular system or between systems). Thus, we cannot reliably translate laboratory findings to clinically relevant information without the second aspect, involving studies in human populations to see if persons with the variant have notably different traits (e.g., metabolic rate, appetite, or simply weight) than those without the variant.

Because we can now genotype large numbers of persons, and large cohorts of well-characterized persons are available to study, it is tempting to forgo the in vitro testing and simply see if a gene variant associates with particular traits in humans. This may be an efficient way to decide which variants are *not* likely to have significant functional alterations, but it may be misleading to assume a variant is the cause of specific traits simply because it associates with them. Because DNA is inherited in large chunks, two variants are often inherited together ("linked"). Thus, traits that appear to associate with the variant we are considering can be caused instead by a different mutation nearby (perhaps one we had not identified, or one we deemed unlikely to be important and thus did not study further). Furthermore, the prevalence of a particular variant may vary significantly in persons of different ethnic or racial backgrounds, such that an apparent association with the variant may actually represent an association with many different genetic influences particular to a specific ethnic group. For these and other reasons, determining how much influence any given genetic variant has on the development of obesity requires consideration of both in vitro and in vivo activity.

Interpreting Reports of Genes That Cause Obesity

Once a gene is identified as possibly influential in the development of obesity, it is now fairly easy to screen the gene for variation in its sequence. As it turns out, most genes have some variation in their sequence. This has resulted in a lot of people with relatively little training or expertise looking for, and finding, polymorphisms in candidate genes. That is fine in itself, but deciding whether a gene variant (polymorphism) has any functional or clinical significance (most do not) can require some thoughtful consideration and some more difficult analyses than many investigators are prepared to do. That, too, is fine in itself, as long as everyone is aware of the limitations of their studies.

Unfortunately, the results are not always presented in a balanced perspective. For this reason the reader must be critical and slightly skeptical of each new report. How many people did they study? Did they replicate it in a different cohort? Were biases introduced by mixing people of differing genetic or social and behavioral backgrounds (e.g., differing races, differing diets)? Is there in vitro data to suggest that this genetic variant could plausibly affect the amount or function of the protein it encodes? Is the known function (and presumed malfunction) of this gene product consistent with all the features seen in persons with this gene variant? Given the function of this gene and the features being attributed to it, are there other features we should expect to see but do not? One would not expect to see all of these issues addressed adequately in a single report. Therefore, one should not believe that a particular gene variant is particularly important until further study is done. We want so much to understand the bases of this terrible problem of obesity that we easily can become overly enthusiastic about new findings. We must remember, however, that many seemingly promising gene variants (for a wide variety of disorders, including obesity) have not panned out after further study.

Adipose Gene Mutations

It is remarkable how much we have learned about adipose tissue in recent years. Impressive work has been done to demonstrate the critical role of transcription factors (CEBP-α and β; PPAR-γ) that control the differentiation of precursor cells into adipocytes and the importance of beta-adrenergic receptors in regulating adipocyte metabolism and fatty acid flux. We are now aware that adipose tissue is an important endocrine organ, as demonstrated by its secretion of leptin that modulates appetite in the hypothalamus. *With the discovery of so many molecules that are so important for adipose development and function, why don't we know all of the adipose gene mutations that lead to obesity?* The simplest answer is that that we have yet to identify more adipose-important molecules, much less screen their genes for mutations. Nonetheless, considerable science is still under way, and more molecules are being identified seemingly every day (e.g., perilipin, resistin, and adiponectin). Though not yet complete, identification and screening of candidate genes is likely to find most or all adipose gene mutations that contribute to many cases of obesity. As suggested earlier, however, the more challenging aspect is to discover what other molecules in *nonadipose* systems throughout the body play important roles in the development of obesity.

Let's consider a hypothetical mutation in a hypothetical gene that is hypothetically expressed only in skeletal muscle tissue. Although only affecting muscle tissue, such a mutation might still lead to greater accumulation of adipose tissue (obesity). Suppose a mutation in the MyoXYZ gene causes stronger, faster muscle contractions than normal, yet expends the same amount of energy per amount of work to accomplish this. This should have no effect on the amount of energy "lost" to work or exercise, and at first glance will have no effect on energy balance. However, stronger, faster contractions could generate normal strength from smaller- than-normal muscles. Thus, lean body mass may be decreased, so the resting metabolic rate would be lower, and the energy balance would thus be tipped toward "saving" energy (as fat). Of course, if the MyoXYZ mutation actually caused stronger, faster contractions while expending *less* energy, the excess energy (and excess fat) would be even greater. It is easy to speculate that such mutations influencing resting metabolic rate may actually exist, not only in muscle but also in the digestive system or any other system.

Therapeutic Context

We have made great strides in our understanding of the genetic influences on obesity in recent years, although obviously we have a long way to go. What we anticipate in the coming years is more of the same, at an even more rapid pace. As with many endeavors, the initial period is the slowest. We have developed good models of obesity and established means of studying important metabolic pathways. Given the number of genes and pathways that we have studied thus far, we are poised to better study the genes and pathways with which they interact, and identify strong candidate genes. The Human Genome Project and technological advances in molecular biology will make identification and screening candidate genes easier than ever. Perhaps the greatest challenge will be putting together the puzzle pieces we are identifying.

While identifying gene variants and establishing persons' genotypes has become easier and more rapid, deciphering exactly what phenotypic traits they influence remains an onerous task. Detailed physiological and molecular characterization of individuals with specific gene variants or combinations of variants—and comparison to "normal" controls—is difficult and time consuming, but may be our best approach. We have just begun to look at combinations of minor effect gene variants to see how they interact. For instance, persons with copies of both variant β3 adrenergic receptor (i.e., 64Arg) and variant PPAR-γ2 (i.e., 12Ala) genes are significantly more obese than persons with either alone (Hsueh et al. 2001). Apparently these variants are synergistic in their effects. Understanding which gene variants affect which—and how—is of obvious importance given our belief that the vast majority of cases of obesity are polygenic in nature. Ultimately, we need to fulfill our promise and provide concrete benefits to patients suffering from (or at risk for) obesity and its sequelae. The notion of "translational research" will become increasingly important as more genetic and physiological information is gathered and the need to translate it into clinically relevant knowledge becomes more evident.

Not long ago, doctors commonly told patients that a "glandular problem" was causing their obesity. While rarely an accurate diagnosis, this certainly was an effective therapy, leading to improved self-esteem and confidence. "It's not my fault that I'm fat; I'm not a lazy, bad person; my doctor said so!" (or my trainer, or my nurse, or any other trusted care provider). We rarely tell patients such things anymore, in part for fear of saying anything that is technically incorrect or potential grounds for a malpractice suit. Perhaps more prominent nowadays is the fear that giving obese persons an excuse will remove guilt as an incentive for them to lose weight (or as a punishment for not losing weight?). Given the paucity of successful weight losers, even among the "guilt feelers," it is doubtful that such an added incentive has been of great significance. Furthermore, the social pressures to look thin and attractive are likely much more powerful motivators in the first place. Obese people will still want to lose weight, even if their care providers tell them they are not lazy, bad people.

Of course, the glandular problem placebo worked primarily because there really are people (albeit relatively few) with weight gain due to hypothyroidism or hypercortisolism. Furthermore, if a specific glandular problem were found to be the cause, then there was hope for an effective therapy for the obesity. The situation with genetic basis for obesity is in some ways quite similar, but in some ways quite the opposite. Both allow patients to shift their anger and frustration from themselves to their "problem." Both provide hope for a treatment "once the specific cause is found." However, obesity is rarely due primarily to a glandular cause that we currently can specifically diagnose and treat. Recognizing that a genetic tendency is much more commonly the cause (compounded by our high-calorie, low-activity environment) has not yet yielded better diagnostic or treatment options. Still, there is reason for hope. New genes and new mutations are being identified daily (literally!), and some of these will be shown to influence the development of obesity. Some of these will lead to more effective therapies. It will take time, but it will happen. Until then, let's rally our patients in a common fight against their "genetic problem" using the best weapons available—a healthy diet, regular exercise, and medication or surgery when appropriate. Experience may suggest that focusing our efforts against "a problem" will not make these weapons much more potent. But experience also tells us that guilt and self-blame are no better, and have a much greater cost.

Summary

At the outset, we stated some goals for this chapter: that readers will be better prepared to (1) understand the importance of looking for genetic influences on obesity, (2) follow the search for those influences, and (3) appreciate why we will need to be patient and thoughtful in that search. Again, we invite those for whom these goals were not met to contact the author or editor. We can advise on how to supplement this chapter and, perhaps more importantly, we can incorporate your experience with this chapter into the design of future chapters.

In terms of the third goal, this chapter has described the complexity of obesity and explained that the biomedical community has only recently begun investigating it in earnest. In many ways, we are entering uncharted waters. We have not yet had many successful explorations into complex, multifactorial, polygenic diseases of adult onset from which to borrow techniques and approaches. Investigators into depression, hypertension, coronary artery disease, diabetes, and of course obesity are all still learning the ropes. Fortunately, we are doing so in an age of great technological advances and are building on the firm foundation laid by those who went before us. There is great promise that we will find most or all of the genetic influences on obesity, and that this knowledge will enable vastly improved prevention and treatment.

References

Farooqi, I.S., Jebb, S.A., Langmack, G., Lawrence, E., Cheetham, C.H., Prentice, A.M., Hughes, I.A., McCamish, M.A., and O'Rahilly, S. 1999. Effects of recombinant leptin therapy in a child with congenital leptin deficiency. *New England Journal of Medicine* 341 (12): 879-884.

Hsueh, W.C., Cole, S.A., Shuldiner, A.R., Beamer, B.A., Blangero, J., Hixson, J.E., MacCluer, J.W., and Mitchell, B.D. 2001. Interactions between variants in the beta3-adrenergic receptor and peroxisome proliferator-activated receptor-gamma2 genes and obesity. *Diabetes Care* 24 (4): 672-677.

Montague, C.T., Farooqi, I.S., Whitehead, J.P. et al. 1997. Congenital leptin deficiency is associated with severe early-onset obesity in humans. *Nature* 387: 903-908.

Stunkard, A.J., Foch, T.T., and Hrubec, Z. 1986. A twin study of human obesity. *Journal of the American Medical Association* 256 (1): 51-54.

Stunkard, A.J., Sorensen, T.I., Hanis, C., Teasdale, T.W., Chakraborty, R. Schull, W.J., and Schulsinger, F. 1986. An adoption study of human obesity. *New England Journal of Medicine* 314 (4): 193-198.

PART II

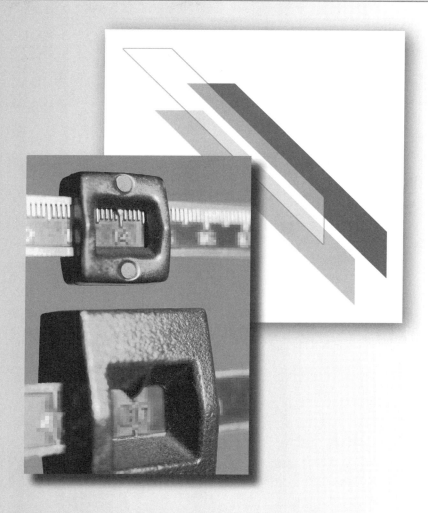

Assessment of the Obese Patient

Chapter 5

Health-Related Quality of Life in Obese Individuals

Kevin R. Fontaine, PhD

Susan J. Bartlett, PhD

Department of Medicine, Division of Rheumatology,
Johns Hopkins School of Medicine

This chapter is a revised and expanded version of a previously published paper: Fontaine, K.R., and Bartlett, S.J. (1998). Estimating the health-related quality of life of obese individuals. Disease Management and Health Outcomes *2: 61-70. Reprinted with the permission of Adis International Limited.*

Overweight and obesity are increasingly prevalent health concerns in the industrialized world (Popkin and Doak 1998). In the United States, an estimated 280,000 to 325,000 deaths a year are attributable to obesity, making it second only to smoking as a preventable cause of death (Allison et al. 1999). Apart from the increased risk of morbidity and mortality associated with excess body fat (Pi-Sunyer 1993, 1999), obesity may also adversely affect an individual's capacity to live a full and active life. That is, it has become increasingly clear that the problems associated with obesity are not restricted to simply causing or exacerbating medical conditions; obesity also appears to have a substantial impact on a person's overall functioning and quality of life (Fine et al. 1999; Fontaine, Bartlett, and Barofsky 2000; Kolotkin, Crosby, and Rhys Williams 2002). In this chapter we will review the impact obesity has on the health-related quality of life (HRQL), illustrate how information on HRQL may inform treatment practices, and suggest directions for future research.

What Is HRQL?

There is no universally accepted definition of HRQL. Conceptual frameworks guide the operationalization and measurement of different dimensions of HRQL. For example, investigators who are interested in the evaluation of the quality of medical care outcomes tend to place greater emphasis on the development of measures that focus on role function and overall well-being (Wan, Counte, and Cella 1997). In contrast, those operating from a medical ethics perspective tend to develop measures assessing the meaning and importance an individual places on the quality of his or her life. As a result, hundreds of tests purport to measure different aspects of quality of life (Fallowfield 1996). However, it is generally accepted that HRQL reflects an individual's subjective evaluation and reaction to health or illness (Fontaine, Cheskin, and Barofsky 1996; Osterhaus, Townsend, and Gandek 1994; Sullivan, Sullivan, and Kral 1987; Wan, Counte, and Cella 1997). HRQL is regarded as a multidimensional construct encompassing emotional, physical, social, and subjective feelings of well-being (Guyatt, Feeny, and Patrick 1993).

Measurement of HRQL

There are two basic approaches to HRQL measurement. The first involves the use of generic instruments that measure broad aspects of HRQL, and the second involves disease-specific or condition-specific HRQL measures.

Generic Instruments

Generic instruments are not designed to assess HRQL relative to a particular medical condition, but rather provide a generalized assessment. The Medical Outcomes Study Short-Form Health Survey (SF-36) (Ware, Snow, and Kosinski 1993) is perhaps the best-known example of such an instrument. It measures HRQL along eight empirically distinct domains: physical functioning, role limitations due to physical problems, bodily pain, general health perception, vitality, social functioning, role limitations due to emotional problems, and mental health. (Table 5.1 presents a number of other generic instruments that have been used to assess the HRQL of obese persons.)

The major advantage of generic HRQL measures is that they allow for comparisons of quality of life across a variety of conditions. Moreover, generic instruments can be administered to different populations to examine the impact of various health care programs on HRQL (Guyatt, Feeny, and Patrick 1993). The major limitation of generic HRQL instruments is that they may not be sensitive enough to detect subtle condition-specific effects on HRQL. For example, an SF-36 assessment on an arthritic patient will not provide information on the intensity, frequency, or duration of the pain and thus may not be sensitive to changes over the course of treatment.

Specific Instruments

The second approach to HRQL measurement involves the use of instruments specific to a disease (e.g., asthma, migraine headache), population (e.g., elderly), or problem (e.g.,

Table 5.1   Generic and Specific HRQL Instruments Used to Assess Obese Persons

Generic Measures

- Medical outcomes study—short form (SF-36)
- Sickness impact profile
- Quality of well-being scale
- Nottingham health profile
- General health index
- Gothenberg quality of life scale
- Symptom checklist (SCL-90)

Specific Measures

- Impact of weight on quality of life scale (IWQOL)
- Impact of weight on quality of life scale—short form (IWQOL-LITE)
- Obesity-specific quality of life scale (OSQOL)
- Heath-related quality of life scale (HRQOL)
- Obesity-related well-being questionnaire (ORWELL)
- Health state preference for persons with obesity scale (HSP)

Reprinted, by permission, from K. Fontaine, 1999, Estimating health related quality of life of obese individuals. In *Managing Obesity*, edited by G. Mallarkey (Auckland, New Zealand: Adis International), 104-106.

sexual function, pain). Measures geared toward specific diseases or populations are likely to be more sensitive and therefore to have greater relevance to practicing clinicians. The Impact of Weight Scale (IWQOL) (Kolotkin, Head, and Hamilton 1995) is an example of a disease-specific HRQL instrument. The IWQOL is a 74-item measure that assesses the effect of weight along eight domains of functioning: health, social and interpersonal, work, mobility, self-esteem, sexual life, activities of daily living, and comfort with food. A brief version of the IWQOL questionnaire, the IWQOL-LITE (see table 5.1 for a selection of obesity-specific HRQL instruments), was recently published (Kolotkin, Crosby, Kosloski et al. 2001).

Helpfulness of HRQL Assessments

Traditionally, those providing medical care (e.g., physicians and nurses) have determined outcomes in medical care largely by objective medical evaluation (e.g., measurable changes in disease status). Increasingly, it has become clear that the perspective of the patient is also a critical variable. As a result, emphasis has shifted toward including subjective evaluations of outcome not only from the perspective of the caregiver, but also from that of the patient (e.g., Guyatt, Feeny, and Patrick 1993; Sullivan, Sullivan, and Kral 1987).

HRQL assessments are of use to clinicians, researchers, administrators, and policy makers. First, they offer a picture of the current state of an individual who is experiencing a particular illness or chronic disease (Barofsky 1996). For instance, HRQL assessments are commonly administered initially to assess the overall impact of a particular condition on functioning and well-being (e.g., Buchwald, Pearlman, Umali et al. 1996; Patrick, Deyo, and Atlas 1995). This provides additional information beyond that offered by traditional medical and clinical measures such as disease stage or progression. Such information is invaluable in helping understand the wide variability in individual responses to similar conditions. For example, some individuals with morbid obesity remain active at work and engaged in social relationships, while others with the same degree of obesity become virtually housebound and isolated. Second, variability on HRQL responses among persons with similar medical conditions allows researchers to determine the relative importance of factors such as age, sex, educational level, duration of illness, and so forth (Fontaine, Cheskin, and Barofsky 1996; Sarlio-Lahteenkorva, Stunkard, and Rissanen 1995; Stewart and Brook 1983). Third, HRQL measures can be used to better assess the efficacy and value of treatment interventions (e.g., Jhingran, Cady, and Rubino 1996; Ware, Bayliss, and Rogers 1996).

The information offered by these assessments may influence treatment decisions in important ways. For instance, a new aggressive oncology treatment may offer a delay in the recurrence of tumors while no treatment results in potentially faster recurrence. However, if patients are aware that the treatment may significantly impair HRQL, they are in a better position to make informed decisions about their care. Thus, HRQL indexes can help clinicians identify treatments that enhance both physical and emotional health. Finally, on a broader level, information on HRQL also may influence the development of clinical pathways, service provision, health care expenditures, and public health policy. Indeed, some managed care organizations are considering HRQL information when making reimbursement decisions (Guyatt, Feeny, and Patrick 1993).

Influence of Obesity on HRQL

Although studies show that obesity adversely affects HRQL (e.g., Sarlio-Lahteenkorva, Stunkard, and Rissanen 1995; Sullivan, Sullivan, and Kral 1987; Seidell 1995), the majority of studies have been restricted to examining the role of obesity in the prevalence of selected chronic diseases or mortality (Allison et al. 2001; National Task Force on the Prevention and Treatment of Obesity 2000). Although interest in the effect of overweight and obesity on HRQL is growing (Fontaine and Barofsky 2001), to date only a handful of empirically based studies have actually investigated the impact of obesity on indexes of functional status and subjective well-being.

Stewart and Brook (1983) found that among a sample of 5,817 people from a general population aged 14 to 61, overweight (defined as a body mass index [BMI: kg/m^2 for men and $kg/m^{1.5}$ for women] of >29.3 for men and >36 for women) was associated with poorer functional status (i.e., capacity to perform a variety of activities such as walking, climbing stairs, working, or participating in sports), pain, worry, a negative general health perception, and restricted activity. In fact, 18% of the overweight respondents reported experiencing at least mild pain that they attributed to their weight, and 18% reported weight-related restrictions in activity. Degree of overweight also appeared to be associated with greater functional impairment.

In a similar study conducted in Holland (Seidell, Bakx, and Deurenberg 1986), obesity (BMI >30) was associated with a variety of complaints (e.g., shortness of breath and musculoskeletal problems) that compromised functional status. By the same token, among the first 1,743 persons sampled in an ongoing national survey of severely obese persons in Sweden (The Swedish Obese Subjects Study [SOS]) (Sullivan, Karlsson, and Sjostrom 1993), elevated levels of anxiety and depression, as well as poorer perceived health, were reported.

In a series of studies to develop and evaluate the psychometric properties of the IWQOL, Kolotkin and colleagues (Kolotkin, Head, and Hamilton 1995; Kolotkin, Crosby, Rhys Williams et al. 2001) found that obese persons reported that their weight had a negative impact on selfesteem and sexual life. Moreover, the impact of weight on HRQL generally worsened as the patients' size increased, and women appeared more prone to experience decrements in self-esteem and sexual life than did men.

By the same token, Mathias, Williamson, and Colwell (1997), using a measure (the HRQOL) containing both global and obesity-specific domains, found that among a sample of 417 obese and normal weight adults, obese individuals reported greater impairment with respect to general health, distress due to obesity, depression, self-esteem, and physical appearance.

Le Pen and colleagues (1998) compared generic (the SF-36) and specific (the obesity-specific quality of life scale [OSQOL]) quality of life measures among a community sample of 500 obese persons residing in mainland France. They found that both assessment instruments were successful at identifying differences between the obese persons and a control group, especially with respect to the physical consequences of obesity. However, subtle differences were obtained between the two forms of HRQL assessment, prompting them to conclude that the instruments are complementary in the sense that they did not refer to exactly the same conceptualization of HRQL.

Our group examined the HRQL, as measured by the Medical Outcomes Study Short-Form Health Survey (SF-36), among 312 obese adults (mean BMI = 38.1) seeking university-based weight loss treatment at our center (Fontaine, Cheskin, and Barofsky 1996). We found that, prior to treatment, our obese patients reported significant decrements in all eight SF-36 domains. Specifically, relative to SF-36 general population norms, they scored significantly lower (i.e., reported greater impairment) on physical functioning, role limitations due to physical problems, bodily pain, general health perception, vitality, social functioning, role limitations due to emotional problems, and mental health. It is important to note that the SF-36 scores of our sample were adjusted for sociodemographic factors and various comorbidities, including depression, to better estimate the unique effect of obesity on HRQL.

The largest effects of obesity on HRQL were with respect to the vitality and bodily pain scales of the SF-36. The low vitality scores suggest that obesity reduces energy levels or "get up and go." Pain also appeared to be an important issue, with 56% of the sample reporting some form of chronic bodily pain. Indeed, compared to other chronic medical conditions (e.g., clinical depression, HIV+, congestive heart failure), patients reported significantly greater impairment on the bodily pain scale of the SF-36. In fact, the level of impairment due to bodily pain was comparable to that reported by patients who suffer from chronic migraine headaches, a disease characterized by severe and debilitating pain.

Subsequent analyses of these data (Barofsky, Fontaine, and Cheskin 1998) revealed that low back pain (50%) and joint pain (28%) were the most prevalent pain complaints. Moreover, in analyses adjusting for sociodemographic characteristics and BMI, compared to patients who did not report pain, those who reported pain displayed significantly greater decrements on all domains of HRQL. That is, pain independent of body weight was a significant contributor to impaired HRQL.

In the largest prospective body weight–HRQL study to date, Fine and colleagues (1999) administered the SF-36 at baseline to over 40,000 participants in the Nurses' Health Study. After categorizing the women into four BMI-defined groups (<25, 25-29.9, 30-34.9, and ≥35), they found a dose-response association between BMI and SF-36 scores. That is, greater BMI was associated with lower scores (i.e., more impairment) on all SF-36 HRQL domains. When the SF-36 was administered four years later, they found that weight gain was associated with decreased physical function and vitality and increased bodily pain regardless of the weight at baseline. Indeed, compared to women who were weight stable, women who gained 9 kg (20 lb) or more over the four years had a seven-unit decline on the SF-36 physical functioning scale. In contrast, weight loss was associated with increased physical function and vitality and decreased bodily pain. They also observed that weight change was more strongly associated with physical health than with mental health SF-36 domains. Finally, age (i.e., <65 versus ≥65) did not appear to influence significantly the weight change–HRQL associations.

A recent SF-36 survey of 5,633 Swedish adults aged 16 to 64 (Larsson, Karlsson, and Sullivan 2002) indicated that both obese men and obese women reported significantly greater impairment on all physically oriented SF-36 scales compared to their normal weight counterparts.

We compared the HRQL of our aforementioned clinic sample with a sample of 89 obese persons who were not currently trying to lose weight (Fontaine, Bartlett, and Barofsky 2000). We found that the obese persons from our clinic sample tended to be heavier (mean BMI of 38 versus 32.5), older, Caucasian, and married, and reported a higher prevalence of diabetes, hypertension, and pain than did the obese persons who were not currently attempting to address their weight. In multivariate analysis, both adjusted and unadjusted for differences on sociodemographic characteristics and comorbid medical conditions, the obese persons from the clinic sample were significantly more impaired on the bodily pain, general health, and vitality scales of the SF-36 than were their non-treatment-seeking counterparts. This suggests that obesity appears to have a pronounced impact on physically oriented HRQL domains independent of whether the person is attempting to lose weight.

In a recent study, Kolotkin and colleagues (2002) evaluated and compared the HRQL, measured by the IWQOL-LITE questionnaire, of overweight and obese persons from different subgroups that varied in treatment seeking and treatment intensity (i.e., overweight/obese people not enrolled in weight loss treatment to gastric bypass patients). They found that HRQL was significantly more impaired among the treatment groups compared to those not seeking treatment. Within treatment groups, they found that HRQL varied by treatment intensity. Specifically, gastric patients were the most impaired, and HRQL was more impaired with increased BMI.

Collectively, studies attempting to estimate the effect of obesity on HRQL indicate that (1) obese persons report significant decrements on HRQL; (2) there appears to be a dose-response relationship between BMI and the degree of HRQL impairment; (3) obesity appears to have a greater impact on physical domains of functioning than on mental health domains; (4) pain appears to be an important comorbid condition that, in and of itself, produces significant impairment in HRQL among obese persons; and (5) there are systematic differences in HRQL as a function of treatment seeking status, treatment modality, and BMI.

Impact of Weight Loss on HRQL

The relationship between weight loss and HRQL among persons who are overweight or obese has recently become a topic of interest to obesity researchers.

Severely Obese Patients

The majority of obesity HRQL-related studies have examined the effect of weight reduction via gastric surgery on functional status and subjective well-being. The results of representative surgical intervention studies are summarized in table 5.2. With the exception of one study (Isacsson et al. 1997), weight reduction via obesity surgery produced dramatic improvements in the majority of HRQL indexes. That is, obese persons who underwent the surgery reported improvements in overall physical functioning and mobility, work capacity, mental health, self-esteem, confidence, sexual activity, social interaction, and general satisfaction with life.

It is important to note that the positive impact of the intervention on HRQL was apparent even taking into consideration the potential adverse effects and complications associated with the surgical procedure itself.

Table 5.2   *Studies Investigating the Effects of Gastric Surgery on Health-Related Quality of Life*

Authors	Sample	Intervention	Weight loss	Follow-Up	HRQL measure	HRQL effect
Dano & Hahn-Pedersen 1977	55 obese patients	Jejunoileal bypass	55 kg	15 mo to 6.5 yr	Study-specific	Improvements in work capacity, sexual activity, adjustment, and leisure time activity
The Danish Obesity Project 1979	130 severely obese and 66 nonsurgery patients	End-to-side jejunoileostomy	42.9 kg at 2 yr postsurgery vs. 5.9 kg nonsurgical group	>3 yr	177-items somatic, psychological symptoms, and social circumstances	Compared to nonsurgery group, considerable improvement in HRQL
Mustajoki et al. 1984	41 morbidly obese patients	Jejunoileal bypass	43 kg	Average of 4.7 yr	Study-specific	Improved HRQL, reduced joint and back symptoms
Carr et al. 1989	42 morbidly obese patients	Vertical banded gastroplasty	Reduction of 14 BMI units	9 to 36 months	Study-specific	Improved self-esteem, confidence, and interpersonal relations
Hafner et al. 1991	83 morbidly obese women	Gastric bypass	35.4 kg at 1 yr	1 yr	Study-specific	Increase in sexual activity and physical activity
Kral et al. 1992	193 morbidly obese and matched controls	Gastric bypass	33 kg	Ongoing	Sickness Impact Profile	Improved mental well-being, perceived health, and social interaction

Study	Sample	Procedure	Weight loss	Follow-up	Instrument	Findings
Larsen 1990	103 morbidly obese patients	Horizontal gastric banding	34.9 kg at 1 yr 31.5 kg at 3 yr	3 yr	SCL90 and study-specific	Enhanced psychosocial functioning, improved HRQL
Isacsson et al. 1997	102 morbidly obese and 74 controls	Vertical banded gastroplasty	not specified	1.5 to 5.5 yr	Gothenberg Quality of Life Scale	Improved self-esteem, no significant improvement in HRQL
Karlsson et al. 1998	487 severely obese patients who underwent gastric surgery and conventionally treated controls	—	N/A	2-year follow-up	Battery of instruments including the Gothenberg Quality of Life Scale	Marked improvement in HRQL among surgical patients. Peak values at 6-12 month postsurgery and moderate decrease at 2-year follow-up
Van Gemert et al. 1999	21 morbidly obese patients	Vertical banded gastroplasty	~36 kg	2 yr	Nottingham Health Profile Part 1 & 2 Visual Analog Scale	
Choban et al. 1999	53 morbidly obese patients	Roux-en-Y gastric bypass	~45 kg	1.5 yr	SF-36	
Weiner et al. 1999	100 morbidly obese patients	Laparoscopic adjustable silicone gastric banding	~45 kg	1.5-2 yr	Study-specific	

Reprinted, by permission, from K. Fontaine, 1999, Estimating health related quality of life of obese individuals. In *Managing Obesity*, edited by G. Mallarkey (Auckland, New Zealand: Adis International), 104-106.

Moreover, the majority of surgical intervention studies have followed the patients for at least one year, suggesting that the effects of weight reduction on HRQL are durable. In addition to the improvement in HRQL, two econometric studies (Hawke et al. 1990; Naslund and Agren 1990) demonstrated that severely obese persons who lose weight via surgery are likely to begin or to return to full- or part-time employment, lessening the economic burden imposed by their severe obesity.

Although weight reduction appears to have a positive impact on HRQL, it is important to keep in mind that these studies were conducted on severely obese patients who were willing to undergo surgery to control their weight. The question arises as to whether weight reduction would have beneficial effects on HRQL among persons who have lower degrees of obesity and undergo a less invasive means of losing weight.

Moderately Obese Patients

We placed 38 mild to moderately obese adults (mean BMI = 31.6) on a lifestyle modification program that included a balanced calorie deficit diet, an emphasis on increasing physical activity, and weekly group meetings focused on modifying behaviors (Fontaine et al. 1999). HRQL was assessed with the SF-36 at baseline and after 12 weeks of treatment. Participants lost an average of 8.6 kg (19 lb). Compared to their baseline SF-36 scores, participants reported significantly improved HRQL with respect to physical functioning, mental health, general health perception, vitality, bodily

pain, social functioning, and role limitations due to physical problems (see figure 5.1). Moreover, the prevalence of self-reported pain decreased from 39 to 13%.

Similarly, Rippe and colleagues (1998) randomly assigned 80 mildly to moderately (i.e., 20 to 50% over ideal body weight) overweight women to either a 12-week intervention program or a control group. The women in the intervention group lost an average of 6 kg (13 lb) on the protocol. They also reported significantly greater improvement in HRQL (relative to their baseline scores) than did the women in the control group. The greatest changes and improvements in HRQL among the intervention group were with respect to the physical functioning, vitality, and mental health scales of the SF-36.

Recently, Kolotkin, Crosby, Rhys Williams, and colleagues (2001) evaluated the effects of weight loss induced by phentermine-fenfluramine and dietary counseling on HRQL. One hundred and forty-one people completed the IWQOL-LITE at baseline and at one-year follow-up. After an average weight loss of nearly 18% of baseline body weight, the researchers found a strong linear association between magnitude of weight loss and changes on the IWQOL-LITE. Specifically, significant changes were observed on the physical function, self-esteem, and sexual life scales relative to baseline.

Collectively, these studies suggest that weight reduction, even a modest reduction, appears to promote significant improvements in HRQL. Hence, it appears that weight reduction is likely to have beneficial effects on HRQL even among those whose weight is not particularly debilitating.

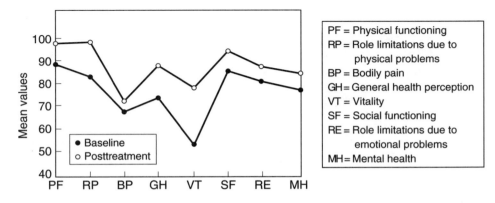

Figure 5.1   Changes in SF-36 scores among moderately obese persons during a 12-week lifestyle modification program.

Reprinted, by permission, from K. Fontaine, 1999, Estimating health related quality of life of obese individuals. In *Managing Obesity*, edited by G. Mallarkey (Auckland, New Zealand: Adis International), 104-106.

Implications of HRQL Assessment for Management of Obesity

As noted, obesity is a complex, multivariate problem strongly related to a variety of factors (e.g., genetic, environmental, and psychosocial). Given this, HRQL assessments of obese patients can potentially be of great benefit in helping practitioners tailor treatments to the particular needs of the individual. For example, as a result of the HRQL assessments of our obese patients we have identified pain as a major concern. As such, we now routinely administer questionnaires to assess pain (e.g., the Brief Pain Inventory) during initial evaluations with new patients. Apart from validating the patients' subjective experience of pain, an assessment of their pain allows us to provide more comprehensive care (i.e., treating their pain in conjunction with a weight reduction intervention).

By the same token, HRQL assessment can help us determine whether a patient's weight is associated with, for example, decreased energy and vitality. In such a case, we would strongly encourage a gradual increase in physical activity not only to facilitate weight reduction, but also to increase energy and overall well-being.

In our view, using HRQL assessments in this way increases the likelihood of providing the level and quality of care required to adequately address a disorder as complicated and multifaceted as obesity.

Limitations and Directions for Future Research

It is important to note that the majority of studies that have examined the HRQL of obese persons were conducted with samples of severely obese persons seeking university- or hospital-based treatment. The recent study by Kolotkin and colleagues (2002) notwithstanding, this raises the possibility that the results may not generalize to obese persons not seeking treatment or to those who lose weight on their own or through less intensive approaches. Indeed, evidence suggests that obese persons who seek university- or hospital-based treatment for their weight exhibit significantly more psychological, affective, and eating disorders (most notably binge eating) than do obese people who do not seek treatment or normal weight controls (e.g., Fitzgibbon, Stolley, and Kirschenbaum 1993;

Higgs, Wade, and Cescato 1997). Although both our study (Fontaine, Bartlett, and Barofsky 2000) and that of Kolotkin and associates (2002) comparing clinic patients with obese persons not currently seeking weight reduction appeared to demonstrate that impairment among obese persons not attempting to lose weight was also substantial, it seems premature to conclude that obesity has a uniform impact on HRQL across treatment seekers and obese persons who do not seek treatment. Additional research is required to obtain more reliable estimates of the impact of obesity on various domains of health status and well-being among non–treatment seekers as well as those who seek commercially based approaches to weight reduction.

Another limitation of current work is that HRQL has been measured with an array of generic- and obesity-specific instruments (e.g., SF-36, Sickness Impact Profile, Gothenburg Quality of Life Scale, IWQOL) that encompass a variety of quality of life domains. This is further complicated by the fact that a number of researchers devise their own measures, which are of uncertain reliability and validity. This makes it very difficult to compare the results across studies, which further undermines our ability to draw definitive conclusions. Consensus on which HRQL measures are most useful with obese individuals would greatly enhance our understanding in this area (Gill and Feinstein 1994).

We believe that the following obesity-HRQL questions need to be satisfactorily addressed to continue to advance our understanding:

- What is the role of HRQL in a person's decision to attempt to lose weight or to seek programmatic weight reduction treatment?
- What impact do weight regain and weight cycling have on HRQL?
- Are obesity-specific HRQL measures superior to generic ones?
- How can HRQL information be used to help us offer treatment to obese individuals that is more compassionate and better tailored to their needs?

Given the dramatic increase in the prevalence of obesity in recent years (e.g., Mokdad et al. 2001) and the personal, social, and economic burden it imposes, it seems vital for workers in this field to continue to pursue this important research.

Summary

Obesity has a significant impact on morbidity and mortality, as well as an individual's capacity to live a full and active life. Traditionally, outcome measures in obesity treatments have emphasized physiological variables such as amount of weight lost and improvements in various health parameters. Increasingly, measures of health-related quality of life (HRQL) are being used to examine the impairment associated with obesity from the patient's point of view, and whether obesity treatment has significantly enhanced functioning and general well-being. Generic measures of HRQL allow clinicians and researchers to compare the negative social, emotional, and physical impact of obesity against other health conditions. Specific measures offer insight into how treatment interventions may positively benefit distinct dimensions of HRQL in overweight persons.

The data are clear: Obesity has a devastating impact on HRQL, especially with respect to physical domains of functioning. Obese persons tend to report that they are severely hampered in their capacity to perform their day-to-day physical activities (e.g., climbing several flights of stairs or carrying groceries), and that these decrements are perceived to limit their personal effectiveness. Musculoskeletal pain is prevalent and also appears to independently impair HRQL. Obesity appears to be associated with substantial decrements in social functioning and mental health, although the magnitude of these relations may be slightly weaker. HRQL also tends to vary considerably as a function of degree of obesity in that severely obese persons (BMI >40) appear to have significantly greater decrements in HRQL relative to persons with lower degrees of obesity.

Collectively, these findings strongly suggest that obesity produces a host of complications, not merely medical ones. Further, many researchers have observed that the psychological burden of obesity may be greater than the physical limitations (Wadden and Stunkard 1987), although the studies conducted by both our group and others (e.g., Fine et al. 1999; Fontaine, Bartlettt, and Barofsky 2000; Fontaine, Cheskin, and Barofsky 1996) have not confirmed this. However, it has been our observation that most obese persons who enter our clinic for treatment report that the impact their weight has on the quality of their lives is one of the primary reasons they are seeking treatment. It may well be that the impairment in obese persons' capacity to live as fully and actively as they desire may be one of the most serious concomitants of obesity.

Although the findings illustrate that obesity has a negative impact on HRQL, weight reduction is associated with improved functional status, reduced pain, and enhanced well-being. Surgical interventions to reduce body weight have been shown to have positive and sustainable effects on HRQL. In fact, among patients who undergo obesity surgery, improved HRQL is consistently reported to be the most important benefit of the weight reduction (Kral, Sjostrom, and Sullivan 1992). Even moderately obese persons who lose a modest amount of weight (i.e., <10 kg or 22 lb) appear to reap the benefits of an enhanced capacity to live a more full and active life (Fontaine et al. 1999).

In sum, although it has long been known that obesity has a negative impact on health, studies of HRQL of obese individuals suggest that it also takes a significant toll on other important aspects of life as well. Greater sensitively to the overall impact of obesity may allow us to provide care to our obese patients that is more compassionate and better tailored to their needs.

Given the difficulties associated with losing weight and keeping it off (e.g., Bartlett et al. 1999; Faith et al. 2000), it seems reasonable that providers of care for obese persons should make greater efforts to provide interventions that address not only their weight, but also the decrements in HRQL. This is consistent with recent conceptualizations of obesity as a chronic disease (Hill, 1998; Stunkard 1996) whose associated health problems (e.g., non-insulin-dependent diabetes or hypertension) can be monitored and controlled rather than cured. To this end, we need to find ways to enhance and sustain positive changes in the HRQL of obese persons, irrespective of whether they are successful at losing weight or maintaining weight loss.

References

Allison, D.B., Fontaine, K.R., Manson, J.E., Stevens, J., and VanItallie, T.B. 1999. How many deaths are attributable to obesity? *Journal of the American Medical Association* 282: 1530-1538.

Allison, D.B., Heo, M., Fontaine, K.R., and Hoffman, D. 2001. Body weight, body composition, and longevity. In *International textbook of obesity,* ed. P. Bjorntrop, 31-48. Sussex, UK: John Wiley & Sons.

Barofsky, I. 1996. Cancer: psychosocial aspects. In *Quality of life and pharmacoeconomics in clinical trials,* ed. Spilker B., 993-1001. Philadelphia: Lippincott-Raven.

Barofsky, I., Fontaine, K.R., and Cheskin, L.J. 1998. Pain in the obese: Impact on health-related quality of life. *Annals of Behavioral Medicine* 19: 408-410.

Bartlett, S.J., Faith, M.S., Fontaine, K.R., Cheskin, L.J., and Allison, D.B 1999. Is the prevalence of successful weight loss and maintenance higher in the general community than the research clinic? *Obesity Research* 7: 407-413.

Buchwald, D., Pearlman, T., Umali, J. et al. 1996. Functional status in patients with chronic fatigue syndrome, other fatiguing illnesses, and healthy individuals. *American Journal of Medicine* 101: 364-370.

Carr, N.D., Harrison, R.A., Tomkins, A. et al. 1989. Vertical banded gastroplasty in the treatment of morbid obesity: Results of three year follow-up. *Gut* 30: 1048-1053.

Choban, P.S., Onyejekwe, J., Burge, J.C., and Flancbaum, L. 1999. A health status assessment of impact of weight loss following Roux-en-Y gastric bypass for clinically severe obesity. *Journal of the American College of Surgery* 188: 491-497.

Dano, P., and Hahn-Pedersen, J. 1977. Improvement in quality of life following jejunoileal bypass surgery for obesity. *Scandinavian Journal of Gastroenterology* 12: 769-774.

Faith, M.S., Fontaine, K.R., Cheskin, L.J., and Allison, D.B. 2000. Behavioral approaches to the problems of obesity. *Behavior Modification* 24: 459-493.

Fallowfield, L.J. 1996. Quality of quality of life data. *Lancet* 348: 421.

Fine, J.T., Colditz, G.A., Coakley, E.H., Moseley, G., Manson, J.E., Willett, W.C., and Kawachi, I. 1999. A prospective study of weight change and health-related quality of life in women. *Journal of the American Medical Association* 282: 2136-2142.

Fitzgibbon, M.L., Stolley, M.R., and Kirschenbaum, D.S. 1993. Obese people who seek treatment have different characteristics than those who do not seek treatment. *Health Psychology* 12: 342-345.

Fontaine, K.R., and Barofsky, I. 2001. Obesity and health-related quality of life. *Obesity Reviews* 2: 173-182.

Fontaine, K.R., Barofsky, I., Andersen, R.E., Bartlett, S.J., Wiersema, L., Cheskin, L.J., and Franckowiak, S.C. 1999. Impact of weight loss on pain and health-related quality of life. *Quality of Life Research* 8: 275-277.

Fontaine, K.R., Bartlett, S.J., and Barofsky, I. 2000. Health-related quality of life among obese persons seeking and not currently seeking treatment. *International Journal of Eating Disorders* 27: 101-105.

Fontaine, K.R., Cheskin, L.J., and Barofsky, I. 1996. Health-related quality of life in obese persons seeking treatment. *Journal of Family Practice* 43: 265-270.

Gill, T.M., and Feinstein, A.R. 1994. A critical appraisal of quality-of-life measurements. *Journal of the American Medical Association* 272: 619-626.

Guyatt, G.H., Feeny, D.H., and Patrick, D.L. 1993. Measuring health-related quality of life. *Annals of Internal Medicine* 118:622-629.

Hafner, R.J., Watts, J.M., and Rogers, J. 1991. Quality of life after gastric bypass surgery for morbid obesity. *International Journal of Obesity and Related Metabolic Disorders* 15: 555-560.

Hawke, A., O'Brien, P., Watts, J.M. et al. 1990. Psychosocial and physical activity changes after gastric restrictive procedures for morbid obesity. *Australian New Zealand Journal of Surgery* 60: 755-758.

Higgs, M.L., Wade, T., Cescato, M. et al. 1997. Differences between treatment seekers in an obese population: Medical intervention vs. dietary restriction. *Journal of Behavioral Medicine* 20: 391-405.

Hill, J.O. 1998. Dealing with obesity as a chronic disease. *Obesity Research* 6 (Suppl.): 34S-37S.

Isacsson, A., Frederiksen, S.G., Nilsson, C. et al. 1997. Quality of life after gastroplasty is normal: A controlled study. *European Journal of Surgery* 163: 181-186.

Jhingran, P., Cady, R.K., Rubino, J. et al. 1996. Improvements in health-related quality of life with sumatriptan treatment for migraine. *Journal of Family Practice* 42: 36-42.

Karlsson, J., Sjostrom, L., and Sullivan, M. 1998. Swedish obese subjects (SOS)—An intervention study of obesity. Two-year follow-up of health-related quality of life (HRQL) and eating behavior after gastric surgery for severe obesity. *International Journal of Obesity and Related Metabolic Disorders* 22: 113-126.

Kolotkin, R.L., Crosby, R.D., Kosloski, K.D., and Williams, G.R. 2001. Development of a brief measure to assess quality of life in obesity. *Obesity Research* 9: 102-111.

Kolotkin, R.L., Crosby, R.D., and Rhys Williams, G. 2002. Health-related quality of life among obese subgroups. *Obesity Research* 10: 748-756.

Kolotkin, R.L., Crosby, R.D., Rhys Williams, G., Hartley, G.G., and Nicol, S. 2001. The relationship between health-related quality of life and weight loss. *Obesity Research* 9: 564-571.

Kolotkin, R.L., Head, S., and Hamilton, M. 1995. Assessing impact of weight on quality of life. *Obesity Research* 3: 49-56.

Kral, J.G., Sjostrom, L.V., and Sullivan, M.B. 1992. Assessment of quality of life before and after surgery for severe obesity. *American Journal of Clinical Nutrition* 55 (Suppl. 2): 611-614.

Larsen, F. 1990. Psychosocial function before and after gastric banding surgery for morbid obesity: A prospective psychiatric study. *Acta Psychiatrica Scandinavica* 359: 1-57.

Larsson, U., Karlsson, J., and Sullivan, M. 2002. Impact of overweight and obesity on health-related quality of life—A Swedish population study. *International Journal of Obesity and Related Metabolic Disorders* 26: 417-424.

Le Pen, C., Levy, E., Loos, F. et al. 1998. "Specific" scale compared with "generic" scale: A double measurement of the quality of life in a French community sample of obese subjects. *Journal of Epidemiology and Community Health* 52: 445-450.

Mathias, S.D., Williamson, C.L., and Colwell, H.H. 1997. Assessing health-related quality of life and health state preference in persons with obesity: A validation study. *Quality of Life Research* 6: 311-322.

Mokdad, A.H., Bowman, B.A., Ford, E.S., Vinicor, F., Marks, J.S., and Koplan, J.P. 2001. The continuing epidemics of obesity and diabetes in the United States. *Journal of the American Medical Association* 286: 1195-1200.

Mustajoki, P., Lempinen, M., and Huikuri, K. 1984. Long-term outcome after jejunoileal bypass for morbid obesity. *International Journal of Obesity and Related Metabolic Disorders* 8: 319-325.

Naslund, I., and Agren, G. 1990. Social effects of gastric restrictive surgery for morbid obesity. *International Journal of Obesity and Related Metabolic Disorders* 14 (Suppl. 2): 159 (abstract).

National Task Force on the Prevention and Treatment of Obesity. 2000. Overweight, obesity, and health risk. *Archives of Internal Medicine* 160: 898-904.

Osterhaus, J.T., Townsend, R.J., and Gandek, B. 1994. Measuring the functional status and well-being of patients with migraine headache. *Headache* 34: 337-343.

Patrick, D.L., Deyo, R.A., and Atlas, S.J. 1995. Assessing health-related quality of life in patients with sciatica. *Spine* 20: 1899-1909.

Pi-Sunyer, F.X. 1993. Medical hazards of obesity. *Annals of Internal Medicine* 119: 655-660.

Pi-Sunyer, F.X. 1999. Comorbidities of overweight and obesity: Current evidence and research issues. *Medicine and Science in Sports and Exercise* 31(Suppl.): S602-S608.

Popkin, B.M., and Doak, C.M. 1998. The obesity epidemic is a worldwide phenomenon. *Nutrition Reviews* 56: 106-114.

Rippe, J.M., Price, J.M., Hess, S.A. et al. 1998. Improved psychological well-being, quality of life, and health practices in moderately overweight women participating in a 12-week structured weight loss program. *Obesity Research* 6: 208-218.

Sarlio-Lahteenkorva, S., Stunkard, A., and Rissanen, A. 1995. Psychosocial factors and quality of life in obesity. *International Journal of Obesity and Related Metabolic Disorders* 19 (Suppl.): 1-5.

Seidell, J.C. 1995. The impact of obesity on health status: Some implications for health care costs. *International Journal of Obesity and Related Metabolic Disorders* 19 (Suppl. 6): 13-16.

Seidell, J.C., Bakx, K.C., and Deurenberg, P. 1986. The relation between overweight and subjective health according to age, social class, slimming behavior and smoking habits in Dutch adults. *American Journal of Public Health* 76: 1410-1415.

Stewart, A.L., and Brook, R.H. 1983. Effects of being overweight. *American Journal of Public Health* 73: 171-178.

Stunkard, A.J. 1996. Current views of obesity. *American Journal of Medicine* 100: 230-236.

Sullivan, M., Karlsson, J., Sjostrom, L. et al. 1993. Swedish obese subjects (SOS): An intervention study of obesity. Baseline evaluation of health and psychological functioning in the first 1,743 subjects examined. *International Journal of Obesity and Related Metabolic Disorders* 17: 503-512.

Sullivan, M.B.E., Sullivan, L.G.M., and Kral, J.G. 1987. Quality of life assessment in obesity: Physical, psychological and social function. *Gastroenterology Clinics of North America* 16: 433-442.

Van Gemert, W.G., Adang, E.M., Kop, M., Vos, G., Greve, J.W., and Soeters, P.B. 1999. A prospective cost-effectiveness analysis of vertical banded gastroplasty for the treatment of morbid obesity. *Obesity Surgery* 9: 484-491.

Wadden, T.A., and Stunkard, A.J. 1987. Psychopathology and obesity. *Annals of the New York Academy of Science* 499: 55-65.

Wan, G.J., Counte, M.A., and Cella, D.F. 1997. A framework for organizing health-related quality of life research. *Journal of Rehabilitation and Outcomes Measures* 1: 31-37.

Ware, J.E., Bayliss, M.S., Rogers, W.H. et al. 1996. Differences in 4-year health outcomes for elderly and poor, chronically ill patients treated in HMO and fee-for-service systems. *Journal of the American Medical Association* 276: 1039-1047.

Ware, J.E., Snow, K.K., and Kosinski, M. 1993. SF-36 health survey: Manual and interpretation guide. Boston: New England Medical Center.

Weiner, R., Datz, M., Wagner, D., and Bockhorn, H. 1999. Quality of life outcome after laparoscopic adjustable gastric banding for morbid obesity. *Obesity Surgery* 9: 539-545.

Chapter 6

Body Composition Assessment in the Obese

Timothy G. Lohman, PhD
University of Arizona at Tucson

Laurie Milliken, PhD
University of Massachusetts at Boston

Estimating body composition in the obese population can be accomplished by both field methods (e.g., skinfolds, bioelectric impedance, and circumferences) and laboratory methods (e.g., underwater weighing, body water, dual-energy X-ray absorptiometry or DXA, and multicomponent models). Laboratory methods offer somewhat smaller errors of estimation, usually between 2 and 3% for percent fat. For field methods the standard errors of estimation are larger (between 3 and 4%). Finally, estimating body fat in overweight and obese individuals from body mass index (BMI) has a standard error ranging from 4 to 6%.

This chapter compares various methods of estimating body composition in obese populations and delineates the advantages and disadvantages of each. It also focuses on estimating changes in body composition with weight loss in the obese population.

Laboratory Methods

The major laboratory methods for assessment of body composition are underwater weighing (UWW), total body water (TBW), dual-energy X-ray absorptiometry (DXA), and various multicomponent approaches (MC) that use two or three methods in the same subjects. For UWW and TBW, the body is as-sumed to be a two-component system with a constant density and water percent of the fat-free mass. For many applications in the adult population, this assumption holds true to a great extent with a water content of 73 ± 2% and a density of the fat-free body of 1.10 ± 0.006 g/cc (Lohman 1981).

Underwater Weighing and Air Displacement Plethysmography

The major assumption of both underwater weighing (UWW) and air displacement plethysmography (ADPl) is that the density of the fat-free body is constant at 1.100 g/c in the adult population. The relationship between body density and percent fat has been well documented in the adult population (Lohman 1981), and results from ADPl are also promising (Dempster and Aikens 1995; Sardinha et al. 1998). The major source of variation in the fat-free body density is the water and mineral content. Research in the past 10 years with multicomponent models that measured the water and mineral content along with body density has shown that both components are maintained at a fairly constant amount throughout the adult years (20 to 70 years of age). The large study by Visser and colleagues (1997) of 668 African American and white subjects age 20 to 95 showed that the density of the fat-free mass varied from 1.0976 to 1.163 in various age, general, and ethnic groups. The two-component model yielded percent fat within 1% of the four-component model (Visser et al. 1997). Thus, the equation of Siri (1961) has wide applicability when used in the adult population.

$$\% \ fat = \frac{495}{D} - 450$$

D = body density from UWW or ADP

The density of the fat-free body in obese individuals may differ from that in the non-obese population because excess adipose tissue leads to a slightly higher water and protein content of fat-free mass (FFM). Although adipose tissue is mostly lipid, additional water and protein contribute to the FFM depending on the degree of adiposity. Womersley and colleagues (1976) estimated obese men to have a fat-free body density of 1.10 and obese women (both younger and older) to be similar to nonobese women.

If the water content of the FFM increases and the bone mineral content of the FFM decreases with increasing levels of obesity due to the hydration effect, then the density of the FFM would decrease and we would expect a greater estimation bias for percent fat from UWW versus percent fat from the multicomponent model with increasing levels of obesity. Bunt, Lohman, and Boileau (1989) directly investigated the effect of water variability in selected women who changed body weight by 2.2 kg (4.8 lb) during a menstrual cycle. Percent fat changed from 24.8 to 27.6% based on UWW of the two-component system, illustrating the effect of higher levels of hydration causing an overestimate of body fatness. If, on the other hand, both total body water (TBW) and total body mineral (TBM) increase in the obese (obese population have a higher bone density), then the hydration effect will be attenuated and less apparent (Prior et al. 1997; Visser et al. 1997).

Research using ADPl in obese subjects has not been published; thus, while the method appears to give comparable results to UWW in the general population, it has not been validated in the obese population.

Total Body Water

The measurement of total body water (TBW) using isotope dilution methods and either infrared or mass spectrometry enables an estimate of body fat assuming a constant hydration level of 73% in FFM (Schoeller 1996; Wang et al. 1999).

$$\% \ fat = \left(1 - \frac{w}{.73}\right)100$$

w = the water content of the body as a fraction of body weight

For a water content of 56% or 0.56 as a fraction of body weight, the estimated fat content would be 23.3%. If an individual were dehydrated (71% water of FFM) or overhydrated (75%, FFM), the percent fat would be overestimated in the former case by 3.3% and underestimated in the latter case by 3.6%. Use of body water as a reference method for body composition is well accepted in the adult population when the level of hydration is fairly constant (Lohman et al. 2000). Lohman and colleagues (2000) addressed the controversy around the level and variation of hydration by presenting evidence that methodological sources contribute to variation in hydration levels. In the obese population, body water is also of use because of evidence that the hydration level in obese individuals is not greatly different from that in nonobese individuals.

Total body water is not often measured by deuterium dilution and, in general, the mass spectrometer produces less variation than the infrared spectrometer. It can also be measured by tritium dilution; however, since tritium is radioactive, it adds small radiation exposure to the body, whereas deuterium is a nonradioactive isotope of hydrogen.

Dual-Energy X-Ray Absorptiometry

Recent review studies by Kohrt (1998) and Lohman and colleagues (2000) indicate that dual-energy X-ray absorptiometry (DXA), using recent versions of software (Hologic 5.64 or above) and Lunar (1.3y extended research version), can be used to estimate the fat content in the body with SEEs (standard errors of estimate) of 2.5 to 3.0% when compared to UWW and MC. Theoretical (Pietrobelli et al. 1996) and empirical (Kohrt 1998; Prior et al. 1997) evidence supports DXA as a reference method for body composition at all ages. With estimates of fat, lean, and bone mineral mass, this method gives body composition estimates that do not depend on the assumptions of the two-component model. Prior and colleagues (1997) have shown that DXA correlates with MC and UWW percent fat estimates with SEEs of 2.8% for both comparisons. Other body composition studies validating DXA as a reference method using recent software show similar SEEs and good agreement between mean values of DXA with the reference methods (Lohman et al. 2000). The exception to this general finding is the work of Clasey and colleagues (1997 and 1999), in which a SEE of 5.0% was found between DXA and MC. In an analysis of the Clasey studies, Lohman and colleagues (2000) found that methodological variation in TBW estimates is a likely source of variation between methods. Prior work by Snead, Birg, and Kohrt (1993); Kohrt (1995, 1998); and Milliken, Going, and Lohman (1996) shows the importance of recent software developments in estimating body composition accurately using DXA.

Two limitations of DXA have been the effects of subject thickness on the accuracy of body composition estimates and body size in obese subjects who fall outside the scan range. The relationship between *R* value and subject thickness is fairly constant from 10 to 25 cm (4 to 10 in.). With an increasing thickness above 25 cm (10 in.), *R* values decline independent of composition (Lohman 1996). Lower *R* values for increasingly thicker subjects could overestimate the body fatness in the obese.

A second limitation is that of body size. Tataranni and Ravussin (1995) proposed a solution to large body size when they found a high correlation between percent fat from the right half of the body and percent fat from the total body. They proposed that very large subjects be scanned on only the right side with some of the left side of the body falling outside the scan area. In our laboratory, we found good agreement (mean difference = 0.1% fat) between right side composition and total body composition with an r^2 of 0.99

and SEE of 0.35% fat. More recently researchers have studied DXA fan beam technology for body composition results and reported validation of this technology (Salamone et al. 2000; Tylavsky et al. 2000; Visser et al. 1999). The advantage of fan beam DXA is the short measurement time (five minutes per scan) for body composition analysis.

Multicomponent Models

Multicomponent models have an advantage over two-component models when variation of the composition of the fat-free body differs from reference man or when, in a given sample, there is more variation in fat-free body composition, or weight loss over time. Heymsfield, Wang, and Withers (1996) outlined various multicomponent approaches, including one of the most popular of which is the use of underwater weighing, total body water, and bone mineral assessment. Various equations have been proposed for estimation of percent fat using the four-component model with slightly different assumptions on the composition of fat-free body components.

One example of a multicomponent model is from Lohman 1986:

$$\% \ fat = \left(\frac{2.747}{D} - 0.714w + 1.146m - 2.0503 \right) 100$$

w = water content relative to body weight,
m = body mineral (osseous and nonosseous mineral) relative to body weight, and
D = body density from UWW

Variation in estimates of osseous (from DXA) and nonosseous mineral (assumed values) have led to different formulations of the original model.

The multicomponent model is especially helpful for following changes in composition with weight loss. Friedl and colleagues (1992) quantified reliable estimates of body fat from the four-component model. They found that when measuring body water, density, and bone mineral, the reliability of the multicomponent model leads to a precision of about 1% fat. Evans and colleagues (1999) used the multicomponent model to study changes in body composition with weight loss in obese women comparing diet and exercise interventions over 16 weeks. They found small differences between the two-component and four-component models.

The disadvantage of the multicomponent model is that it requires an accurate assessment of body density using UWW as well as accurate measurements of body water and bone mineral. The work of Clasey and colleagues (1997) showed that methodological variation in body water reduces the validity of the MC approach and leads to inaccurate conclusions (Lohman et al. 2000).

Field Methods

Field methods for estimating fatness tend to be relatively inexpensive tools that are widely applicable to large populations. However, these tools also include errors that are higher than those of laboratory methods. The accuracy of field methods is established by comparing estimates of fatness for a given population to more accurate values obtained from laboratory techniques. Several statistical tools are used to assess the level of agreement between the field and laboratory methods. Mean values of fatness for the field method and the laboratory method can be compared to determine statistical differences. The relationship between the two fatness values (correlation coefficient, r) along with the error associated with this relationship (SEE) can also be determined. Finally, Bland-Altman plots can identify whether the differences between the two fatness values ($Fatness_{criterion} - Fatness_{field method}$) (residual scores) are affected by the absolute level of fatness. In general, the two techniques, on good agreement, should show small mean differences, a strong association (r), low errors (SEE), and no relationship between the residual scores and the absolute level of fatness (Going and Davis 1998; Lohman 1992). In general, body composition methods that have SEEs greater than 5.0% are not recommended for assessing body composition of the individual (Lohman 1992) (see table 6.1).

Body Mass Index

Height, weight, and various combinations of different exponents of height and weight have been used to estimate percent fat in both obese and nonobese populations. One of the best studies to evaluate various weight–height relationships in the assessment of obesity is

Table 6.1 *Subjective Rating for Percent Fat Standard Errors of Estimate*

Standard error of estimate, percent fat	Subjective rating
5.0	Not recommended
4.5	Fair
4.0	Fairly good
3.5	Good
3.0	Very good
2.5	Excellent
2.0	Ideal

that by Womersley and Durnin (1977), who compared various ratios of weight (w) and height (h) including w/h^2 (Quetelet's index or BMI), w/h, and w/h^3 (ponderal index), as well as others. Underwater weighing (UWW) was used as the criterion method in men and women ranging from 20 to 76 years of age. In each age group, correlations were lower and SEEs were higher (except in lowest age group) for men than for women (see table 6.2). For men, the SEEs ranged from 4.8 to 5.6% fat and for women from 3.8 to 6.1% fat. Over a wide age range, the SEEs for men were 5.9% compared to 5.4% for women. Jackson and Pollock (1985) and Smalley and colleagues (1990) also found larger SEEs for men (5.7%) than for women (5.1%) in adult samples over a wide age range. Deurenberg, Westrate, and Seidell (1991) also examined the BMI-percentage fat relationship in 747 males and females aged 16 to 83 years and found that BMI, age, and sex predicted percentage fat well ($r = 0.89$, SEE = 4.1%). However, in obese subjects in this sample, BMI slightly overestimated percentage fat.

Using the equations of Womersley and Durnin (1977), we can show the relation of BMI to percent fat in both men and women. We can see that a BMI of 27 corresponds to percent fat of 23.7% for men and 33.5% for women using these equations (see tables 6.3 and 6.4).

The studies of both Smalley and colleagues (1990) and Curtin and colleagues (1997

Table 6.2 **Conditions and Standard Errors of Estimate for Indices of Height and Weight With Percent Fat From UWW**

Age group	Indices	Women		Men	
		r	SEE	*r*	SEE
20-29 years	*w/h*	0.68	6.1	0.50	5.5
	w/h²	0.71	6.1	0.55	5.0
	w/h³	0.70	6.1	0.56	4.8
30-39 years	*w/h*	0.89	3.8	0.54	5.6
	w/h²	0.91	3.9	0.56	5.6
	w/h³	0.91	3.9	0.55	5.6
40-49 years	*w/h*	0.81	3.8	0.60	5.5
	w/h²	0.84	3.9	0.62	5.4
	w/h³	0.83	3.8	0.57	5.6
50-76 years	*w/h*	0.86	4.3	0.51	5.4
	w/h²	0.88	4.3	0.53	5.4
	w/h³	0.87	4.3	0.56	5.6

Data from Womersley and Durnin 1977.

Table 6.3 **Percent Fat From BMI in Men and Women Using the Overall Equation**

Sample	Equation	SEE percent fat	*N*
Women (17-68 years)	Percent fat = 1.37 × BMI − 3.47	5.4	324
Men (17-76 years)	Percent fat = 1.34 × BMI − 12.47	5.9	245

Data from Womersley and Durnin 1977.

Table 6.4 **Percent Fat From BMI Values**

BMI	Percent fat	
	Women	Men
20	23.9	14.3
25	30.8	21.8
27	33.5	23.7
30	37.6	27.7
35	44.5	34.4
40	51.3	41.1

Data from Womersley and Durnin 1977.

showed high specificity but low to moderate sensitivity (a large fraction of false negatives) when they compared BMI to a specific cutoff point of percent fat. Recent evidence in postmenopausal women suggests that a lower obesity cutoff point for BMI (24.9 versus 30.0, which is currently recommended by the National Institutes of Health) improved the performance of BMI as a diagnostic tool for obesity (Blew et al. 2002). In this study, a BMI of 24.9 corresponded to a sensitivity (true-positive rate) of 84.4% compared to only 25.6% using a cutoff point of 30.0. The false-positive rate was 14.6% and 0.7% for BMIs of 24.9 and 30.0, respectively.

Anthropometric Measurements

Skinfold thicknesses are practical measurements routinely used to estimate body composition. The measurement of subcutaneous fat is used in the prediction of total body fatness because about 50 to 70% of total body fat is located subcutaneously and this fat is related to overall fatness (Lohman 1981). The SEEs associated with the prediction of percent fatness from skinfold measurements in the general population range from 3.0 to 4.5, making skinfolds an acceptable technique to estimate fatness (Lohman 1981).

The errors associated with skinfold measurements are considerably higher for the determination of body fatness in the obese (Gray et al. 1990) than in leaner populations. In very obese subjects, the size of the calipers is often too small to measure the thickness of the entire skinfold, especially at the abdomen and thigh. Biological differences between the lean and obese can also affect the relationship between subcutaneous fat and overall fatness. The compressibility of the fold may vary among people and, in the obese, may result in improper placement of the caliper on the fold because the subcutaneous fat cannot be lifted from the underlying muscle (Gray et al. 1990).

Generalized equations have been developed for the prediction of body density from skinfold measurements (Durnin and Womersley 1974; Jackson and Pollock 1978; Jackson, Pollock, and Ward 1980) with percent body fat calculated from body density using the equation by Siri (1961). These equations were developed on large populations of males and females who varied widely in age and body fatness. As is the case with any equation, a larger error may result when the equation is applied to populations that differ from the population in which the equation was initially validated.

For example, Jackson, Pollock, and Ward (1980) developed an equation for the prediction of body density from the sum of three skinfolds in women. The subjects included in this validation study were women between the ages of 18 and 55 (mean = 31.4 ± 10.8 years) and were 4 to 44% body fat (mean = 24.1 ± 7.2% fat) as measured by hydrostatic weighing. This study included relatively few obese women over 40 years of age. When this equation was applied to a population 52.9 years of age (range = 21-72 years) and 36.9% fat (range = 30-48%), percent body fat was significantly underestimated compared to the criterion (Heyward et al. 1992). The r's and SEEs in the original investigation were >0.80 and <3.8%, respectively, while Heyward and colleagues (1992) found $r = 0.59$ and SEE = 3.4%. In addition, the correlation between the residual scores and the criterion percent fat was positive and significant, indicating that the difference between the predicted percent fat and the criterion percent fat was greater at higher levels of fatness.

Researchers have also documented significant positive relationships between the residual scores and the level of fatness when using the equation by Durnin and Womersley (1974) (Fogelholm et al. 1997; Fuller, Sawyer, and Elia 1994; Gray et al. 1990). However, in a more obese population the relationship between the predicted and criterion percent fat was stronger, the SEE lower, and the mean difference between the predicted and criterion smaller when using the equation by Durnin and Womersley (1974) than when using the equations by Jackson and colleagues (1978, 1980) (Gray et al. 1990). In a sample of 21 obese females (mean = 46.9 ± 6.5%) who were of a similar age to the Gray (1990) sample, the correlation between the criterion body fat and the body fat using the Jackson, Pollack, and Ward (1980) and then the Durnin (1974) equation was lower ($r = 0.38$ and 0.22, respectively) with a higher SEE (4.6 and 5.1%, respectively). The ability of skinfold equations to predict body fatness was less successful in obese individuals than in nonobese individuals.

An alternative anthropometric technique to predict body fatness is the use of circumference or girth measures. Although this technique is of limited usefulness in lean and athletic populations where larger girths can be due to increased lean mass, in obese populations, larger girth measurements are typically due to larger amounts of fat. Tran and Weltman (1989) developed an equation to predict the body density of 482 women 15 to 79 years of age and 12.7 to 63.1% fat. When compared to hydrostatic weighing, $r = 0.89$ and SEE = 4.2% fat. The authors later cross-validated this equation and found SEEs of 3.6% and 2.9%, respectively. Katch and McArdle (1973) also developed a girth equation and found $r = 0.64$ and SEE = 4.3% when compared to the criterion. Upon cross-validation, the r and SEE were 0.68 and 3.3% fat, respectively, with a mean difference of 0.58%. Girth equations have errors similar to skinfold equations in the nonobese and are more useful in the very obese, especially when assessing changes in body fatness. Further cross-validation efforts are needed in this population. Also, the ability of this technique to determine changes in body composition is limited, especially when lean mass is increased such as in strength training.

Bioelectrical Impedance Analysis (BIA) Measurements

BIA is a rapid, noninvasive technique used to estimate body composition and requires little technician skill. A weak electrical current is introduced into the body through electrodes placed at the hands and feet. The impedance (composed of resistance and reactance) to the flow of this current relates to the amount of body water present. FFM, fat mass, and percent fat can be calculated given that the water content of FFM is constant at 73%. SEEs for the prediction of FFM in the general population range from 2.1 to 3.6 kg (4.6 to 7.9 lb) (Lohman 1992).

Because BIA depends on the measurement of body water and assumes that water is 73% of FFM, larger errors can occur when hydration levels vary. Deurenberg (1996) discussed three factors that can affect the validity of BIA for the obese: (1) relative total body water tends to be increased causing body fat to be underestimated; (2) extracellular water may also be increased, which would result in an underestimation of body fat; and (3) differences in body geometry in the obese (such as increased abdominal adiposity) compared to the lean may affect impedance independent of differences in FFM and would result in an overestimation of body fat.

Despite these concerns, the SEEs for FFM from a variety of equations ranged from 2.0 to 3.5 kg (4.4 to 7.7 lb) for obese women and from 3.0 to 5.1 kg (6.6 to 11 lb) for obese men (Carella et al. 1997; Fogelholm et al. 1997; Gray et al. 1989, 1990; Heyward et al. 1992; Kushner et al. 1990; Kushner and Schoeller 1986; Stolarczyk

et al. 1997; van der Kooy et al. 1992). This does not mean that Deurenberg's concerns are not well founded. Careful examination of several validation and cross-validation studies reveals that, in every study in which Bland-Altman analysis was performed, a significant positive association existed between the residual scores for percent fat and the absolute level of fatness. There was a significant underestimation of percent fat from BIA as the obesity level of the subjects increased.

Many generalized equations exist to estimate body fatness using BIA, including those that are preprogrammed with impedance analyzers. Generalized BIA equations typically suffer from the limitations outlined previously and will result in significant underestimations of body fat when applied to an obese population. The fatness-specific equations of Gray and colleagues (1990) and Segal and colleagues (1988) provide good alternatives for body composition assessment. Gray and colleagues (1990) developed an equation for women >48% fat, while Segal's equation (1988) is for women >30% and men >20% fat. The errors associated with these equations tend to be lower (2.0 to 3.7 kg or 4.4 to 8.1 lb FFM) than generalized equations applied to obese subjects (2.6 to 5.06 kg or 5.7 to 11.1 lb FFM). Mean differences between the criterion and BIA using the Segal equation tend to be relatively small (-2.1 to 0.7 kg or -4.6 to 1.5 lb), while for Gray and colleagues (1989), mean differences were higher (0.4 to 6.2 kg or 0.9 to 13.6 lb).

One limitation to the use of the fatness-specific equations of Segal and colleagues (1988) is that these equations require a prior knowledge of body fatness to categorize the subjects as obese or nonobese. Stolarczyk and colleagues (1997) determined in a large population diverse in ethnicity and fatness that the average of body fat from the generalized and fatness-specific equations provides an alternative to prior classification of obesity. The average of the two Segal equations compared well to hydrostatic weighing as well as other BIA equations. For women, the r, SEE, and mean difference for BIA versus the criterion were 0.93, 2.2 kg (4.8 lb), and 0.21 kg (0.5 lb), respectively. For men, their r, SEE, and mean difference for BIA versus the criterion were 0.94, 3.6 kg (7.9 lb), and 0.51 kg (1.1 lb), respectively.

A final concern when using BIA is the effect of ethnicity. Many equations have been validated and cross-validated on ethnically homogenous samples. Jakicic, Wing, and Lang (1998) showed that BIA underestimates FFM in Caucasian women but overestimates FFM in African American women. An ethnic-specific equation was proposed but has not been cross-validated.

Assessment of Body Composition Changes

The measurement of body composition changes with weight loss is an important aspect of body composition assessment. Changes in fat, muscle, and bone density are important aspects to quantify especially when significant weight loss takes place. Using the two-component model (UWW or TBW) assumes that the fat-free body composition does not change, and thus, estimates of muscle versus bone cannot be made. Recently, researchers have applied multicomponent models to weight loss studies, enabling estimates of fat-free body composition changes.

Evans and colleagues (1999) provided separate estimates of water, mineral, and protein mass for subjects who lost weight from diet only versus subjects who lost weight from diet and exercise over 16 weeks. The results using a four-component model indicate a similar loss between groups in fat mass, but a larger weight, fat-free mass, and water loss in the diet-only group (see table 6.5).

These results showing the benefits of exercise and diet in maintaining the composition of fat-free mass are rarely shown in weight loss studies because of the failure to use multicomponent models. Future studies using DXA or multicomponent models are essential for the proper assessment of compositional change with weight loss.

In terms of weight loss and changes in bone density, early work found that weight loss and bone mineral loss were closely associated. However, more recent research indicates less change in bone density with modest weight loss (Van Loan, Johnson, and Barbieri 1998).

Assessing body composition changes at the individual versus the group level often is misunderstood. Evans and colleagues (1999) pointed out that assessing change by various methods leads to variation of 2% in body fatness (standard deviation of the difference). This variation includes both methodological and biological variation due to variations in individuals' body fat changes over time. The biological variation is due partly to genetics and partly to genetics combined with environmental factors. Evans and colleagues (1999) stated that to detect an actual change in percent fat with 95% confidence for the individual, body fat would have to change 4%. Several misconceptions can arise from this statement.

First, we can say that some individuals change more than others and, therefore, this source of variation included in the 2% standard deviation is not of methodological origin and should not be charged against a given method. Second, since different methods measure different aspects of body composition changes, the 2% standard deviation does not include the lack of validity in a given method to measure change. The variation between the multicomponent model estimate of change and a given method in question is an estimate of this change. In measuring change in body fatness over time, Houtkooper and colleagues (2000) found, in general, a correlation of 0.5 between DXA and UWW changes.

In the case of Evans and colleagues (1999), we are not given the error (SEE) between the multicomponent method and the methods in question and cannot estimate the error of each method

Table 6.5   *Changes in Body Composition With Diet Only and Diet and Exercise Groups Using Multicomponent Model*

Weight loss	Diet only (kg)	Diet and exercise (kg)
Body mass	−7.2	−3.9
Fat mass	−4.2	−3.6
Fat-free mass	−3.0	−0.3
Water mass	−1.9	−0.4
Protein mass	−1.1	0.0

Data from Evans et al. 1999.

to measure changes in the individual as compared to the multicomponent approach.

Finally, it is important to distinguish between group changes, which usually have a small measurement error, and individual changes, which have a larger error of measurement. While an individual change of 2.0% body fat cannot be reliably assessed (within methods), a group change can be more reliably assessed, and with 10, 16, and 25 subjects per group, the standard error of the mean change is 0.6%, 0.5%, and 0.4%, respectively. Thus, we can distinguish between interventions, a difference of 1% body fat if sample sizes are 16 or greater per group. This within-method of analysis does not include the between-method or validity aspects of the method to accurately measure the body composition changes that take place. Thus, a given method may be a reliable measure of body composition change as found by Evans and colleagues (1999) for several methods. However, it may not be a valid method; for example, the mean change in body composition by BMI does not discriminate between interventions as to the actual changes in fat, water, and muscle.

Body composition changes in the general population are difficult to assess using the field techniques described here. The relatively low reproducibility of measurements from day to day results in the limited ability to detect small changes over time in response to interventions. To determine the minimum amount of change that can be detected, researchers would have to measure several people twice in one week and calculate the difference between day 1 and day 2. The standard deviation of the differences in this situation is the minimum level of change that can be detected in that population using a given technique. The standard deviation of the differences will vary from one field method to another and from one population to another. For example, if the skinfold technique was used in a population of obese subjects and the technician had difficulty reproducing measurements from day to day, the standard deviation of the differences would be high and the minimum detectable amount of change would be large. If a technician can more easily reproduce skinfold measurements in a lean population, the amount of change detected will be smaller. Indeed, highly precise and reproducible techniques such as DXA allow the detection of very small amounts of change.

Several studies have focused on the measurement of body composition changes in the obese. Most of these studies indicate that both BIA and skinfolds underestimate the amount of fat loss in obese subjects (Carella et al. 1997; Fogelholm et al. 1997; Kushner et al. 1990; van der Kooy et al. 1992), although some do report that BIA may be useful (Kushner et al. 1990; Ross et al. 1989). The changes in body water during weight loss (Deurenberg 1996) or the disproportionate loss of intra-abdominal fat relative to subcutaneous fat (Gray et al. 1990) may account for the underestimations associated with BIA and skinfolds, respectively.

Summary

In this chapter, we reviewed laboratory and field methods for assessing body composition in the obese population and for assessing body composition changes with weight loss. Body mass index (BMI), a frequently used measure of obesity, has the largest estimation error (SEE is 4 to 6% for the individual) and is not accurate for individual assessment. In addition to the large prediction error, BMI cutoff points lead to a low to moderate degree of sensitivity, with a large number of false negative cases. Field methods of body fatness yield SEEs of 3 to 4% for the individual and provide a better indicator of body fatness than BMI. Equations cross-validated on the obese population are recommended for skinfolds, circumferences, and bioelectric impedance. Laboratory methods using the two-component model are appropriate for the obese and UWW, ADPl, and TBW are recommended (SEEs between 2 and 3%). In addition, DXA and multicomponent model are recommended when an accurate estimate of fatness is needed (MC) or for assessment of fat distribution (DXA).

Measuring changes in body fatness over time in response to different interventions requires the use of multicomponent models to accurately assess water, fat, and lean tissue changes. We carefully reviewed the limitations of field methods and laboratory methods using the two-component system to assess body composition changes, and examined the misconceptions related to the accuracy of individual versus group changes.

References

Blew, R.M., Sardinha, L.B., Milliken, L.A., Teixeira, P.J., Going, S.B., Ferreira, D.L., Harris, M.M., Houtkooper, L.B., and Lohman, T.G. 2002. Assessing the validity of body mass index standards in early postmenopausal women. *Obesity Research* 10 (8): 799-808.

Bunt, J.C., Lohman, T.G., and Boileau, R.A. 1989. Impact of total body water fluctuation on estimation of body fat from body density. *Medicine and Science in Sports and Exercise* 21 (1): 96-100.

Carella, M.J., Rodgers, C.D., Anderson, D., and Gossain, V.V. 1997. Serial measurements of body composition in obese subjects during a very-low-energy diet (VLED) comparing bioelectrical impedance with hydrodensitometry. *Obesity Research* 5 (3): 250-256.

Clasey, J.L., Hartman, M.L., Kanaley, J., Wideman, L., Teates, C.D., and Bouchard, C. 1997. Body composition by DEXA in older adults: Accuracy and influence of scan mode. *Medicine and Science in Sports and Exercise* 29 (4): 560-567.

Clasey, J.L., Kanaley, J.A., Wideman, L., Heymsfield, S.B., Teates, C.D., Gutgesell, M.E., Thorner, M.O., Hartman, M.I., and Weltman, A. 1999. Validity of methods of body composition assessment in young and older men and women. *Journal of Applied Physiology* 86 (5): 1728-1738.

Curtin, F., Morabia, A., Pichard, C., and Slosman, D.O. 1997. Body mass index compared to dual energy X-ray absorptiometry: Evidence for a spectrum bias. *Journal of Clinical Epidemiology* 50 (7): 837-843.

Dempster P., and Aikens, S. 1995. A new air displacement method for the determination of human body composition. *Medicine and Science in Sports and Exercise* 27 (12): 1692-1697.

Deurenberg, P. 1996. Limitations of the bioelectrical impedance method for the assessment of body fat in severe obesity. *American Journal of Clinical Nutrition* 64 (3 suppl.): 449S-452S.

Deurenberg, P., Westrate, J.A., and Seidell, J.C. 1991. Body mass index as a measure of body fatness: Age- and sex-specific prediction formulas. *British Journal of Nutrition* 65 (2): 105-114.

Durnin, J.V.G.A., and Womersley, J. 1974. Body fat assessed from total body density and its estimation from skinfold thickness: Measurements on 481 men and women aged from 16 to 72 years. *British Journal of Nutrition* 32 (1): 77-97.

Evans, E.M., Saunders, M.J., Spano, M.A., Arngrimsson, A.A., Lewis, R.D., and Cureton, K.J. 1999. Body-composition changes with diet and exercise in obese women: A comparison of estimates from clinical methods and a four-component model. *American Journal of Clinical Nutrition* 70 (1): 5-12.

Fogelholm, M.G., Sievanen, H.T., van Marken Lichtenbelt, W.D., and Westerterp, K.R. 1997. Assessment of fat-mass loss during weight reduction in obese women. *Metabolism* 46 (8): 968-975.

Friedl, K.E., DeLuca, J.P., Marchitelli, L.J., and Vogel, J.A. 1992. Reliability of body-fat estimations from a four-component model by using density, body water, and bone mineral measurements. *American Journal of Clinical Nutrition* 55 (4): 764-770.

Fuller, N.J., Sawyer, M.B., and Elia, M. 1994. Comparative evaluation of body composition methods and predictions, and calculation of density and hydration fraction of fat-free mass, in obese women. *International Journal of Obesity Related Metabolic Disorders* 18 (7): 503-512.

Going, S.B., and Davis, RL. 1998. Body composition assessment. In *American college of sports medicine resource manual for guidelines for exercise testing and prescription*, 3rd ed., 378-386. Baltimore: Williams & Wilkins.

Gray, D.S., Bray, G.A., Bauer, M., Kaplan, K., Gemayel, N., Wood, R., Greenway, F., and Kirk, S. 1990. Skinfold thickness measurements in obese subjects. *American Journal of Clinical Nutrition* 51 (4): 571-577.

Gray, D.S., Bray, G.A., Gemayel, N., and Kaplan, K. 1989. Effect of obesity on bioelectrical impedance. *American Journal of Clinical Nutrition* 50 (2): 255-260.

Heymsfield, S.B., Wang, Z.M., and Withers, R.T. 1996. Multicomponent molecular level models of body composition. In *Human body composition*, eds. A.F. Roche, S.B. Heymsfield, and T.G. Lohman, 129-147A. Champaign, IL: Human Kinetics.

Heyward, V.H., Cook, K.L., Hicks, V.L., Jenkins, K.A., Quatrochi, J.A., and Wilson, W.L. 1992. Predictive accuracy of three field methods for estimating relative body fatness of non-obese and obese women. *International Journal of Sports Nutrition* 2: 75-86.

Houtkooper, L., Lohman, T., Going, S., and Sproul, J. 2000. Comparisons of models for assessing body composition changes over 1 year in postmenopausal women. *American Society for Clinical Nutrition* 72: 401-406.

Jackson, A.S., and Pollock, M.L. 1978. Generalized equations for predicting body density of men. *British Journal of Nutrition* 49: 497-504.

Jackson, A.S., and Pollock, M.L. 1985. Practical assessment of body composition. *The Physician and Sports Medicine* 13: 76-84.

Jackson, A.S., Pollock, M.L. and Ward, A. 1980. Generalized equations for predicting body density of women. *Medicine and Science in Sports and Exercise* 12 (3): 175-181.

Jakicic, J.M., Wing, R.R., and Lang, W. 1998. Bioelectrical impedance analysis to assess body composition in obese adult women: The effect of ethnicity. *International Journal of Obesity Related Metabolic Disorders* 22 (3): 243-249.

Katch, F.I., and McArdle, W.D. 1973. Prediction of body density from simple anthropometric measurements in college-age men and women. *Human Biology* 45 (3): 445-455.

Kohrt, W. 1995. Body composition by DEXA: Tried and true? *Medicine and Science in Sports and Exercise* 27: 1349-1353.

Kohrt, W. 1998. Preliminary evidence that DEXA provides an accurate assessment of body composition. *Journal of Applied Physiology* 84: 372-377.

Kushner, R.F., Kunigk, A., Alspaugh, M., Andronis, P.T., Leitch, C.A., and Schoeller, D.A. 1990. Validation of bioelectrical impedance analysis as a measurement of change in body composition in obesity. *American Journal of Clinical Nutrition* 52 (2): 219-223.

Kushner, R.F., and Schoeller, D.A. 1986. Estimation of total body water by bioelectrical impedance analysis. *American Journal of Clinical Nutrition* 44 (3): 417-424.

Lohman, T.G. 1981. Skinfolds and body density and their relationship to body fatness: A review. *Human Biology* 53: 181-225.

Lohman, T.G. 1986. Applicability of body composition techniques and constants for children and youth. In *Exercise and sport sciences review,* ed. K.B. Pandolf, 325-357. New York: MacMillan.

Lohman, T.G. 1992. Body density, body water, and bone mineral: Controversies and limitations of the two-component systems. In *Advances in body composition assessment,* 3-4, 15. Champaign, IL: Human Kinetics.

Lohman, T.G. 1996. Dual energy X-ray absorptiometry. In *Human body composition,* eds. A.F. Roche, S.B. Heymsfield and T.G. Lohman, 63-78. Champaign, IL: Human Kinetics.

Lohman, T.G., Harris, M., Teixeira, P.J., and Weiss, L. DXA. 2000. Assessing body composition and body composition changes—Another look. *Annals of the New York Academy of Sciences* 904: 45-54.

Milliken, L.A., Going, S.B., and Lohman, T.G. 1996. Effects of variations in regional composition on soft-tissue measurements by dual-energy X-ray absorptiometry. *International Journal of Obesity Related Metabolic Disorders* 20 (7): 677-682.

Pietrobelli, A., Formica, C., Wang, Z.M. and Heymsfield, S.B. 1996. Dual-energy X-ray absorptiometry body composition model: Review of physical concepts. *American Journal of Physiology* 271 (6 Pt 1): E941-E951.

Prior, B.M., Cureton, K.J., Modlesky, C.M., Evans, E.M. et al. 1997. In vivo validation of whole body composition estimates from dual-energy X-ray absorptiometry. *Journal of Applied Physiology* 83 (2): 623-630.

Ross, R., Leger, L., Martin, P., and Roy, R. 1989. Sensitivity of bioelectrical impedance to detect changes in human body composition. *Journal of Applied Physiology* 67 (4): 1643-1648.

Salamone, L.M., Fuerst, T., Visser, M., Kem, M., Lang, T., Cauley, J.A., Nevitt, M., Tylavsky, F., and Lohman, T.G. 2000. Measurement of fat mass and leg fat mass using fan beam dual-energy x-ray absorptiometry: A validation study in elderly adults. *Journal of Applied Physiology* 89: 345-352.

Sardinha, L.B., Lohman, T.G., Teixeira, P.J., Guedes, D.P., and Going, S.B. 1998. Comparison of air displacement plethysmography with dual-energy X-ray absorptiometry and three field methods for estimating body composition in middle-aged men. *American Journal of Clinical Nutrition* 68 (4): 786-793.

Schoeller, D.A. 1996. Hydrometry. In *Human body composition,* eds. A.F. Roche, S.B. Heymsfield, and T.G. Lohman, 25-44. Champaign, IL: Human Kinetics.

Segal, K.R., Van Loan, M., Fitzgerald, P.I., Hodgdon, J.A., and Van Itallie, T.B. 1988. Lean body mass estimation by bioelectrical impedance analysis: A four-site cross-validation study. *American Journal of Clinical Nutrition* 47 (1): 7-14.

Siri, W.E. 1961. Body composition from fluid spaces and density. In *Techniques for measuring body composition,* eds. J. Broznek and A. Henschel, 223-244. Washington, DC: National Academy of Sciences.

Smalley, K.J., Knerr, A.N., Kendrick, Z.V., Colliver, J.A., and Owen, O.E. 1990. Reassessment of body mass indices. *American Journal of Clinical Nutrition* 52 (3): 405-408.

Snead, D.B., Birg, S.J. and Kohrt, W.M. 1993. Age-related differences in body composition by hydrodensitometry and dual energy X-ray absorptiometry. *Journal of Applied Physiology* 74 (2): 770-775.

Stolarczyk, L.M., Heyward, V.H., Van Loan, M.D., Hicks, V.L., Wilson, W.L., and Reano, L.M. 1997. The fatness-specific bioelectrical impedance analysis equations of Segal et al: Are they generalizable and practical? *American Journal of Clinical Nutrition* 66 (1): 8-17.

Tataranni, P.A., and Ravussin, E. 1995. Use of dual-energy x-ray absorptiometry in obese individuals. *American Journal of Clinical Nutrition* 62 (4): 730-734.

Tran, Z.V., and Weltman, A. 1989. Generalized equation for predicting body density of women from girth measurements. *Medicine and Science in Sports and Exercise* 21 (1): 101-104.

Tylavsky, F.A., Fuerst, T. et al. 2000. Measurement of changes in soft tissue mass and fat mass with weight change: Pencil- versus fan-beam dual-energy X-ray absorptiometry. Health ABC Study. *Ann N Y Acad Sci* 904: 94-97.

van der Kooy, K., Leenan, R., Deurenberg, P., Seidell, J.C., Westerterp, K.R., and Hautvast, J.G. 1992. Changes in fat-free mass in obese subjects after weight loss: A comparison of body composition measures. *International Journal of Obesity Related Metabolic Disorders* 16 (9): 675-683.

Van Loan, M.D., Johnson, H.L., and Barbieri, T.F. 1998. Effect of weight loss on bone mineral content and bone mineral density in obese women. *American Journal of Clinical Nutrition* 67 (4): 734-738.

Visser, M., Fuerst, T. et al. 1999. Validity of fan-beam dual-energy X-ray absorptiometry for measuring fat-free mass and leg muscle mass. Health, Aging, and Body Composition Study--Dual-Energy X-ray Absorptiometry and Body Composition Working Group. *Journal of Applied Physiology* 87 (4): 1513-1520.

Visser, M., Gallagher, D., Deurenberg, P., Wang, J., Pierson, R.N., Jr., and Heymsfield, S. 1997. Density of fat-free body mass: Relationship with race, age, and level of body fatness. *American Journal of Physiology* 272 (5 Pt 1): E781-E787.

Wang, Z., Deurenberg, P., Wang, W., Pietrobelli, A., Baumgartner, R.N., and Heymsfield, S.B. 1999. Hydration of fat-free body mass: Review and critique of a classic body-composition constant. *American Journal of Clinical Nutrition* 69 (5): 833-841.

Womersley, J., and Durnin, J.V.G.A. 1977. A comparison of the skinfold method with extent of "overweight" and various weight-height relationships in the assessment of obesity. *British Journal of Nutrition* 38 (2): 271-284.

Womersley, J., Durnin, J.V.G.A., Boddy, K., and Mahaffy, M. 1976. Influence of muscular development, obesity, and age on the fat-free mass of adults. *Journal of Applied Physiology* 41 (2): 223-229.

Chapter 7

Clinical Evaluation of the Obese Patient

Samuel C. Durso, MD
Johns Hopkins School of Medicine

Obesity, or excess total body fat, is extraordinarily common in highly industrialized societies and is increasing in both incidence and prevalence (Gortmaker et al. 1987; Kuczmarsk et al. 1994; Morbidity and Mortality Weekly Report 1994). Physicians are regularly called on to evaluate and treat obese patients. Although some of these patients will seek medical treatment primarily for their obesity, most will be seen for disease indirectly associated with or possibly incidental to their obesity. This means that all physicians, regardless of specialty, must develop expertise in the clinical examination of obese persons. This expertise includes quantifying and characterizing excess body fat for the purpose of assessing its contribution to health risks, developing proficiency in performing the physical exam of obese persons, and recognizing alterations in the physiological state created by the burden of excess weight.

The examination of the obese patient presents four distinct challenges for the clinician. First, obesity often interferes with the physical assessment. Increased size and limited mobility create a barrier to performance of the physical exam. For instance, blood pressure may be overestimated and recorded as spuriously elevated if measured with a cuff that is too small relative to the patient's arm. In addition, increased chest wall and abdominal fat may impair effective auscultation and palpation of these anatomical areas.

The second challenge facing the clinician is to be aware of the fact that obese patients are at increased risk for a host of diseases, many of which will not be recognized prior to the clinical evaluation. Many conditions affecting the patient are clinically silent and require appropriate screening for early detection. Early stages of diabetes and hyperlipidemia are two examples. The third challenge for the clinician is to recognize genetic syndromes and endocrine disease that may be causing obesity. Such conditions, although uncommon (e.g., Prader-Willi and Cushing's disease), must be recognized in order to implement effective therapy. Fourth, physicians must keep in mind that primary eating disorders, such as bulimia, are increasingly present in obese patients. These conditions can affect successful weight management and produce adverse health consequences in their own right.

Clinical Exam

The clinical exam of obese patients includes the usual elements of the history and physical as well as recognition of comorbid conditions and diseases more prevalent in overweight patients. Special skill in the interview and physical examination and a few accommodations in the examining room are all that are necessary to accomplish this goal.

Approach to the Patient

Physicians should strive to establish an open and nonjudgmental relationship with all patients, particularly obese patients. Obese persons often encounter social prejudice and ridicule, perhaps not surprising in a culture that values thinness (Foster and Wadden 1994). From youth through adulthood, the obese person is more likely to be judged as stupid, lazy, dishonest, and unattractive (Harris, Harris, and Bochner 1982; Staffieri 1967). Unfortunately, caregivers are not immune from applying these stigmata to overweight patients. Physicians are more likely to assign negative attributes to obese patients than to those of normal weight, seeing the obese as weak-willed, ugly, and awkward (Maddox and Liederman 1969). Needless to say, judgments such as these will interfere with a healthy doctor–patient relationship.

Furthermore, it is important for the physician to inquire about and focus appropriately on the patient's concerns. While neglecting to discuss obesity-related health questions is a breach of professional responsibility, focusing prematurely on a person's obesity when that person has come with a different concern is insensitive. For instance, the obese patient, perhaps frustrated by years of unsuccessful attempts to lose weight, will not be comforted during a visit seeking relief from acute foot pain to hear a long discussion about the association between obesity and gout. Although an association exists between gout and obesity, obese patients with pain, like all patients, will want pain relief first, after which they may be receptive to discussing long-range health goals. Obesity treatment, as with other complex behavioral endeavors, requires that the physician establish trust and rapport—something to be developed over time.

Outfitting the Exam Room

Given the prevalence of obesity, all physicians' offices should be well outfitted with equipment that permits an optimal examination of overweight patients. Offices should be equipped with scales for measuring weight and height. Examining rooms should be designed to accommodate large patients. Ideally, each room should have an ophthalmoscope, large blood pressure cuff, a dressmaker's tape measure for measuring waist circumference, a 128-Hz tuning fork or #10 monofilament for diabetic sensory screening, and an adequate range of vaginal specula for gynecologic exams. A heavy Queen's Square reflex hammer, consisting of a rubber tire on the end of a stick, often works better than the typically light "tomahawk" reflex hammers.

A body mass index (BMI) chart in each examining room facilitates recording the BMI and enhances patients' appreciation of the association between obesity and increased health risks. (The American College of Physicians produces an attractive, laminated BMI chart that can be displayed [800-523-1546 ext. 2600].) A low examining table or ideally an electric lift table in at least one examining room is a great assistance to severely obese patients. Sturdy wall-mounted grab bars next to an examination table are useful for patients with hampered mobility including the very obese. Large gowns are available and should be provided as well.

The Clinical History

The patient's experience with obesity provides important therapeutic and prognostic information. Information regarding the age of onset of obesity, the family history, and past medical history creates a context for assessing the health risks. A history of dieting and current nutritional intake can simultaneously reveal information about the patient's food knowledge, emotional responses to eating and dieting, as well as the reasons for past failures with dieting. This information helps the clinician plan weight loss strategies and set reasonable weight reduction goals. The clinical history, too, will alert the physician to higher-than-usual risks for genetic, medical, and psychological disorders that may complicate obesity treatment or worsen its adverse health consequences.

Age of Onset and Family History

A combination of genetic and environmental factors influences a person's tendency to become obese (Hewitt 1997; Teasdale, Sorensen, and Stunkard 1990). Studies of monozygotic twins reared apart indicate that the genetic influence promoting obesity is quite strong, perhaps accounting for about 50% of body weight variation. However, lifestyle and behavior probably account for the sharp upward increase in obesity witnessed in recent decades (Rosser 1987).

The age at which obesity begins is prognostically important. Childhood obesity constitutes a silent epidemic with immediate and long-term health risks (Diamond 1998; Morbidity and Mortality Weekly Report 1998). Obese children are more likely to become obese adults (Kotani et al. 1997; Whitaker et al. 1997) and carry increased risk for diabetes mellitus, coronary artery disease, and orthopedic and respiratory disease into adulthood (Dietz 1998; Srinivasan and Berenson 1995; Webber et al. 1995).

Because childhood obesity characteristically results in a hyperplastic fat mass, adults who became obese as children often fail to attain ideal body weight since successful dieting does not result in a reduced number of fat cells. These same adults tend to regain weight more quickly when no longer dieting (Wadden and Foster 1992).

Most obese adults, however, become so during adulthood, and both men and women tend to gain weight as they age (Dwyer 1994). Mild adult-onset obesity is characterized by a hypertrophic fat mass. People who become moderate to severely obese, corresponding to 40% or more overweight, develop a combined hypertrophic and hyperplastic fat cell mass. Therefore, adults below 40% overweight have more success achieving normal weight, as dieting results in reduced fat cell size, but not fat cell number (Wadden and Foster 1992).

Patients are usually aware of an association between reaching certain milestones in life and weight gain. Often this is linked to changes in lifestyle as well as physiological events. Pregnancy and menopause are important influences for women. Many adult men and women note increasing weight coinciding with the completion of education and settling into a career or marriage—all corresponding to a more sedentary lifestyle.

Stopping smoking is another event associated with an average weight gain of approximately 10 lb (4.5 kg), although some is gradually lost during the following one to five years (Froom, Melamed, and Benbassat 1998; Klesges et al. 1998; O'Hara et al. 1998).

Eating History

A careful diet history is important in assessing current eating habits and past experience with dieting. Knowing the patient's eating pattern,

food preferences, and physical activity are essential to understanding the factors sustaining obesity. Furthermore, cultural food preferences and the time and location of meals in relation to the patient's daily schedule will provide important information that must be incorporated into a therapeutic plan. Clinicians quickly learn that a diet failing to take this information into account will not achieve long-term success. Interviews with dieticians, structured recall, and prospective food diaries are often illuminating. Reviewing these records with the patient during the initial and subsequent examinations creates an opportunity for patient education, sensitizes the patient to his or her food intake, and builds rapport.

Methods for evaluating a patient's dietary habits include a 24-hour dietary recall, dietary history, and a prospective three-day food record. Information from these three sources provides an estimate of the patient's daily caloric intake and food preferences, as well as meal composition, nutritional adequacy, eating times, and eating settings (McNulty 1992).

Reviewing food records aids in determining the degree to which the patient's obesity is sustained by excess calories and fat. While food records do not help establish precise caloric balance due to patients' tendencies to underestimate food intake, small daily variances in an overall positive calorie balance and periodic overeating uncover much qualitative information (Dwyer 1994). Patients who report a relatively low caloric intake may have low energy requirements that can be confirmed by measuring their resting metabolic rate (Feurer and Mullen 1986). Patients with low metabolic rates benefit more from increased physical activity than from further calorie restriction (McNulty 1992).

Reviewing food records can help the clinician understand and correct commonly held misunderstandings the patient may have about the caloric value of various food types. For example, some patients mistakenly consume or feed their children foods such as granola bars, fruit juice, and dried fruits and nuts, assuming that these are inherently healthy. Patterns of excessive intake of high-caloric fatty foods, desserts, and alcoholic beverages may emerge. Reviewing the times and location of eating can be instructive as well. Common patterns include large meals eaten on weekends with family or in social settings, high caloric meals of convenience foods eaten during lunch breaks, or excessive snacking when alone or during the evenings. Eating in response to stress or depression and binge eating may become apparent from inspecting a food record; such revelations offer an opportunity to tactfully ask the patient about these behaviors, which many patients will affirm.

The physician should become acquainted with the energy expenditure of the common household chores and recreational activities listed in table 7.1. This information can be used to reinforce goals for incorporating regular exercise to help sustain a healthy

Table 7.1   *Caloric Expenditure for Common Recreational and Occupational Tasks*

Category	Self-care or home	Occupational	Recreational	Physical conditioning
Very light <4 kcal/min	Washing, shaving, dressing, desk work, writing, washing dishes, driving auto	Sitting (clerical, assembly), standing (clerk, bartender), driving truck, operating crane	Shuffleboard, horseshoes, bait casting, billiards, archery, golf (cart)	Walking (2 mph), stationary bicycle (very low resistance), very light calisthenics
Light 4-6 kcal/min	Cleaning windows, raking leaves, weeding, power lawn mowing, waxing floors (slowly), carrying objects (15-30 lb or 7-14 kg)	Stocking shelves (light objects), light welding, light carpentry, machine assembly, auto repair, paper hanging	Dancing (social and square), golf (walking), sailing, horseback riding, volleyball (6 man), tennis (doubles)	Walking (3-4 mph), level bicycling (6-8 mph), light calisthenics
Moderate 6-8 kcal/min	Easy digging in garden, level lawn mowing, climbing stairs (slowly), carrying objects (30-60 lb or 14-27 kg)	Carpentry (exterior home building), shoveling dirt, using pneumatic tools	Badminton (competitive), tennis (singles), snow skiing (downhill), light backpacking, basketball, skating (ice or roller), horseback riding (racing)	Walking (4.5-5 mph), bicycling (9-10 mph), swimming (breast stroke)
Heavy 8-10 kcal/min	Sawing wood, heavy shoveling, climbing stairs (moderate speed), carrying objects (60-90 lb or 27-40 kg)	Tending furnace, digging ditches, pick and shovel	Canoeing, mountain climbing, fencing, paddleball, touch football	Jogging (5 mph), swimming (crawl), rowing machine, heavy calisthenics, bicycling (12 mph)
Very heavy >10 kcal/min	Carrying loads upstairs, carrying objects (<90 lb or 40 kg), climbing stairs (quickly), shoveling heavy snow, shoveling 10 min (16 lb or 7 kg)	Lumberjack, heavy labor	Handball, squash, ski touring over hills, vigorous basketball	Running (≥6 mph), bicycle (≥13 mph or up steep hills), rope jumping

Reprinted from *Heart disease: A textbook of cardiovascular medicine*, 4th edition, E. Braunwald, Copyright 1999, with permission from Elsevier Science.

weight. Likewise, the physician should have a working knowledge of the caloric, nutrient, and fiber content of food both for assessing the patient's diet and for reinforcing patient education.

It is often necessary to tie information about smoking cessation with dietary therapy. Because cessation often results in weight gain, obese patients who smoke may question the benefits of stopping in the face of this predictable outcome. The physician must reassure the patient that the benefits of not smoking outweigh the risks of weight gain and be prepared to help the patient meet this challenge.

Details about the patient's previous experiences with self-guided diets, professional weight loss programs, or participation in groups such as Overeaters Anonymous helps the physician plan for a successful experience for future weight loss.

Eating Patterns

Most obese persons do not appear to eat differently from nonobese persons. There is no evidence that the speed of eating, bite size, or time chewing contributes significantly to obesity. It is clear, however, that a subgroup of obese persons binge eat (O'Neil and Jarrell 1992). Binge eating, a distinctive pattern of overeating during a discrete period of time followed by intense guilt, affects as many as 30% of obese persons seeking treatment for obesity (Wadden 1995). While obese patients who do not binge eat have psychological profiles similar to nonobese persons, as many as 50% of obese patients who binge eat suffer with depression and other psychological disorders. These conditions are likely to interfere with weight loss management and need specific treatment in their own right.

Purging through self-induced vomiting, laxative abuse, and diuretic abuse is less common in overweight binge eaters compared to those of average weight. Nevertheless, one should consider this possibility as it constitutes an inherent medical danger and a contraindication to a very low calorie diet (Wadden and Bartlett 1992).

A cyclical history of weight loss and gain, so called "yo-yo" dieting, has been suggested to adversely affect body composition, metabolism, or weight loss, although this has not been clearly substantiated (Atkinson 1992). Nevertheless, such cycling can have an understandably negative impact on the obese person's self-esteem. Multiple attempts to achieve normal weight followed by weight regain can make a person feel defeated and humiliated. The problem for some may be that they tend to seek short-term and unrealistically low weights and thus set themselves up for failure. The clinician should take this reaction into consideration and help the patient to set realistic weight loss goals.

Review of Systems

A thorough review of systems is a necessary part of a traditional interview for all new patients. Examples of questions included in the review of systems can be found in standard textbooks of physical diagnosis. Because mild obesity, particularly if it occurs in a gynecoid or lower body distribution, does not appear to carry an increased risk for morbidity or mortality, physicians can pursue a review of systems used for average-risk patients. Moderate to severe obesity, however, is associated with a number of health risks, which are listed in table 7.2. For these patients, physicians should focus the review of systems on these conditions.

The high prevalence and severe consequence of cardiovascular and pulmonary disease in moderate to severely obese patients necessitates that the clinician focus on antecedent conditions such as hypertension, hyperlipidemia, diabetes mellitus, left ventricular hypertrophy, pulmonary embolism, and sleep apnea. When untreated, these conditions can lead to congestive heart failure, angina, myocardial infarction, stroke, respiratory failure, and sudden death.

The presence of hypertension alone, certainly when mild, does not produce symptoms. Some patients will experience headache, dizziness, and blurry vision with severe hypertension. A past history of elevated blood pressure may indicate long-standing hypertension with a greater risk of congestive heart failure and atherosclerosis.

Angina, transient ischemic attacks, and claudication of the extremities typically indicate advanced atherosclerotic vascular disease.

Physicians should ask patients about a previous history of pancreatitis or recurrent attacks of severe epigastric pain that may be a clue to severe hypertriglyceridemia, although causes such as alcohol abuse and cholelithiasis may be more common.

Polydipsia, polyphagia, polyuria, sudden unexplained weight loss, dizziness, stocking-glove sensory loss, and vaginal or skin infection are frequent presenting symptoms of

Table 7.2   *Medical Risks Associated With Obesity*

Endocrine—metabolic

Hyperglycemia, hyperinsulinemia, insulin resistance

Hypertriglyceridemia, hypercholesterolemia, ($\uparrow$ VLDL, $\uparrow$ LDL, $\downarrow$ HDL)

$\uparrow$ Cortisol production but normal plasma cortisol, diurnal rhythm urine-free cortisol, and overnight dexamethasone suppression test

Early menarche, menstrual abnormalities, hirsutism

$\downarrow$ Sympathoadrenal activity

$\downarrow$ SHBG and $\uparrow$ total or free androgens

$\downarrow$ Growth hormone, basally and after provocative stimuli

Hyperuricemia, gout

Cardiovascular

Hypertension

Coronary artery disease

Congestive heart failure

Varicose veins

Cerebrovascular disease

Pulmonary

Hypoventilation (e.g., Pickwickian) syndromes

Sleep apnea syndrome

Chronic respiratory infections

Gallbladder

Cholelithiasis (cholesterol) stones

Musculoskeletal

Osteoarthritis

Chronic orthopedic problems

$\downarrow$ Ambulation

Renal

Nephrotic syndrome (normal or nonspecific biopsy)

Oncology

Endometrial, breast carcinoma (postmenopausal women), prostate, colon

Dermatologic

Acanthosis nigricans

Chronic skin infections

Psychosocial

Depression, loss of self-esteem

$\downarrow$ Employability

Pregnancy

Worsen underlying hypertension, diabetes mellitus

$\uparrow$ Maternal mortality

Surgery (especially under general anesthesia)

Increased perioperative morbidity and mortality

Adapted, by permission, from M.R. Blackman, 1999, Obesity. In *Principles of ambulatory medicine*, 5th ed. (Baltimore: Lippincott, Williams, and Wilkins).

diabetes mellitus. Those with milder diabetes may be asymptomatic, and so their condition may only be discovered with screening.

Exertional dyspnea, orthopnea, and edema may indicate congestive heart failure. However, these symptoms are not specific. Poor physical conditioning and varicose veins, both of which are common in obese persons, may produce exertional dyspnea and dependent edema in the absence of heart failure.

The clinician should ask about unilateral lower extremity swelling. This sign may indicate lower extremity venous insufficiency that often begins more prominently in one leg before affecting both. However, acute unilateral lower extremity swelling with or without pain may be due to venous thrombosis or thrombophlebitis. Because the obese are at increased risk of pulmonary emboli, attacks of chest pain and dyspnea, sometimes accompanied by wheezing, should suggest the possibility of pulmonary emboli.

Excessive daytime drowsiness and prominent snoring are common presenting symptoms of obstructive sleep apnea. The clinician should ask the patient if he or she experiences inadequate rest after sleep or daytime sleepiness. The patient should also ask his or her partner if the patient exhibits nocturnal apnea or restless thrashing during sleep.

Less dangerous but important conditions affecting obese patients are heartburn; biliary colic; intertrigenous skin infections; hydradinitis suppurativa; acanthosis nigricans, fallen arches, heel spurs, or gout producing painful feet and ankles; and knee, hip, and back pain secondary to osteoarthritis, ligamentous strain, and herniated intervertebral discs.

Obese men and women who are more than 40% overweight are at increased risk for cancer mortality (Lew and Garfinkel 1979). Excess cancer mortality in men is attributable primarily to cancer of the colon and rectum. Severely obese women have increased mortality from cancer of the breast, cervix, endometrium, ovaries, gallbladder, and biliary passages. Symptoms or change in function of these organ systems should be considered and appropriately evaluated. Increased risk of colorectal, breast, and cervical cancer for which effective screening has been shown to reduce mortality should be taken into consideration when making age-appropriate screening recommendations.

The clinical history should include questions screening for depression and physical and emotional abuse. Even when depression is not clinically overt, symptoms of low self-esteem or self-image may have an important impact on subsequent medical therapy. Obese children and adolescents are more likely than their normal weight peers to have low self-esteem (Braet, Mervielde, and Vandereycken 1997; Pierce and Wardle 1997).

Medications

The clinician should record a detailed accounting of all medications, both prescription and over-the-counter. Medications of both types can be abused in the quest for weight loss. Prescription drugs such as diuretics are sometimes taken from family or friends, with or without their knowledge, to achieve these purposes. Laxatives are used by some for short- and long-term weight loss. Herbal products are often considered innocuous and may not be reported along with medications unless the clinician asks about these specifically. All of these drugs can have profound metabolic and physical consequences, including electrolyte imbalance, hypotension, bowel dysfunction, and cardiac arrhythmia.

All medications should be continuously reviewed during weight loss. Some medications, such as antihypertensives, may need to have the dose adjusted downward as the patient loses weight.

Medications may be responsible for iatrogenic obesity. These include insulin, corticosteroids, tricyclic antidepressants, phenothiazines, oral contraceptives, mood stabilizers (e.g., lithium), anticonvulsants (e.g., valproic acid), and cyproheptadine. When available, an alternative medication less prone to stimulate weight gain should be substituted.

Physical Exam

Clinicians must become proficient in using standard techniques for measuring body fat and assessing the health risks that result from obesity. Furthermore, increased fat mass affects the interpretation of many aspects of the physical exam. Finally, clinicians examining obese patients should be alert for signs of disease and syndromes associated with obesity.

General

The physical examination of the obese patient is fundamentally the same as that of nonobese patients. Increased subcutaneous and visceral fat, however, often interferes with palpation, percussion, and auscultation of the underlying structures. In many instances clinicians can overcome these limitations by using ingenuity and taking an extra measure of care. Extreme obesity can also limit the patient's mobility, making positioning and examination of the trunk and extremities challenging. Too often, though, clinicians abort a difficult exam before attempting to overcome these limitations. When obesity precludes an adequate examination, the physician should note this.

Imaging methods such as X ray, CAT scans, echocardiogram, and abdominal ultrasound can be judiciously used to overcome the limitations of a physical exam. However, the quality of these studies can be impaired by excess fat as well. In some cases the patient's physical size itself will preclude access to machines such as the closed MRI.

An important aspect of the physical exam is accomplished when the physician first greets the patient. Dress, demeanor, stature, and gait are but a few features that should be readily apparent. Obesity itself will be self-evident, and the physician should note whether its distribution is primarily android or gynecoid, the former being associated with higher cardiovascular risks. In addition, certain endocrine and genetic syndromes will suggest themselves because of the characteristic appearance of the face or other features.

Weight, height, waist circumference, and blood pressure measurements are essential elements of the patient's risk assessment.

Obtaining an accurate blood pressure is crucial to assessing the obese patient's risk for cardiovascular disease. The blood pressure should be measured when the patient is comfortably seated with the arm supported so that the blood pressure cuff is at heart level. The cuff width should be two-thirds of the distance from the axilla to the antecubital space, and the cuff bladder should encircle at least 80% of the arm (Petrie et al. 1986). The standard 23-cm or larger 35-cm cuffs will be too small for most obese patients, who will require a 42-cm cuff. Another common obstacle to obtaining an accurate blood pressure measurement is failure to remove constricting garments from around the patient's upper arm. Also, many obese patients have conical-shaped upper arms that interfere with good cuff placement. In the latter case the blood pressure can sometimes be measured by placing the cuff around the forearm and listening over the radial artery. If this technique is not satisfactory, digitally obtained blood pressures may be an alternative (Kaplan 1994).

The BMI and the waist-to-hip ratio (WHR) are the easiest and most reliable methods of estimating body fat in the office. The BMI is strongly correlated with total body fat, although it may overestimate fat content in very muscular individuals. The WHR contributes additional risk stratification when the BMI is between 25 and 34.9. If the BMI appears to be excessively high (e.g., a very muscular athlete may have a BMI of 32), a normal WHR will indicate that total body fat is probably normal.

The BMI is calculated by dividing the weight in pounds by the height in inches squared or correspondingly using the weight measured in kilograms and the height in meters squared. Nomograms or tables are more convenient and have the added benefit of presenting a figure relative to normal values that will demonstrate to the patient the increased risks secondary to obesity.

The WHR is obtained by measuring the minimal circumference of the waist and dividing that by the maximal circumference of the hips while the patient is standing. A WHR of 1.0 or greater for men or 0.85 or greater for women imparts increased health risks. Patients with mild to moderate lower body obesity do not appear to be at increased risk for metabolic or cardiovascular disease as are those with upper body obesity. Morbidity and mortality risks are evident when the BMI is 30 or greater or when the WHR is elevated for a BMI below 30.

Measuring the WHR accurately and consistently can be difficult. Many favor measuring the waist circumference alone. When the BMI is below 35 kg/m^2, a waist circumference >102 cm (>40 in.) in men and >88 cm (>35 in.) in women imparts increased relative health risk as shown in chapter 1 (see table 1.1).

Eyes

Examination of the ocular fundi should be performed routinely in the evaluation of obese patients. This may reveal arteriosclerotic narrowing and arteriolar-venous nicking, hypertensive or diabetic hemorrhages, or occasionally cholesterol emboli (Hollenhorst plaques) indicative of carotid atherosclerosis. Papilledema, indicative of increased intracranial pressure, may point to a mass of the hypothalamus or pituitary gland, or pseudotumor cerebri. Visual fields should be tested by direct confrontation. Finding bilateral homonymous hemianopsia suggests the presence of a pituitary tumor compressing the optic chiasm, although other scotoma or ocular palsies may result from tumors in or around the hypothalamic and pituitary area.

Oropharynx

When examining the oropharynx, the physician should note the condition of the patient's enamel. Chronic gastric acidic reflux may cause noticeable erosion of the tooth's surface—a condition that may result from gastroesophageal reflux or self-induced vomiting.

Craniofacial abnormalities, including abnormal oral development, are seen with Prader-Willi, Cohen, and Carpenter syndromes (Bray 1995).

A small posterior pharyngeal space produced by hypertrophic tonsils and fat may increase the patient's risk for developing obstructive sleep apnea.

Neck

Neck structures are commonly hidden by subcutaneous fat. This obscures landmarks such as the belly of the sternocleidomastoid muscle and suprasternal notch. The thyroid gland, carotid arteries, and internal and external jugular veins are all more difficult to examine. A large or asymmetrical thyroid gland may be more easily appreciated if inspection is performed while the neck is gently extended under tangentially directed light. Palpation is easier if the patient is given water to swallow while the clinician carefully feels the gland between and behind the sternocleidomastoid muscles.

The carotid arteries can usually be palpated without difficulty. Likewise, bruits are usually audible, but may be reduced in intensity. Their presence may indicate local carotid artery atherosclerosis, and is associated with a high risk of coronary atherosclerosis.

Visualizing the internal jugular venous waves or the level of internal or external jugular venous distention in an obese person is not always possible. Too often, however, a failure to observe the jugular venous pulsation is attributable to improper technique. Viewing the neck under tangentially directed light while the neck is gently extended allows adequate visualization more often than not.

Chest

Increased fat over the chest wall, reduced respiratory excursion, and general immobility often limit accurate assessment of the intrathoracic structures. Lung and heart sounds are often diminished in intensity. This can be partially overcome by using a good stethoscope in a quiet room. Palpation and percussion of the chest and heart of severely obese patients is often difficult. Asking the patient to stand for auscultation and percussion of the chest reduces fat folds and lowers the diaphragm, making this part of the exam easier.

Auscultation of the first and second heart sounds may be more difficult in the severely obese than in the nonobese patient, but this is highly variable. Most often the heart sounds are best heard with the patient supine. When this is not satisfactory, one can turn the patient to the left to better palpate and auscultate the heart at the cardiac apex. Occasionally asking the patient to stand and lean forward brings the heart closer to the anterior chest wall and may aid auscultation, particularly over the figurative "sash" from the right upper sternal border to the cardiac apex. The left lateral position and leaning forward are also recommended for optimally hearing mitral and aortic murmurs, respectively.

Special attention to the cardiac rhythm may reveal ectopy, a finding that is more frequent in the severely obese with hypertrophic hearts or patients with electrolyte imbalance. Auscultation over the left second interspace may reveal an increased intensity of the pulmonic component of the second heart sound that is indicative of pulmonary hypertension. A left-sided third heart sound (S3), although normal in some children, is abnormal in adults over the age of 40, while a left-sided fourth heart sound (S4) is almost invariably abnormal (the exception being trained athletes and the elderly). The S3 typically indicates decreased myocardial contractility, myocardial failure, and volume overload, and the S4 corresponds to decreased left ventricular compliance often due to hypertension, coronary artery disease, and cardiomyopathy—conditions commonly found in obese patients (Bickley and Hoekelman 1999). Right-sided third and fourth heart sounds may signal pulmonary hypertension.

Because chest compliance is reduced in obese patients, atelectasis, producing bibasilar rales, is common. This is not usually important, except when immobility supervenes. Thus, obese patients who are immobile postoperatively or during acute illness are prone to pneumonia and hypoxia. Basilar rales detected on a routine physical exam most often clear by having the patient stand and take a deep breath (Guenter 1977).

Abdomen

The abdomen is a preferential location for subcutaneous and visceral fat deposition, especially for patients with an android body habitus. An apron of fat may hang below the inguinal ligaments. Skin underlying this apron may be macerated and inflamed. The umbilicus is typically inverted and prone to infection.

Percussion of the fatty panniculus dulls the usual abdominal tympany. This may limit the examiner's ability to appreciate a change from between dullness and tympany at the border of the liver's lower edge. The liver edge too is more difficult to palpate because of the fat abdominal wall. It is worth remembering that an enlarged liver in very obese patients, particularly those with diabetes, may be the result of fatty infiltration.

Regions of tenderness, guarding, and rebound are detected in obese patients with about the same efficiency as they are in thinner patients. However, underlying masses, whether inflammatory, vascular, neoplastic, or physiological, are frequently harder to feel.

One technique that aids palpating the obese abdomen is to press gently with two hands, one on top of the other, using the finger pads of the lower hand to feel underlying structures. By pressing a little more deeply with abdominal muscle relaxation following each exhalation, the examiner can feel successively more deeply.

Firm or irregular masses, depending on their size, are typically easier to appreciate than soft or smooth-surfaced masses. Thus, a uterine fibromyoma or a polycystic ovary may be easier to feel than a more subtle mass such as a simple ovarian cyst. Even a significantly enlarged uterus, massive ovarian cyst, or distended bladder can be missed in the very obese patient. These can be difficult to palpate because their margins are often smooth and indistinct. In addition, the presence of abdominal wall scarring or unrelaxed abdominal rectus muscles may further complicate the exam. However, if the clinician is alert and palpates carefully, he or she can usually appreciate a distinctive firmness not confused with a soft, abdominal fat pad. Percussion too will produce a dullness that cannot be accounted for by the usual anatomy. In these cases an ultrasound of the abdomen and pelvis or catheterization of the bladder will resolve the questions.

An abdominal aneurysm is more difficult to feel through an obese abdominal wall, and the abdominal wall thickness must be considered when estimating its size. If an expansile mass is suspected, abdominal ultrasound or CT scan should be performed (Lederle and Simel 1998).

The presence of abdominal ascites, even if large, may be quite difficult to determine in severely obese patients. If diagnostic paracentesis is contemplated, an abdominal ultrasound may be necessary both to detect and to localize fluid.

Pelvis, Rectum, and Genitalia

Both pelvic and rectal exams are more difficult to perform in obese patients. Large thighs and redundant tissue in the perineum make inspection of this area difficult. Often, excess tissue closes in around the speculum interfering with visualization of the vagina and cervix. Using an adequate-sized speculum and having an assistant hold redundant soft tissue apart can help. Bimanual palpation of the uterus is as difficult as most of the abdominal exam. The same technique of pressing successively deeper with each exhalation, as with the exam of the abdomen, can help. Typically, the smaller adnexal structures are not palpable in very obese patients. When they are, the physician should suspect a mass.

The rectal exam in females is usually performed as part of the pelvic exam while the patient is in the lithotomy position. It can be performed while the female patient lies on her side. The rectal exam of very obese males is made easier by having the patient bend over the examining table while supporting his trunk on the table. The patient or an assistant can then separate the patient's buttocks. This greatly assists the digital examination of the anal and rectal canals.

Android obesity should raise the possibility of testicular failure in men and Stein-Leventhal syndrome in women. Atrophic testes are smaller than 4.0 × 3.0 cm (1.6 × 1.2 in.) and are soft rather than firm. Polycystic ovaries are firm, enlarged, and irregular.

Musculoskeletal Exam

Examination of all joints, including the peripheral joints of the hands and feet, is made more difficult by increased subcutaneous fat. Peripheral features of osteoarthritis or classic gout in the first metacarpophalangeal joint are recognizable in the presence of obesity. However, palpation of the ankle, knee, shoulder, hip, and back structures, difficult under normal circumstances, is much more so in the severely obese. Even when one has difficulty appreciating the presence of a joint effusion because of overlying fat, warmth to the back of the examiner's hand can indicate joint or periarticular inflammation. Sometimes one can infer bony or ligamentous problems simply by noting abnormalities in posture and position, as with scoliosis or inverted ankles. Genu valgus and varus abnormalities can suggest cartilage loss due to osteoarthritis of the knees. Flattened arches and inverted ankles are readily apparent when observing the patient stand.

Skin

Perhaps the most common skin abnormality of obese patients is maceration of the intertriginous skinfolds. Skin under the breast, in the groin, and between the buttocks easily becomes irritated by friction and infected with yeast, dermatophytes, and staphylococci. Obese patients with diabetes are even more prone to these infections. Acanthosis nigricans can be seen in patients with Cushing's syndrome, polycystic ovary disease, and diabetes. A milder form is seen in obese patients

without these disorders. Areas of skin inflammation and rash may appear prominent due to the tendency for obese persons to overheat easily and sweat (McLaren 1993).

Inspection of the knuckles and the dorsum of the fingers may reveal callused skin in patients who engage in repeated self-induced vomiting.

Breasts

The breasts may become quite large in obese women, producing considerable pain due to the pendulous mass. Shoulder and back pain, often accompanied by exaggerated kyphosis, is common. Bra straps may produce marked grooves across the shoulders, causing pain.

The clinical breast exam is difficult if the breasts are very large. First, the breasts should be inspected for asymmetry, skin retraction, nipple crusting, discharge, and galactorrhea. Palpation should be performed when the patient is both upright and supine. Masses palpated while the patient is upright may be missed while the same person is supine and vice versa. A thorough breast examination takes several minutes per breast. This includes a systematic palpation of the entire teardrop structure radiating from the aeriolae to and including the axillae while the patient is supine and gently palpating the entire breast between the pads of the fingers of both hands while the patient is upright.

Gynecomastia in men, a true increase in breast tissue, should be differentiated from pseudogynecomastia, an increase in subareolar fat. From a clinical point of view, this can usually be done by palpation since breast tissue is more firm than fat, although occasionally a mammogram is necessary to make the distinction. A nontender, firm, glandular disk of tissue less than 5.0 cm (2 in.) in diameter is common in obese men and warrants no more evaluation than the usual history and physical exam (Santen 1995).

Secondary Causes of Obesity

Obesity secondary to endocrine disorders is relatively rare. The importance of recognizing these forms of secondary obesity lies in the necessity of treating the underlying disorder. These conditions include hypercortisolism, growth hormone deficiency, hypogonadism, polycystic ovary (Stein-Leventhal) syndrome, and syndrome X (hyperlipidemia, hypertension, hyperinsulinemia, glucose intolerance, and insulin resistance). Patients with these syndromes characteristically exhibit increased upper body fat.

Physical findings in the patient with hypercortisolism may include a plethoric, round face; hypertension; a central fat distribution accompanied by a increased intrascapular fat pad; muscle loss in the proximal extremities; increased fine facial hair; and purple abdominal striae. These findings, however, are not invariably present or may be subtle.

Growth hormone deficiency results in increased body fat that is reversible with replacement. An age-related decline in growth hormone likely accounts for the increased adiposity so typically seen in older people. Studies suggest that growth hormone supplementation may reverse this fat accumulation as well (O'Conner, Stevens, and Blackman 1996).

A decidedly rare cause for obesity, disease of the hypothalamus, appears to result in reduced satiety and hyperphagia. Neoplasm, trauma, and infection are the most common causes.

Hyperinsulinism resulting from endogenous tumor production, as occurs with pancreatic islet cell tumors, is reported to produce obesity. These rare benign or malignant tumors may cause overeating to compensate for recurring hypoglycemia.

The association of upper body obesity, hyperlipidemia, hypertension, hyperinsulinemia with glucose intolerance, and insulin resistance has been referred to as syndrome X (Reaven 1988). Neither the genetic nor the metabolic abnormality accounting for this cluster of findings is well understood. Therapy is directed at optimizing blood glucose and lipids and controlling blood pressure.

Young women with hirsuitism (but not virilization), irregular menses, and enlarged ovaries suggest polycystic ovary (Stein-Leventhal) syndrome. Polycystic ovary syndrome is not rare and may occur in 5 to 10% of premenopausal women. As many as 50% of these women develop android obesity, and some have type 2 diabetes (Goudas and Dumesi 1997).

The causes and presentations of male hypogonadism are many. Male hypogonadism should be suspected in prepubertal or pubertal boys who fail to develop secondary sex characteristics or in men who develop a gradual loss of male secondary sex characteristics and libido. Replacement therapy corrects the disproportionate fat gain.

Hypothyroidism does not typically account for obesity. Most often it is discovered incidentally or in screening obese patients who seek an explanation for their obesity. When hypothyroidism is detected and corrected in an obese person, it rarely leads to a loss of more than 10 lb (4.5 kg) of excess weight, most of which is fluid.

While most obesity is polygenic and strongly influenced by environmental factors, rare genetic syndromes such as Prader-Willi syndrome, characterized by childhood-onset obesity, hyperphagia, mental retardation, short stature, and hypogonadism, will usually be recognized in childhood. Other genetic syndromes (Bardet-Biedl, Ahlstrom, Cohen, and Carpenter) are notable for distinctive physical features as well (Bray 1995).

Laboratory Studies

Laboratory testing is often driven by clinical suspicion of underlying disease based on the history and physical exam. A fasting blood glucose and lipid panel (triglycerides, total, and LDL and HDL cholesterol) should be part of the routine screening panel for moderate to severely obese patients and probably those with upper body obesity.

As noted earlier, significant obesity is not attributable to hypothyroidism, although it may be suspected on other clinical grounds. Nevertheless, many patients will be reassured only by confirmatory blood test. A thyroid-stimulating hormone (TSH) is considered to be the best single screening test for hypothyroidism.

Normal results of an overnight dexamethosone suppression test or 24-hour urinary-free cortisol test will adequately rule out endogenous hypercortisolemia when this is suspected. A mildly elevated serum testosterone will add support to the diagnosis of Stein-Leventhal syndrome when suggested by the history and physical. When a clinician suspects hypothalamic-pituitary disease, she should usually refer the patient for specialized serological test and neuroimaging.

Summary

Although challenging to perform due to the physical impediment of increased fat, the clinical examination of the obese patient, as with other patients, is worthwhile to master. The challenge is to perform a skillful exam, while always preserving the patient's dignity, and to use the information gained to the patient's benefit.

References

Atkinson, R.L. 1992. Medical evaluation and monitoring of patients treated by severe caloric restriction. In *Treatment of the seriously obese patient*, eds. T.A. Wadden and T.B. VanItallie, 273-289. New York: The Guildford Press.

Bickley, L.S., and Hoekelman, R.A. 1999. The cardiovascular system. In *Bates' guide to the physical examination and history taking*, 277-332. Philadelphia: Lippincott.

Braet, C., Mervielde, I., and Vandereycken, W. 1997. Psychological aspects of childhood obesity: A controlled study in a clinical and nonclinical sample. *Journal of Pediatric Psychology* 22 (1): 59-71.

Bray, G.A. 1995. The syndrome of obesity: An endocrine approach. In *Endocrinology*, ed. L.J. DeGroot, 3rd ed., 2624-2662. Philadelphia: W.B. Saunders Company.

Diamond, F.B., Jr. 1998. Newer aspects of the pathophysiology, evaluation, and management of obesity in childhood. *Current Opinion in Pediatrics* (4): 422-427.

Dietz, W.H 1998. Childhood weight affects adult morbidity and mortality. *Journal of Nutrition* 128 (2 Suppl.): 411S-414S.

Dwyer, J.T. 1994. Medical evaluation and classification of obesity. In *Obesity pathophysiology, psychology and treatment*, eds. G.L. Blackburn and B.S. Kanders, 9-38. New York: Chapman and Hall.

Feurer, I.D., and Mullen, J.L. 1986. Measurement of energy expenditure. In *Clinical nutrition*, eds. J. Rombeau and M. Caldwell, 224-236. Philadelphia: Saunders.

Foster, G.D., and Wadden, T.A. 1994. The psychology of obesity, weight loss and weight regain: Research and clinical findings. In *Obesity, pathology and treatment*, eds. G.L. Blackburn and B.S. Kanders, 140-166. New York: Chapman and Hall.

Froom, P., Melamed, S., and Benbassat, J. 1998. Smoking cessation and weight gain. *Journal of Family Practice* 46 (6): 460-464.

Gortmaker, S.L., Dietz, W.H., Sobol, A.M. et al. 1987. Increasing pediatric obesity in the United States. *American Journal of Diseases of Childhood* 141: 535-540.

Goudas, V.T., and Dumesi, D.A. 1997. Polycystic ovary syndrome. *Endocrinology and Metabolic Clinics of North America* 26 (4): 893-912.

Guenter, C.A. 1977. Abnormalities of the chest wall. In *Pulmonary medicine*, eds. C.A. Guenter and M.H. Welch, 502-512. Philadelphia: Lippincott.

Harris, M.B., Harris, R.J., and Bochner, S. 1982. Fat, four-eyed and female: Stereotypes of obesity, glasses and gender. *Journal of Applied Sociology and Psychology* 12: 503.

Hewitt, J.K. 1997. The genetics of obesity: What have genetic studies told us about the environment? *Behavior Genetics* 27 (4): 353-358.

Kaplan, N.M. 1994. Measurement of blood pressure. In *Clinical hypertension*, 23-45. Baltimore, Williams & Wilkins.

Klesges, R.C., Ward, K.D., Ray, J.W. et al. 1998. The prospective relationship between smoking and weight in a young, biracial cohort: The Coronary Artery Risk Development in Young Adults Study. *Journal Consulting and Clinical Psychology* 66 (6): 987-993.

Kotani, K., Nishida, M. et al. 1997. Two decades of annual medical examination in Japanese obese children: Do obese children grow into obese adults? *International Journal of Obesity and Related Metabolic Disorders* 21 (10): 912-921.

Kuczmarsk, R.J., Flegal, K.M., Campbell, S.M. et al. 1994. Increasing prevalence of overweight among U.S. adults. *Journal of the American Medical Association* 272: 205-211.

Lederle, F.A., and Simel, D.L. 1998. Does this patient have an abdominal aortic aneurysm? *Journal of the American Medical Association* 281 (1): 77-82.

Lew, E.A., and Garfinkel, L. 1979. Variations in mortality by weight among 750,000 men and women. *Journal of Chronic Disease* 32: 563-567.

Maddox, G.L., and Liederman, V. 1969. Overweight as a social disability with medical implications. *Journal of Medical Education* 44: 214.

McLaren, D.S. 1993. Cutaneous lesions in nutritional, metabolic, and heritable disorders. In *Dermatology in general medicine*, eds. T.B. Fitzpatrick, A.Z. Eisen et al., 1815-1826. New York: McGraw-Hill.

McNulty, S. 1992. Nutritional counseling during severe calorie restriction and weight maintenance. In *Treatment of the seriously obese patient*, eds. T.A. Wadden and T.B. VanItallie, 331-353. New York: The Guilford Press.

Morbidity and Mortality Weekly Report. 1994. Centers for Disease Control and Prevention: Prevalence of overweight among adolescents—United States, 1988-91. 43: 818-821.

Morbidity and Mortality Weekly Report. 1998. Prevalence of overweight among third and sixth-grade children—New York City, 1996. 47 (45): 980-984.

O'Conner, K.O., Stevens, T.E., and Blackman, M.R. 1996. GH and aging. In *Growth hormone in adults*, eds. A. Juul and J.O.L. Jorgensen, 323. Cambridge, UK: Cambridge University Press.

O'Hara, P., Connett, J.E., Lee, W.W. et al. 1998. Early and late weight gain following smoking cessation in the Lung Health Study. *American Journal of Epidemiology* 148 (9): 821-830.

O'Neil, P.M., and Jarrell, M.P. 1992. Psychological aspects of obesity and dieting. In *Treatment of the seriously obese patient*, eds. T.A. Wadden and T.B. VanItallie, 252-270. New York: The Guilford Press.

Petrie, J.C., Obrien, E.T., and Lettler, W.A. et al. 1986. Recommendations on blood pressure measurement. *British Medical Journal* 293: 611-615.

Pierce, J.W., and Wardle, J. 1997. Cause and effect beliefs and self-esteem of overweight children. *Journal of Child Psychology and Psychiatry* 38 (6): 645-650.

Reaven, G.M. 1988. Banting Lecture 1988. Role of insulin resistance in human disease. *Diabetes* 37: 1595.

Rosser, S. 1987. Childhood obesity and adulthood consequences. *Acta Paediatrica* 87 (1): 1-5.

Santen, R.J. 1995. Gynecomastia. In *Endocrinology*, ed. L.J. DeGroot, 2474-2484. Philadelphia: Saunders.

Srinivasan, S.R., and Berenson, G.S. 1995. Childhood lipoprotein profiles and implications for adult coronary artery disease: The Bogalusa Heart Study. *American Journal of Medical Science* 310 (Suppl. 1): S62-67.

Staffieri, J.R. 1967. A study of social stereotype of body image in children. *Journal of Personality and Social Psychology* 7: 101.

Teasdale, T.W., Sorensen, T.I., and Stunkard, A.J. 1990. Genetic and early environmental components in sociodemographic influences on adult body fatness. *British Medical Journal* 300 (6740): 1615-1618.

Wadden, T.A. 1995. Obesity. In *Comprehensive textbook of psychiatry*, eds. H.I. Kaplan and B.J. Saddock, 1481-1490. Baltimore: Williams & Wilkins.

Wadden, T.A., and Bartlett, S.J. 1992. Very low calorie diets: An overview and appraisal. In *Treatment of the seriously obese patient*, eds T.A. Wadden and T.B. VanItallie, 44-79. New York: The Guilford Press.

Wadden, T.A., and Foster, G.D. 1992. Behavioral assessment and treatment of markedly obese patients. In *Treatment of the seriously obese patient*, eds. T.A Wadden and T.B. VanItallie, 290-330. New York: The Guilford Press.

Webber, L.S., Wattigney, W.A., Srinivasan, S.R. et al. 1995. Obesity studies in Bogalusa. *American Journal of Medical Science* 310 (Suppl. 1): S53-61.

Whitaker, R.C., Wright, J.A., Pep, M.S. et al. 1997. Predicting obesity in young adulthood from childhood and parental obesity. *New England Journal of Medicine* 337 (13): 869-873.

Chapter 8

Dietary Intake: Recording and Analyzing

Judith M. Ashley, PhD, MSPH, RD

Vicki H. Bovee, MS, RD

Department of Nutrition and School of Medicine,
University of Nevada

To assess individuals' nutritional adequacy (energy, nutrients, and other food components) and eating patterns (mealtimes, food groups, and serving sizes), clinicians must obtain intake information on the different foods and beverages consumed. Intake information should also include dietary supplements, including vitamins, minerals, and herbs. In the clinical setting, documentation and analysis of a patient's usual dietary intake is useful in designing nutrition care plans and in evaluating the effectiveness of counseling. However, no ideal method exists for assessing food or nutrient intakes. The choice depends primarily on the type of information needed, time limitations, the objective of the analysis, and the expertise of the professional staff, as well as the resources available (Serdula et al. 2001; Sugerman, Eissenstat, and Srinith 1989). For example, the instrument chosen in the treatment of obesity should target caloric intake as well as dietary adequacy. Dietary assessment in obese or overweight patients also needs to fulfill several counseling purposes, including (1) establishing baseline eating patterns to design an individualized intervention, (2) encouraging self-monitoring of changes in targeted areas, and (3) providing feedback to the patient (Oneil 2001). In addition, since dietary intake will be assessed over a long period of time, patient burden or inconvenience is often a primary consideration. Thus, during the intervention clinicians may use a variety of instruments from the simple to the complex to increase patient compliance. Internet dietary assessment tools, which are growing in popularity, also constitute a convenient and feasible assessment method for patients (Boeckner et al. 2002).

Methods of Determining Dietary Intake

Methods of determining dietary intake involve instruments that can be categorized as either *retrospective*, requiring recall of the foods and beverages eaten, or *prospective*, requiring record keeping concurrent with eating (Thompson and Byers 1994). Both methods require nutritional analysis based on the data collected (see table 8.1).

Several nutritional analysis software programs available today can be adapted to meet a variety of needs, from evaluating the disease risk of an individual to comparing intake to a special population or age group. These programs range from the more expensive research-based programs, in which higher accuracy and precision require extensive food databases, to the more moderately priced systems suitable for patient use in a clinical practice. Databases

Table 8.1   *Retrospective and Prospective Dietary Intake Methods*

Method	Advantages	Disadvantages
24-hour food recall	Minimizes respondent burden. Quick to administer—20 to 40 min. Reduces likelihood that respondent will modify intake.	Requires trained staff to administer. Relies on memory of respondent for accuracy. One day may not be representative of typical day or influences of weekends, holidays, etc.
Food frequency questionnaire	Self-administered with minimal instruction. Reduces respondent burden. Covers a longer time span so infrequently consumed foods are included.	May require computer software to scan responses. Forms may not include specific foods since the food lists are based on general population intake.
Food history	Differentiates between weekday and weekend eating. Identifies meals away from home and food selections. Documents food intake over a long period of time.	Interviewer requires high level of skill and expertise. Needs to be followed up with a prospective food record.
Food record	Individual can receive instruction in advance, thus relying less on memory. Reveals usual eating patterns.	Requires greater respondent burden, motivation, and education. Act of recording may alter usual food intake. Analysis can be labor intensive and expensive even with computer software.
	Modified food record: Low respondent burden. Can target single nutrient.	Inappropriate for those following unconventional diets. Single nutrient target does not evaluate overall adequacy or variety of the diet.

used to calculate nutrients are derived primarily from the updates of the USDA food composition tables and additional information from food manufacturers, fast food and convenience food companies, foreign food composition tables, and research published in scientific journals (Grossbauer 1994). In general, databases that contain more foods are considered better since analysis will involve fewer substitutions during data entry. However, computerized diet analysis programs vary in quality and operating features (Lee, Nieman, and Rainwater 1995; McCullough et al. 1999).

Retrospective Methods

Three retrospective methods are used in dietary assessments. Each is presented here with its respective strengths and weaknesses.

24-Hour Food Recall (Multiple or Single Days)

For a food recall, a trained staff member conducts a face-to-face or telephone interview with a patient or subject. For the 24-hour recall, the person is asked to remember everything she or he had to eat and drink for the past one-day period, from midnight to midnight. The interviewer asks the time of day that any meals (breakfast, lunch, or dinner) or snacks were eaten. A two-pass method is used to help capture all of the data. First, the person is asked to reconstruct the overall eating events of the previous day, along with the main food and beverage items consumed, but not the exact amounts. In the second pass, the interviewer reads back what was recorded and prompts for more complete information (portions, condiments, brand names, additional items, and preparation and cooking methods) and for estimates of quantities based on household measures using cups, spoons, ruler sizes, and counts (the number of each item consumed). Three-dimensional food models or two-dimensional illustrations of portion sizes are often used as visual memory aids for quantitative estimates. Details of recipes or mixed-dish ingredients are collected for special foods prepared at home or eaten out. For most persons, approximately 20 to 40 minutes are needed to complete the interview. The recall can be done at a preset time or unannounced, with no prior knowledge of which day will be picked.

Strengths and weaknesses. The 24-hour recall method has the advantage of reducing respondent burden (inconvenience) by being reasonably quick to administer (Biro et al. 2002). Because the interview asks about the previous day, respondents are more likely to remember their dietary intake. Computer analysis systems are now available that facilitate recording the diet recall directly into the program for analysis. Use of the unannounced recall method also minimizes the tendency of the respondent to modify food habits for the recall (Smith, Jobe, and Mingay 1991). Although a single day's recall may not accurately represent a person's usual intake, it can give a useful overview of the diet if it is a typical day. Administering several 24-hour dietary recalls in succession has been shown to increase the validity of the information collected (Kabagambe et al. 2001), but its use in a clinical setting is limited because of the amount of time required of the clinician to make the phone calls.

However, the 24-hour recall is primarily based on the memory of the respondent and the accuracy of the respondent's recall. A person must be aware of the details of what was eaten and be able to estimate portion sizes accurately. Some respondents may recall an "ideal diet" by including only the foods that are perceived as healthy and omitting foods such as high-fat desserts or alcoholic drinks. The 24-hour days chosen may not represent the usual day-to-day intake of an individual, especially over a longer period. This method also may not account for the influence of weekends, seasons, and holidays. Although large food intakes are frequently underestimated, small intakes are often overestimated by the recall method (Guthrie 1984). Thus,

the success of the 24-hour-recall depends on the respondent's memory and ability to accurately estimate portion sizes consumed, as well as the persistence and skill of the interviewer, who must be careful to avoid leading questions and judgmental comments.

Food Frequency Questionnaires

Several commercial food frequency questionnaires are available that were first developed for diet analysis in epidemiological studies. They are designed to capture a respondent's usual food consumption over a period of time (months to years) using preformatted lists of food items that act as memory prompts. After each food item a set of options is given for choosing the usual frequency or consumption for the specified period of time. Some food frequency questionnaires use an extensive list of the most commonly eaten items (usually over a hundred food items) in the general population. These longer lists generally take about 45 minutes to complete. However, the list of foods can be brief if only one or a few nutrients of food groups are of interest (e.g., calcium) (Montomoli et al. 2002), provided the dietary components are concentrated in a relatively small number of foods. These simplified and shorter questionnaires have applicability in clinical practice for a more rapid assessment of the usual food components of interest (Svilaas et al. 2002). Food frequency questionnaires have also been developed for specific ethnic (Kim, Chan, and Shore 2002) and age groups (Buzzard et al. 2001), so that the food items listed take into account specific dietary patterns that are tailored to the patients of interest.

Food frequency questionnaires are considered *quantitative* if they ask only about the number of servings of foods consumed, and *semiquantitative* if they also ask questions about portion sizes (e.g., small, medium, or large). Some semiquantitative questionnaires contain pictures or photographs to aid in estimating serving or portion sizes (Kumanyika et al. 1996). The nutrient analysis of the intakes is derived from the reported frequency and portion size of each food. The food frequency questionnaires are usually self-administered with minimal instructions. A trained staff member can quickly review the questionnaire for missing items or duplications. If the person requires more assistance (e.g., the elderly), an interviewer can administer questionnaires.

Many food frequency questionnaires also include general questions to distinguish usual choices with different calorie or fat levels (e.g. whole, 2%, 1%, or skim milk) and preparation details. The list of foods can also be adapted to include specific foods important in certain populations (e.g., ethnic- or age-specific groups). The longer, research-quality food frequency questionnaires are available in scannable form for rapid analysis, but the software program itself is not always available for analysis. The individual scannable forms must be purchased, filled out individually, and sent in for scanning and analysis. For some, a shorter version containing fewer entries is available that focuses on a few foods or nutrients targeted to change behaviors specific to disease prevention or risk. Some have been calibrated against the longer instrument for accuracy (Block et al. 1989; Feskanich et al. 1994). They can be more easily and quickly administered and are useful in a variety of settings, including clinical practice.

Strengths and weaknesses. The two main advantages of food frequency questionnaires are reduced respondent burden and lower cost for limited data collection and processing (Block 2001). Because they ask about intake over a longer period of time, they can also identify foods that are consumed less often. Food frequency questionnaires can be used to rank which foods or food groups are usually eaten. They are not limited to recent dietary changes resulting from illness or lifestyle changes, so they are useful in determining patients' prior food intake. However, their limitations include the use of patients' long-term memories, and their inability to estimate the usual portion sizes. Food frequency questionnaires require a standardized food intake during the period in question. In addition, since the list of foods and beverages is usually limited to those of the general population, these questionnaires can miss getting information on some of the regional or cultural dietary items of an individual.

Food Histories

The food history method is one of the first interview methods developed that attempted to estimate the usual food intake over a relatively long period of time (Burke 1947). Determining usual intake requires considerable experience and skill on the part of the staff interviewer (Westerterp and Goris 2002). In this method, it is especially important that the interviewer be as nonjudgmental as possible in order to get an accurate food history. The interviewer needs to avoid any leading questions or comments about the adequacy of the diet described. A typical beginning question about eating habits would be, "What time do you usually first eat in the morning, and what do you usually eat?" As the interviewer develops the list of foods and beverages typically eaten throughout the day, she asks questions about the details depending on the selection. For example, if the patient mentions only cereal and fruit as a typical breakfast, additional questions would include, "Do you add anything to your cereal?" and "Do you usually drink any beverage at breakfast?" Portion size estimates can be done using a variety of usual techniques, including common utensils, commercial plastic food models, or two-dimensional models. Questions also include preparation and cooking methods as well as brand names.

Strengths and weaknesses. The food history facilitates questions about typical and atypical days, including the difference between weekend and weekday eating, as well as eating out frequency and selections. Some general information can also be obtained about seasonal and holiday changes. Depending on the skill of the staff interviewer and the information needed, the food history can be brief or labor intensive. In general, diet histories provide more qualitative than quantitative information on diet and nutrient intakes and require experienced interviewers. In the clinical setting, they are useful in documenting basic information and are best followed by a prospective food record for review at a follow-up visit.

Prospective Methods

Prospective methods require the recording of food intake as it is consumed, or food records. Considered the original "gold standard" of dietary intake, food records or diaries have the patient or subject record all food and beverages consumed on a prospective basis over a designated time period varying from days to weeks (Biro et al. 2002). Weekend days are usually included to account for the potential difference in food intake from weekdays. Food records may be kept by someone other than the patient or subject, who may be too young or impaired to keep his or her own record. Convenient-sized booklets or preprinted sheets are provided for recording, along with written instructions and examples. Instructions (verbal and written) emphasize the importance of complete and "honest" recording with detailed descriptions and accurate quantities. When the record is turned in, a trained staff member reviews it for completeness and asks about any inconsistencies or other details that were omitted.

Strengths and weaknesses. The strength of food records is that the person can be instructed about record keeping well in advance and is not relying on memory. The patient or subject is less likely to forget or omit foods when they are recorded as they are consumed. In addition, less staff time is required initially for the recording since the patient is writing down the foods consumed. In the clinical setting, reviewing food records with the patient can help in identifying eating habits and patterns to identify appropriate areas for behavior change. However, detailed record keeping involves a greater respondent burden and motivation and a higher level of education. Although longer records may be desirable to reveal usual eating patterns, they are more tedious to continue for all but the most highly committed, and time constraints may favor shorter versions in the clinical setting. In addition, the act of recording foods as they are eaten can influence the types of foods chosen and the quantities consumed by some people. The costs of nutritional analysis are higher when staff time to review and enter the records is calculated, even with the assistance of computerized analysis programs.

There are many variations of food records, primarily to reduce the burden of recording every dietary item, or to emphasize a particular food group or nutrient. The most common modification is based on the USDA Food Guide Pyramid (FGP). The person is asked to write down in general which foods are eaten, but then to concentrate on determining the number of servings from each food group—for example, the number of servings of grains, fruits, vegetables, milk products, and meats or meat alternatives (and usually glasses of wa-

ter). Intake is compared to the recommended servings per day based on the FGP, and overall diet adequacy and caloric intake is emphasized. However, the FGP approach may not be appropriate for those on less conventional diets, such as liquid or supplemental formula regimens, and scores are only an estimate of actual nutrient values.

Other common modifications are based on targeting single nutrients, such as fat intake for cardiovascular disease diets or carbohydrate intake for diabetic diets. The person is asked to write down in general which foods are eaten, but then to calculate only the fat grams or carbohydrate grams consumed at each eating event for the day. Targeting single nutrients requires that the person have a book or tables that list the nutrient(s) of interest for a large number of commonly eaten foods. However, good record modifications that target only single nutrients have the limitation of not evaluating the overall adequacy or variety of the diet.

Guidelines for Selecting an Appropriate Method

One issue with both retrospective and prospective methods of recording is that people tend to underreport actual energy intake. All methods are subject to problems such as changes in food intake to simplify recording or choosing not to eat foods that may be seen as unhealthy, neglecting to record foods or amounts of foods that may have been consumed in excessive quantities, difficulty determining actual portion size, and memory lapses (Kretsch, Fong, and Green 1999). Other variables that influence underreporting are literacy, percentage of body fat, BMI, and depression (Kretsch, Fong, and Green 1999; Kubena 2000). Adults, particularly women, with a BMI greater than 27.3 underreported energy intake more than adults with a lower BMI.

Keeping a diet record requires motivation. Typically the validity of diet records decreases when the number of days increases. For a dietary assessment, the number of days recorded is usually limited to four because of the burden to the patient and the time and cost of analyses (Craig et al. 2000). For ongoing dietary weight loss treatment, the best indicator of weight loss throughout the first year is the number of food records kept per week. In one study, the number of days recorded at six months was the most powerful indicator of weight loss, and those keeping five or more days of food records per week consistently lost the most weight (Streit et al. 1991).

Food Record Instruction and Review

Adequate instruction delivered by trained staff will help decrease the errors in food recording. (Figure 8.1 summarizes some key points of food record instruction.) Individuals consuming processed foods, fast foods, restaurant meals, and meals prepared away from home are likely to have more difficulty recording intake because of unknown food composition and the difficulty of estimating portion sizes (Streit et al. 1991). Using commercial plastic food models or household measuring tools will enhance the ability to estimate food portions for some, but not all, food items (Bolland, Yuhas, and Bolland 1988).

Individuals should be instructed to write down everything they eat and drink for the day beginning at midnight. They should be encouraged not to change their eating habits for the day, but to eat as they normally would eat and record the food as soon as they consume it. Foods added at the table, such as

condiments, need to be included. Standard measuring cups and measuring spoons, actual food scale weights, package weights, and food labels are tools used to determine portion sizes. A complete description of the food, cooking methods, recipe ingredients, and amounts should be included in the food intake record. A detailed description of the food (e.g., 3-oz boneless, skinless, broiled chicken breast) will help eliminate assumptions by the intake reviewer. (Figure 8.2 shows the details required for accurate food intake recording.) Individuals can also be instructed to record the locations of meals eaten, such as at home in front of the television, at a restaurant, or at someone else's home.

Food intake should be reviewed for completeness of details by the clinician. Figures 8.3 and 8.4 provide examples of incomplete and complete food intake records. Individuals should include all meals, note if a meal was skipped, list portion sizes in standard measurements, provide complete descriptions of foods and preparation methods, and include food labels for unusual food items.

Satisfactorily completed food intake records can be assessed for nutritional adequacy, nutrient composition, caloric intake, and eating patterns using several methods. Computer software for nutrient analysis is readily available. These programs determine single nutrient intake and diet adequacy compared to the U.S. RDA guidelines, and break down the intake into the food exchange lists. Entering the data and completing the analysis for a three- to four-day record usually takes one to two hours. The clinician can review the food intake record with the individual by comparing the intake to the USDA Food Guide Pyramid or by using food exchange lists.

Strategies for Converting a Food Record Into a Meal Plan

Patient input for meal planning is essential for eating and behavior changes to occur. Eating patterns such as time of day, usual foods, amounts eaten, and location of the meal or snack are factors to be considered. Building on current habits and making small changes a few at a time will promote successful change. For example, cardiology patients are often asked to reduce the amount of fat in their

---

Key Points for Food Record Instruction

1. Write down everything you eat or drink beginning at midnight.

2. Eat what you would normally eat; don't change your eating habits.

3. Describe the food completely including brand names and preparation method.

4. Record the portion size eaten in standard measurements using standard measuring cups and spoons or a food scale.

5. Be sure to include any foods added at the table such as condiments, sauces, sweeteners, etc.

6. Record the food as you eat it.

7. For recipes include the ingredients and amounts, preparation method, and number of servings the recipe made.

Figure 8.1 Key points for food record instruction.

Beverages—recorded in fluid ounces
Coffee/tea—caffeinated or decaffeinated, brewed or instant, flavored
Creamers—liquid or powder, milk or cream, low fat or regular fat, flavored
Sweeteners—sugar or sugar substitute
Sodas—regular or diet, caffeinated or decaffeinated
Alcohol—mixed drink, hard liquor, beer, or wine; low calorie or regular
Cocoa—type, sugar free, fat free, made with milk or water

Breads and bread products—recorded in weight, slice, or piece
White, whole wheat, rye, cracked wheat, raisin, etc.
Homemade, store-bought, bakery item
Diameter of bagel, muffin, or roll
Added toppings such as butter or margarine, cream cheese, jellies, jams, peanut butter

Cereals—recorded in cups or weight
Hot cereal—regular or instant, flavored, type of liquid added for cooking, added fat or sweetener
Cold cereal—specific brand name and type, sweetener added

Grain products—recorded in cups
Pasta—prepared mix or plain product, preparation method, sauces or fat added
Rice—white or brown, prepared mix or plain product, preparation method, fat or sauces added
Waffles/pancakes—type or flavor; homemade, mix, or frozen; syrup toppings or added fats
Tortillas—size; flour or corn; regular, low fat, or fat free
Other grain products such as couscous, bread stuffing, kasha—prepared mix or homemade; added fat, sauces, or gravy

Dairy products—recorded in fluid ounces for liquids, cups or weight for solid food
Milk—percent fat, condensed, evaporated, dry, flavored
Cheese/cottage cheese—type of cheese; regular, reduced fat, fat free, or percent fat
Ice cream, ice milk, frozen treats—flavor; regular, light, or fat free; sugar free; added toppings
Yogurt—flavor; regular, light, or fat free; sugar free
Cream cheese/sour cream—regular, low fat, or fat free; flavor
Whipped toppings—regular, low fat, or fat free
Puddings/custard—homemade, mix, or ready-to-serve; low calorie or fat free; type of milk used in preparation

Fats—recorded in teaspoons or tablespoons
Butter—whipped, stick, or light; salted or unsalted
Margarine—regular, low fat, or fat free, stick or tub
Oil—type
Commercial salad dressing/mayonnaise—flavor; regular, light, or fat free; low sodium
Peanut butter—regular or reduced fat; low sodium

Fruit—recorded in cups or size of piece
Dried
Fresh
Frozen—sugar added
Canned—water, juice, or syrup pack; drained or undrained

(continued)

Figure 8.2 Food record details.

Juice—recorded in fluid ounces
Fresh—calcium fortified
Frozen, bottled, or canned—sugar added, calcium fortified
Juice drink—flavor

Vegetables—recorded in cups or size of piece
Fresh or raw—added fat such as a dip
Frozen/canned—added fat or sauces, preparation method

Meat—recorded in ounces, cooked, with or without bone specified
Fish—type, preparation methods, fat or sauces added
Poultry—type; white or dark meat; skin eaten; preparation method; fat, sauce, or gravy added
Red meat—type; cut of meat; percent of fat for ground meat; preparation method; fat, sauce, or gravy added
Cold cuts and processed meats—kind of meat; regular, low fat, or fat free

Other protein foods—recorded in cups
Beans—dried or canned, preparation method, fat added
Nuts—regular, dry, or honey roasted; salted or unsalted
Eggs and egg substitute—method of preparation, fat or salt added

Snack foods—recorded in weight or cups
Type—chips, pretzels, crackers, popcorn, etc.
Brand name—flavor; regular, reduced fat, or fat free; low sodium

Sweets and desserts—recorded in size of piece or number of pieces
Brownies—homemade or store-bought, nuts, frosting
Cakes—flavor; homemade or store-bought; frosting or toppings; regular, low fat, or fat free
Candy—hard candy or chocolate, brand name
Cookies—homemade or store-bought; brand name; type; regular, reduced fat, or fat free
Donuts/pastries—type, homemade or store-bought, nuts, toppings, regular or reduced fat
Pies—homemade or store-bought, double crust, meringue or crumb topping, whipped topping or a la mode
Gelatin desserts—regular or sugar-free; added fruit, nuts, or toppings

Soups—recorded in cups
Ready-to-serve, homemade, diluted, or condensed; made with water or type of milk

Prepared foods (frozen dinners, pizza, package mixes, etc.)—recorded in cups or piece
Brand name
Description
Preparation method

Mixed dishes—recorded in cups
Recipe ingredients using previous checklists
Preparation method

Restaurant meals
Name of restaurant
Name of menu item
Preparation method
Condiments added at the table

Figure 8.2 (Continued)

Location/time	Amount	Food/description
Home—7 A.M.	1 bowl	Cold cereal
	1/2 cup	Milk
	1	Banana
Work—noon	1	Roast beef sub sandwich
	1 bag	Potato chips
	large	Pepsi
Home—6 P.M.	1 piece	Roasted chicken
	1/2 cup	Mashed potatoes
	1 large bowl	Tossed salad with dressing
Home—9 P.M.	2 handfuls	Wheat Thins™
	1 glass	Orange juice

Figure 8.3 Sample of incomplete food intake.

diets. Assessing a patient's current eating pattern will enable the clinician to gauge the extent of change needed to achieve the therapeutic goal. If the patient frequently eats high-fat foods, the transition to lower-fat foods should happen gradually based on food preferences. Interviewing the patient about the details of the recorded food intake can also reveal the extent of the patient's knowledge of fat sources in different foods. Patients may range from very informed to uninformed, so nutrition education needs will vary accordingly.

The clinician should ask the patient to look at the food record and determine the strengths and weaknesses of eating patterns and food selections. It is critical to remain nonjudgmental with the responses. Patients should be asked what they would like to change and how that change would benefit them. Exploration of obstacles

Location/time	Amount	Food/description
Home—7 A.M.	1 1/2 cups	Bowl of cereal
	1/2 cup	1% milk
	1 medium	Banana
	12 oz	Brewed caffeinated coffee
	1 tbsp	Fat-free liquid coffee creamer
Work—noon	1 6-in. sub sandwich from Subway	White roll, roast beef, provolone cheese, lettuce, tomato, onions, vinegar, oil, mayonnaise
	15 chips	Potato chips
	16 oz	Diet soda
Work—3 P.M.	1 small	Fresh apple
Home—6 P.M.	1 medium	Roasted chicken breast, skin not eaten
	1/2 c	Instant mashed potatoes made with regular margarine and 1% milk
	1/2 c	Gravy made with meat drippings
	2 c	Packaged iceberg salad mix
	1 small	Fresh tomato
	3 tbsp	Regular ranch dressing
	8 oz	White wine
Home—9 P.M.	1 c	Regular Wheat Thins
	8 oz	Orange juice, calcium fortified

Figure 8.4 Sample of complete food intake.

will help the patient identify potential barriers. Changes should be slow and gradual to enhance long-term changes. For example, patients who may benefit from increased fruit and vegetable intake may show a less-than-average intake of these items on their food records. Adding more fruits and vegetables will require a restructuring of their eating habits that is rarely done overnight. Many patients have a limited number of fruits or vegetables that they commonly eat. Although increasing the variety of selections would be helpful, it is often met with resistance. When the patient is an active partner in making changes, success is more likely. Once the patient has achieved the smaller changes, he or she is more likely to feel that larger changes are possible.

Summary

In the clinical setting, it is often important to assess the usual dietary intake of patients and how it might influence the prevention or treatment of health problems. There are a variety of dietary intake methods that can be used by the clinician to assess the food or nutrient intake of patients. It is important that the clinician become familiar with the advantages and disadvantages of these different methods, which include the 24-hour food recall, food frequency questionnaire, food history, and food record. In general, the ideal method would require the least amount of time for both the patient and clinician to complete, while giving the key results needed to design better nutrition care plans and to evaluate the effectiveness of patient counseling.

References

Biro, G., Hulshof, K.F., Ovesen, L., and Amorim Cruz, J.A. 2002. Selection of methodology to assess food intake. *European Journal of Clinical Nutrition* 56 (Suppl. 2): S25-S32.

Block, G. 2001. Invited commentary: Another perspective on food frequency. *American Journal of Epidemiology* 154 (12): 1089-1099.

Block, G., Clifford, C., Naughton, M.D., Henderson, M., and McAdams, M.A. 1989. A brief dietary screen for high fat intake. *Journal of Nutrition Education* 21: 199-207.

Boeckner, L.S., Pullen, C.H., Walker, S.N., Abbott, G.W., and Block, T. 2002. Use and reliability of the World Wide Web version of the Block Health Habits and History Questionnaire with older rural women. *Journal of Nutrition Education and Behavior* 34 (Suppl. 1): S20-24.

Bolland, J.E., Yuhas, J.A., and Bolland, T.W. 1988. Estimation of food portion sizes: Effectiveness of training. *Journal of the American Dietetic Association* 88: 817-821.

Burke, B.S. 1947. The dietary history as a tool in research. *Journal of the American Dietetic Association* 23: 1041-1046.

Buzzard, I.M., Stanton, C.A., Figueiredo, M.. Fries, E.A., Nicholson, R., Hogan, C.J., and Danish, S.J. 2001. Development and reproducibility of a brief food frequency questionnaire for assessing the fat, fiber and fruit and vegetable intakes of rural adolescents. *Journal of the American Dietetic Association* 101 (12): 1438-1446.

Craig, M.R., Kristal, A.R., Cheny, C.C.L., and Shattuck, A.L. 2000. The prevalence and impact of 'atypical' days in 4-day food records. *Journal of the American Dietetic Association* 100: 421-427.

Feskanich, D., Marshall, J., Rimm, E.B., Litin, L.B., and Willett, W.C. 1994. Simulated validation of a brief food frequency questionnaire. *Annals of Epidemiology* 4: 181-187.

Grossbauer, S. 1994. Using computers in communications. In *Communicating as professionals*, 2nd ed., ed. R. Chernoff, Chicago: American Dietetic Association.

Guthrie, H.A. 1984. Selection and quantification of typical food portions by young adults. *Journal of the American Dietetic Association* 84: 1440-1448.

Kabagambe, E.K., Baylin, A., Allan, D.A., Siles, X., Spiegelman, D., and Campos, H. 2001. Application of the method of triads to evaluate the performance of food frequency questionnaires and biomarkers as indicators of long-term dietary intake. *American Journal of Epidemiology* 154 (12): 1126-1135.

Kim, J., Chan, M.M., and Shore, R.E. 2002. Development and validation of a food frequency questionnaire for Korean Americans. *International Journal of Food Science and Nutrition* 53 (2): 129-142.

Kretsch, M.J., Fong, A.K.H., and Green, M.W. 1999. Behavioral and body size correlates of energy intake underreporting by obese and normal-weight women. *Journal of the American Dietetic Association* 99: 300-306.

Kubena, K.S. 2000. Accuracy in dietary assessment: On the road to good science. *Journal of the American Dietetic Association* 100: 775-776.

Kumanyika, S., Tell, G.S., Fried, L., Martel, J., and Chinchilli, V.M. 1996. Picture-sort methods for administering a food frequency questionnaire to older adults. *Journal of the American Dietetic Association* 96: 137-144.

Lee, R.D., Nieman, D.C., and Rainwater, M. 1995. Comparison of eight microcomputer dietary analysis programs with the USDA Nutrient Data Base for Standard Reference. *Journal of the American Dietetic Association* 95: 858-867.

McCullough, M.L., Karanja, N.M., Lin, P.H., Obarzanek, E., Phillips, K.M., Laws, R.L., Vollmer, W.M., O'Connor, E.A., Champagne, C.M., and Windhauser, M.M. 1999. Comparison of 4 nutrient databases with chemical composition data from the Dietary Approaches to Stop Hypertension trial. DASH. *Journal of the American Dietetic Association* 99 (8 Suppl.): S45-53.

Montomoli, M., Gonnelli, S., Giacchi, M., Mattei, R., Cuda, C., Rossi, S., and Gennari, C. 2002. Validation of a food frequency questionnaire for nutritional calcium intake assessment in Italian women. *European Journal of Clinical Nutrition* 56 (1): 21-30.

Oneil, P.M. 2001. Assessing dietary intake in the management of obesity. *Obesity Research* 9 (Suppl. 5): 361S-366S.

Serdula, M.K., Alexander, M.P., Scanlon, K.S., and Bowman, B.A. 2001. What are preschool children eating? A review of dietary assessment. *Annual Review of Nutrition* 21: 475-498.

Smith, A., Jobe, J.B., and Mingay, D.J. 1991. Question-induced cognitive biases in reports of dietary intake by college men and women. *Health Psychology* 10: 244-251.

Streit, K.J., Stevens, N.H., Stevens, V.J., and Rossner, J. 1991. Food records: A predictor and modifier of weight change in a long-term weight loss program. *Journal of the American Dietetic Association* 91: 13-216.

Sugerman, S.B., Eissenstat, B., and Srinith, U. 1989. Dietary assessment for cardiovascular disease risk determination and treatment. In *Cardiovascular nutrition: Strategies and tools for disease management and prevention,* eds. P. Kris-Etherton and J.H. Burns. Chicago: American Dietetic Association.

Svilaas, A., Strom, E.C., Svillas, T., Borgejordet, A., Thoresen, M., and Ose, L. 2002. Reproducibility and validity of a short food questionnaire for the assessment of dietary habits. *Nutrition Metabolism and Cardiovascular Disease* 12 (2): 60-70.

Thompson, F.E., and Byers, T. 1994. Dietary assessment resource manual. *Journal of Nutrition* (Suppl.): 2245S-2317S.

Westerterp, K.R., and Goris, A.H. 2002. Validity of the assessment of dietary intake: Problems of misreporting. *Current Opinion Clinical Nutrition and Metabolic Care* 5 (5): 489-493.

Chapter 9

Assessment of Physical Activity and Energy Expenditure

Michael J. LaMonte, PhD, MPH

Division of Cardiology, University of Utah School of Medicine and LDS Hospital

Barbara E. Ainsworth, PhD, MPH

Department of Epidemiology and Biostatistics and Department of Exercise Science, Norman J. Arnold School of Public Health, University of South Carolina at Columbia

Catrine Tudor-Locke, PhD

Department of Exercise and Wellness, Arizona State University East

Obesity occurs when energy intake chronically exceeds energy expenditure. Some researchers postulate that reduced daily energy expenditure (EE) associated with low levels of habitual physical activity (PA) may be of particular importance to sustained positive energy balance given that consumption of high-fat, energy-dense food makes equivalent compensatory reductions in energy intake nearly impossible (Hill and Melanson 1999). Therefore, increasing population levels of PA may be a primary public health strategy to overcome the current obesity epidemic.

Regular PA plays an important role in the maintenance of body weight and composition, and in the regulation of skeletal muscle and adipose tissue metabolism (American College of Sports Medicine 1998, 2001; Blair 1993; Grundy et al. 1999; Klem et al. 1997; Schmitz et al. 1998). Higher levels of PA correlate with better cross-sectional weight status (Ching et al. 1996; Macera and Pratt 2000), attenuated long-term weight gain (Ching et al. 1996; Schmitz et al. 1998), and maintenance of long-term weight loss (Klem et al. 1997). Two recent consensus statements (Grundy et al. 1999; National Heart, Lung, and Blood Institute 1998) recognized the role of PA in the prevention and treatment of obesity and its related adverse health sequellae. Current public health recommendations suggest that moderate PA performed for at least 30 minutes on most days of the week is sufficient to confer protection against several chronic diseases, many of which are associated with overweight and obesity (Pate et al. 1995). This amount of PA is equivalent to an EE of approximately 150 kcal day^{-1} or 2 kcal kg of body weight^{-1} × day^{-1} (American College of Sports Medicine 1998, 2001; U.S. Department of Health and

Human Services 1996). Unfortunately, the prevalence of meeting recommended levels of PA is substantially lower for obese (BMI ≥30 kg/m²) compared with nonobese (BMI <25 kg/m²) U.S. adults (19.7% versus 30.1%, respectively) (Macera and Pratt 2000). Fundamental to furthering current knowledge of the role PA plays in the etiology, prevention, and treatment of obesity is the degree to which PA can be accurately measured at the population level.

Precise assessment of free-living PA is critical for accurate descriptive epidemiology of the PA-obesity relationship, for designing appropriate interventions aimed at modifying body composition and related risk factors, and for promoting lifestyle change. However, because PA is a complex, multidimensional behavior, precise measurement remains a challenge for practitioners, researchers, and health care providers, especially among free-living populations (Ainsworth, Montoye, and Leon 1994; LaMonte and Ainsworth 2001). Feasibility considerations both in terms of expense and administrative burden result in the need for low-cost, indirect methods of assessing PA levels as part of a holistic approach to population-based treatment of obesity and related health conditions. The purpose of this chapter is to provide an overview of methods used to assess PA and EE in a variety of settings.

Physical Activity (PA) and Energy Expenditure (EE)

It is important to differentiate between PA and EE (see figure 9.1). PA is a behavior defined as body movement produced by skeletal muscle contraction, whereas EE is a result of the PA and reflects the net transfer of energy required to support the skeletal muscle contraction (LaMonte and Ainsworth 2001). PA is traditionally defined in terms of the frequency (number of sessions) and duration (minutes per session) of specified activities. Additional categorization can be based on the intensity or rate of EE attributed to a defined activity. EE is commonly expressed in terms of kilocalories (kcal) or kilojoules (kJ) of expended energy per unit time of observation. Because EE is closely related to body size, it is preferable to express the energy cost of a specific activity in units that account for body mass such as kcal kg⁻¹ × hr⁻¹ or METs (work metabolic rate/resting metabolic rate; 1 MET ~ 1 kcal × kg⁻¹ × hr⁻¹). Hence, PA may be classified by purpose, such as sports, occupation, and home care, or by intensity, as in light, moderate, and vigorous.

The term *energy expenditure* is used to quantify the total amount or *volume* of physical activity performed. Energy expenditure for individual activities can be estimated by mul-

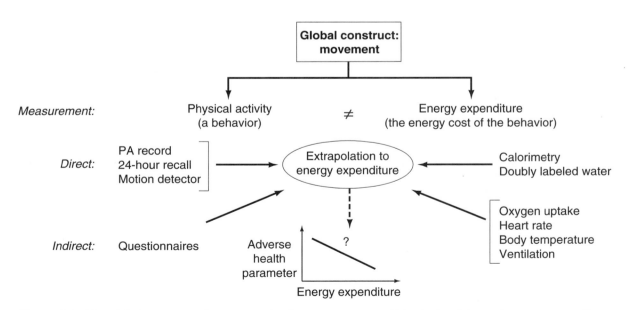

Figure 9.1 The global construct of movement for the measurement of physical activity and energy expenditure.

tiplying the frequency, duration, and intensity (e.g., energy cost of a specific activity) of the activity. Total EE for combined activities can be estimated by summing the EE estimates of each individual activity. Ainsworth and associates published a Compendium of Physical Activities (Ainsworth, Haskell et al. 2000) in an attempt to provide researchers and practitioners with a standardized linkage among specific activities, their purpose, and their estimated energy cost expressed in METs. For example, suppose a 75-kg (165-lb) individual walked for 30 minutes at a pace of 3.5 mph (93.8 meters $\times$ min^{-1}). Using the compendium, one would find that brisk walking on level ground at 3.5 mph carries an estimated energy cost of 3.3 METs. By multiplying the activity intensity (3.3 METs) by its duration (30 minutes), one would arrive at an energy expenditure of 99 MET-minutes (MET-min) during this bout of PA. To convert MET-min to kcal, one would multiply MET-min (99 MET-min) by the individual's body mass divided by 60 kg (60 kg, or 132 lb, is an assumed constant for the MET values in the compendium; 75 kg $\div$ 60 kg = 1.25) and compute a caloric expenditure of about 124 kcal (99 MET-min $\times$ 1.25). Available evidence suggests that the volume of activity (e.g., total daily EE) is more important than the specific type of activity with respect to weight loss and prevention of weight regain (American College of Sports Medicine 2001; Grundy et al. 1999). The exact amount of EE required to achieve these outcomes is, however, currently unknown.

The utility of a standard approach to linking PA and EE is predicated on accurate and precise measures of both variables. Several direct and indirect methods exist to assess PA and EE in laboratory and field settings (Ainsworth, Montoye, and Leon 1994; LaMonte and Ainsworth 2001) (see figure 9.1). Direct measures of PA include the use of PA records, logs, 24-hour recalls, and mechanical or electronic motion sensors to obtain the frequency, duration, and pattern of physical activities performed over a defined observation period. Direct PA assessment methods can be interviewer- or self-administered, or involve wearing a motion sensor device during a defined period of observation. Direct PA measures collect detailed information pertaining to individual PA behaviors as the activities are being performed, and consequently impose a fair amount of administrative burden to the researcher and the respondent. Indirect PA measures involve the use of questionnaires that require respondents to recall their usual PA habits during some time in the far or recent past. Indirect methods, which can be interviewer- or self-administered, typically provide less detail than direct PA measures, but offer substantially less administrative burden.

Energy expenditure is more difficult to measure precisely without the use of expensive laboratory procedures involving metabolic chambers and radioactive isotope tracers (Ainsworth, Montoye, and Leon 1994). The energy cost of movement can be estimated from field measures of physiological variables or PA (LaMonte and Ainsworth 2001); however, most indirect methods have yet to be refined for application outside the context of controlled research settings.

A primary goal of measuring PA and EE is to obtain a reliable and accurate estimate of the energy expended during a given activity or series of activities. The EE can then be interpreted within the context of recommended PA or EE levels required to achieve a defined health-related outcome (e.g., weight loss or glycemic control). Although one can estimate EE from surrogate measures of PA, an inherent level of imprecision will exist due to factors influencing EE (e.g., sex, age, body mass, skeletal muscle morphology, mechanical efficiency, or fitness) that are not accounted for in these PA measures (Montoye et al. 1996). Further, the ability of respondents to accurately recall their PA patterns introduces another source of error into the estimation of EE from self-reported measures of PA (Durante and Ainsworth 1996; Lichtman et al. 1992).

A number of published resources describe detailed methods used to measure PA and EE that have been used in various settings. The reader is referred to books and journal publications included in the reference section of this chapter (Ainsworth, Montoye, and Leon 1994; American Association for Active Lifestyles and Fitness 2000; Kriska and Casperson 1997; LaMonte and Ainsworth 2001; Montoye et al. 1996).

Measurement of Physical Activity

Because PA influences or is influenced by a variety of other health parameters, accurate

PA assessment is necessary in many research, clinical, and intervention settings. Clinicians can measure PA using methods that range in precision from crude categorization of activity status (e.g., sedentary or active) to detailed descriptions of activities (e.g., type, duration, or frequency) and their estimated energy costs. Following is an overview of some direct and indirect methods that have been used to assess PA (see figure 9.1) in various research and clinical settings.

Direct Physical Activity Assessment Methods

Direct measures of PA attempt to characterize the actual type, duration, and intensity of movement during a period of PA. Methods such as PA records and motion sensors are used to collect PA information while (or immediately after) an individual engages in various activities (see figure 9.2). PA logs collect similar information at the end of a defined observation period (e.g., at the end of a day). While none of these methods is adequate alone to characterize total PA, they are considered objective quantitative measures of activity exposure. Therefore, direct measures of PA are often used to validate PA surveys and other subjective indexes of PA.

PA Records

PA records are ongoing detailed accounts of sources and patterns of PA that individuals record in diary format during a defined time frame (Ainsworth, Montoye, and Leon 1994). Their level of detail ranges from recording each activity and its associated duration (Ainsworth et al. 1999) to recording activities performed at specified time intervals (e.g., every 15 minutes) (Bouchard et al. 1983). Ainsworth and colleagues (Ainsworth et al. 1999; Ainsworth, LaMonte et al. 2000; Conway et al. 1999; Irwin et al. 2000; LaMonte et al. 2001; Wilcox et al. 2001) and others (Fogelholm et al. 1998) have used PA records in field settings to obtain detailed accounts of all physical activities performed during several days to weeks.

The PA record is a pocket-sized booklet wherein subjects record information about

Time began	Position (circle one)	Description (What are you doing?)	How hard? (circle one)	Activity group (circle one)	(leave blank) Code	Mins
8:05 AM PM	Recline Sit Stand Walk	walk in house to fix breakfast	Light Moderate Vigorous	SC HH PAR TRANS OCC WALK INAC LG EC MISC	17150	1
8:06 AM PM	Recline Sit Stand Walk	fix breakfast	Light Moderate Vigorous	SC HH PAR TRANS OCC WALK INAC LG EC MISC	05050	4
8:10 AM PM	Recline Sit Stand Walk	eat breakfast	Light Moderate Vigorous	SC HH PAR TRANS OCC WALK INAC LG EC MISC	13030	5
8:15 AM PM	Recline Sit Stand Walk	gather things to leave home	Light Moderate Vigorous	SC HH PAR TRANS OCC WALK INAC LG EC MISC	09071	3
8:18 AM PM	Recline Sit Stand Walk	walk to car	Light Moderate Vigorous	SC HH PAR TRANS OCC WALK INAC LG EC MISC	17161	2
8:20 AM PM	Recline Sit Stand Walk	drive car to work	Light Moderate Vigorous	SC HH PAR TRANS OCC WALK INAC LG EC MISC	16010	

a. Physical activity record

ID# ______ Day of the week __________ Day # ________ Date ____/____/____

Amount of Time

			Hours	Minutes
Household				
Indoors				
Cooking	Yes	No	____	____
Cleaning up	Yes	No	____	____
Laundry	Yes	No	____	____
Shopping	Yes	No	____	____
Dusting	Yes	No	____	____
Scrubbing	Yes	No	____	____
Vacuuming	Yes	No	____	____
Home repair	Yes	No	____	____
Mopping	Yes	No	____	____
Washing car	Yes	No	____	____
Other	Yes	No	____	____
Outdoors				
Mowing lawn	Yes	No	____	____
Raking lawn	Yes	No	____	____
Weeding	Yes	No	____	____
Sweeping	Yes	No	____	____
Shoveling	Yes	No	____	____
Pruning	Yes	No	____	____
Chopping wood	Yes	No	____	____
Other	Yes	No	____	____
Care of Others				
Bathing	Yes	No	____	____
Feeding	Yes	No	____	____
Playing	Yes	No	____	____
Lifting	Yes	No	____	____
Pushing wheelchair	Yes	No	____	____
Transportation				
Drive car	Yes	No	____	____
Ride in car	Yes	No	____	____
Walking				
To get places	Yes	No	____	____
For exercise	Yes	No	____	____
With the dog	Yes	No	____	____
Work breaks	Yes	No	____	____

			Hours	Minutes
Dancing				
In church	Yes	No	____	____
For pleasure	Yes	No	____	____
Other	Yes	No	____	____
Sports				
Golf	Yes	No	____	____
Team sports	Yes	No	____	____
Other	Yes	No	____	____
Conditioning				
Aerobics	Yes	No	____	____
Jogging	Yes	No	____	____
Swimming	Yes	No	____	____
Bicycling	Yes	No	____	____
Stretching	Yes	No	____	____
Weight lifting	Yes	No	____	____
Other	Yes	No	____	____
Inactivity				
Watching TV	Yes	No	____	____
Read or sew	Yes	No	____	____
Use computer	Yes	No	____	____
Other				
Occupation				
Sitting task	Yes	No	____	____
Standing tasks	Yes	No	____	____
Walking tasks	Yes	No	____	____
Heavy labor	Yes	No	____	____
	Yes	No	____	____
Volunteer				
Sitting tasks	Yes	No	____	____
Standing tasks	Yes	No	____	____
Walking tasks	Yes	No	____	____
Heavy labor	Yes	No	____	____

Monitors
Time put ON ____________ A.M.
Time taken OFF ____________ P.M.
Steps taken ________________

b. Physical activity log

Figure 9.2 Instruments used in the assessment of physical activity and energy expenditure: *(a)* a physical activity record and *(b)* a physical activity log.

the type (e.g., walking, cooking, or gardening), purpose (e.g., transportation and home care), duration (e.g., minutes), perceived intensity (light, moderate, vigorous), and body position (reclining, sitting, standing, walking) for every activity completed within a defined time frame (typically 24 hours) (see figure 9.2a for a sample PA record). PA records can be kept for one day or several weeks and across seasons to obtain information about habitual physical activity levels and patterns and related seasonal variations in these behaviors (Levin et al. 1999).

PA records are scored using the Compendium of Physical Activities (Ainsworth, Haskell et al. 2000) to link a MET intensity score with the type and purpose of the activity performed as previously described. Once scored, the PA record provides a detailed account of the minutes spent and estimated energy expended in various types, intensities, and patterns of PA. Thus, PA records allow practitioners to assess individual or population-specific PA prevalence estimates (e.g., percentage of respondents who engage in 30 minutes of moderate PA on five or more days per week) as well as recommended levels of health-related EE (e.g., ≥ 2 kcal $\times$ $\text{kg}^{-1} \times \text{hr}^{-1}$).

Conway and colleagues (1999) reported a mean difference of $7.9 \pm 3.2\%$ between seven-day PA records and doubly labeled water estimates of free-living activity-related EE in men. Using PA records, Ainsworth and colleagues (1999) identified that African American and Native American women living in the southeastern and southwestern regions of the United States, respectively, spent approximately 1 1/2 hours per day in moderate-intensity (3-6 METs) physical activities. The primary activities performed were household chores, occupation, walking for exercise, childcare, and lawn and garden activities. In contrast, fewer than 5 minutes per day were spent in sport and conditioning activities. Interestingly, despite spending essentially no daily time in sport or conditioning activities, over 45% of the African American women met recommended (Pate et al. 1995) amounts of moderate PA. This prevalence estimate is a striking contrast to the 25% of African American women who reported meeting the moderate PA recommendation in leisure time on a recent cycle of the National Health Interview Survey (Jones et al. 1998).

The difference in the prevalence of African American women meeting the moderate PA recommendation in these two studies illustrates the utility of the PA records over traditional PA surveys in identifying relevant population-specific sources of PA that may contribute to health-related levels of EE. More important, precise and complete assessment of *habitual* daily PA levels may serve as the referent point for prescribing additional levels of EE required to modify body composition or metabolic fitness levels.

In another analysis of PA records from the same study sample reported on by Ainsworth and colleagues (1999), researchers observed that women tended to overestimate the time spent in PA perceived as vigorous intensity and underestimate the time spent in activities perceived as light intensity (Wilcox et al. 2001). This information may be useful to understand how patients may perceive the intensity of PA in contrast with the true metabolic cost of the activity, which is the variable of interest for PA interventions aimed at modifying body composition (American College of Sports Medicine 1998, 2001). Together with population-specific focus groups (Henderson and Ainsworth 2000), PA records may provide the information necessary to plan PA interventions that are culturally and geographically relevant to the target population in order to optimize a program's effect on targeted health-related outcomes (e.g., weight loss).

Similar to their dietary counterpart aimed at assessing energy intake (Willett 1998), PA records have many applications in assessing sources and patterns of PA. Their feasibility, however, is limited by cost, the potential for altered behavior, and administrative burden on the practitioner and participant. PA records require participants to be highly motivated in order to write every PA they perform into the record book immediately after completing the activity. Further, since a daily PA record may have from 25 to 250 different activities recorded, the records require considerable time and patience of the study staff to edit, code, score, and summarize. For these reasons, PA records may best be suited for use in small-scale epidemiological studies of PA, small PA intervention trials, or as a criterion measure for validating simpler field surveys of PA.

PA Logs

PA logs aim to provide a detailed account of habitual daily activities and their associated duration (Ainsworth, Montoye, and Leon 1994). The PA log is structured as a checklist of specified activities usually developed from population-specific PA focus groups (Ainsworth, Montoye, and Leon 1994; Henderson and Ainsworth 2000) or from targeted behaviors being tracked in a research or clinic setting (e.g., walking or specific exercises). PA logs are generally one page in length and may be formatted in various ways to meet the specific needs of researchers and practitioners. The Bouchard PA Log (Bouchard et al. 1983) was designed for respondents to check the type and intensity of activity they are performing every 15 minutes during a specific period. The Ainsworth PA Log (Ainsworth, Bassett et al. 2000) is a modifiable form that includes a list of 20 to 50 activities that reflect population-specific PA interests (see figure 9.2b). At the end of the day, respondents identify the type and duration of activities performed that day. The PA log takes only a few minutes to complete and provides information about the type, time, and estimated energy cost of physical activities performed during specified periods. PA logs are useful for determining whether recommended PA levels are being met by assigning intensity values from the compendium of PA to the activity items selected by the respondent and computing intensity-specific (e.g., moderate or vigorous) PA summary scores in terms of MET-min $\times$ day^{-1} or kcal $\times$ day^{-1}.

PA logs may be more convenient to complete and process than PA records as they are less time consuming for the respondent and contain less information for data processing. Alternatively, PA logs may be of limited value if participants engage in activities other than those listed on the log.

PA Recalls

Unlike the diary format of the PA record, PA recalls are typically interviews (telephone or in person) aimed at detailing an individual's PA level during the past 24 hours or longer (Ainsworth, Montoye, and Leon 1994). PA recalls are similar to PA records in that they can identify the type, duration, purpose, and estimated intensity of activities performed in a specified period. The PA recall is patterned after methods used in 24-hour dietary recalls and takes from 20 to 45 minutes to complete (Matthews et al. 2000; Matthews et al. 2002; Willett 1998). Matthews and colleagues (2000) recently used multiple random 24-hour PA recalls conducted with telephone interviews to profile activity patterns and estimate EE among adults in a one-year cohort study of blood lipid variability Test-retest reliability was higher for men ($R = 0.26$ to 0.58) than it was for women ($R = 0.22$ to 0.26). Larger criterion validity correlations between total MET-hr $\times$ day^{-1} from the 24-hour PA recall and activity counts $\times$ min^{-1} $\times$ day^{-1} from an Actillume (Ambulatory Monitoring, Inc., Ardsely, NY) accelerometer were also observed among men ($r = 0.74$) than were observed among women ($r = 0.32$). The researchers suggested that given the feasibility, reasonable reliability and validity, minimal participant effort, and potential reductions in response bias and altered activity patterns during assessment, 24-hour recalls may be an attractive population-based method of assessing PA.

Although the 24-hour PA recall method seems practical and has the potential to obtain detailed PA information, this method may not be suitable in populations with limited telephone access and may be hampered by individuals who are unwilling or unable to complete the phone interview when they are called. Further, the 24-hour recall time frame may be unrepresentative of a person's true habitual PA pattern or level, which may limit its use in some research or clinical settings. Additional testing of the 24-hour PA recall method in large, diverse populations is required to substantiate its validity for use in population-based studies of PA.

Motion Detectors

Motion detectors are mechanical and electronic devices worn on the body to provide a direct measure of PA. Energy expenditure is often extrapolated from the PA data under the assumption that movement (or acceleration) of the limbs and torso is closely related to whole-body EE (Freedson and Miller 2000; Haskell et al. 1993). There are several types of motion detectors that differ in technological sophistication and in the type of movement data generated.

Pedometers. Pedometers are small, inexpensive devices (~ $20) used to quantify walking activity directly in terms of accumulated steps per unit time (e.g., per day) (Ainsworth, Montoye, and Leon 1994; Tudor-Locke and Myers 2001). Prior to 1980, many of the mechanical pedometers relied on spring-loaded devices to register steps (Montoye et al. 1996). These devices were found to have unacceptable accuracy and reliability due to stretching of the springs and lack of a suitable calibration mechanism (Bassey et al. 1987; Gayle, Montoye, and Philpot 1977; Washburn, Chin, and Montoye 1980). Recent technological advances have resulted in the development of electronic pedometers (e.g., Yamax Digiwalker) that are smaller and may be more reliable than earlier models.

Worn at the waist, electronic pedometers are triggered by vertical forces that cause a horizontal spring-suspended lever arm to move up and down. Movement of the lever arm opens and closes an electrical circuit. Each time the circuit closes, a "step" is counted. Step registration, in theory, should reflect the vertical forces of footstrike; however, essentially any vertical force through the hip area can trigger the device. An estimate of distance walked is obtained by calibrating the pedometer to an individual's stride length during a short walking trial over a known distance.

Researchers recommend that the raw "steps" data be used to represent ambulatory activity as a continuous variable (Rowlands, Eston, and Ingledew 1999; Tudor-Locke and Myers 2001).

The Yamax Digiwalker (Model DW-500) has demonstrated reasonable precision for use in research and clinical settings where walking is the primary type of PA (Bassett et al. 1996; Nelson, Leenders, and Sherman 1998; Welk, Differding et al. 2000). The Digiwalker was accurate to within 2% of actual steps taken during self-paced over-ground walking (Bassett et al. 1996), and within 3 to 5% of actual steps taken during a trial of walking and jogging (Welk, Differding et al. 2000). Error in step counting is higher at slow walking paces (Bassett et al. 1996; Welk, Differding et al. 2000). Another study (Shepherd et al. 1999) reported slightly higher error in step counting among individuals with a BMI >30 kg/m^2, which may have been due to slower self-paced walking or altered device triggering

due to increased adiposity or higher ground reaction forces among obese compared to normal weight individuals. Other researchers have observed a relationship between body size and pedometer counts (Welk, Differding et al. 2000). Estimates of EE derived from pre-programmed regression equations and stride length tend to be imprecise when compared with objective measures of EE (Bassett et al. 2000; Nelson, Leenders, and Sherman 1998; Rowlands, Eston, and Ingledew 1997; Tudor-Locke and Myers 2001). Compared with indirect calorimetry, the Digiwalker precisely estimated EE during a very limited range of walking speeds (2.0-3.5 mph or 53.6–93.8 m $\times$ min^{-1}) (Nelson, Leenders, and Sherman 1998).

Although the Digiwalker provides an objective and accurate measure of ambulatory PA, individual variability in step counts can be large. Potential sources of individual variability in step counting appear to be related to walking pace and body size. Digiwalker steps have been inversely related with walking pace over a fixed distance, and with body weight and stride length at a fixed walking pace (Bassett et al. 1996; Washburn, Chin, and Montoye 1980; Welk, Differding et al. 2000). Welk and colleagues (Welk, Differding et al. 2000) identified a potential concern with using pedometers in obese populations by showing positive associations ($r = 0.55$ to 0.66) between step counts at a constant pace and percent fat in a field study of middle-aged adults.

Ambulatory physical activity has been consistently related to body composition variables in observational studies. Tudor-Locke and colleagues (2001) found steps $\times$ day^{-1} were inversely related to BMI and percent body fat ($r = -0.30$, and $r = -0.27$, respectively, $p < 0.01$) in 109 healthy middle-aged adults. This finding is consistent with data from other adult and child populations (McClung et al. 2000; Rowlands, Eston, and Ingledew 1999). Finally, steps $\times$ day^{-1} and BMI were inversely related ($r = -0.27$, $p < 0.01$), and significant differences ($F = 2.96$, $p < 0.05$) in steps $\times$ day^{-1} were observed between health-related BMI categories (National Heart, Lung, and Blood Institute 1998) among adults with type 2 diabetes (Tudor-Locke et al. 2002). These data suggest that ambulatory activity patterns are different between individuals categorized by weight status, and therefore may support the use of pedometers to monitor or promote walking activities in obese populations.

It is currently impossible to identify an empirically based threshold level of steps × day⁻¹ to achieve national health-related physical activity goals (Pate et al. 1995). Preliminary evidence suggests that individuals with values greater than approximately nine thousand steps per day are more frequently classified as normal weight, whereas those with values less than around five thousand steps per day are more frequently classified as obese (Tudor-Locke et al. 2001). The average steps × day⁻¹ reported for women enrolled in a weight loss trial was 9,155 (range = 3,916 to 15,383) (Fogelholm et al. 1998). A recent field study (Welk, Differding et al. 2000) showed that participants reporting involvement in structured vigorous PA had an average of 11,603 steps × day⁻¹ and an average of 8,265 steps × day⁻¹ when only unstructured light to moderate PA was reported. Japanese researchers (Hatano 1993; Yamanouchi et al. 1995) have used the Digiwalker to advocate walking for health and suggest that taking at least 10,000 steps × day⁻¹ in ambulatory activities is equivalent to an EE of ~ 300 kcal × day⁻¹. The only published study to document weight loss with a pedometer-based intervention reported that successful subjects averaged 19,200 steps × day⁻¹ (Yamanouchi et al. 1995), substantially more than the recommended 10,000 steps × day⁻¹.

The use of pedometers as a motivational adjunct to PA intervention is promising; however, their use as objective PA monitors is limited by issues pertaining to device calibration and the inability to differentiate type, frequency, duration, and intensity of PA. Variability in activity patterns and a lack of empirical evidence to define threshold levels of pedometer steps × day⁻¹ that are related with favorable health outcomes make it very difficult to establish pedometer-based PA guidelines that equate to existing public health PA recommendations. Used in conjunction with a detailed self-report of PA (e.g., PA log), pedometers can provide a simple, cost-effective way to monitor both the quantity and quality of certain types of PA.

Accelerometers. Accelerometers are battery-operated electronic motion sensors that, in theory, measure the rate and magnitude of displacement of the body's center of mass during movement. Generally, these devices assess PA by sensing the acceleration forces during movement. The absolute value and frequency of acceleration forces is integrated and summed over a defined observation period and reported as an activity "count." Energy expenditure can be estimated from the integral of "counts" (accelerations) using regression equations derived from controlled laboratory experiments and measured oxygen uptake (Freedson, Melanson, and Sirard 1998; Hendelman et al. 2000; Montoye et al. 1983; Swartz et al. 2000).

Accelerometers are typically worn at the waist and measure movement in single (uniaxial; Caltrac™, MTI) or multiple planes (triaxial; Tritrac) by way of piezoelectric signaling. Manufacturers of the MTI and Tritrac suggest that these monitors filter out accelerations with frequencies outside the range of human movement, thereby minimizing the influence of artifact due to involuntary movement. Activity or EE data is either displayed for hand recording (Caltrac) or stored in solid-state memory for computer downloading and processing at a later time (MTI, Tritrac).

Caltrac accelerometer. The Caltrac accelerometer (Muscle Dynamics Fitness Network, Torrance, CA) was first described for use as an objective PA measure during laboratory-based studies performed in the early 1980s by Montoye and colleagues (1983). The device estimates resting EE using sex, age (yr), height (in.), and weight (lb) as follows (Hemokinetics, Inc., Madison, WI):

Men: kcal × min⁻¹ = [(473 × Wt) + (982 × Ht) − (531 × Age) + 4686] / 100,000

Women: kcal × min⁻¹ = [(331 × Wt) + (351 × Ht) − (352 × Age) + 49,854] / 100,000

As accelerations or "counts" are recorded during movement, EE is estimated from oxygen uptake ($\dot{V}O_2$) using the following equations that assumes 5 kcal for every 1 L O_2 uptake (Montoye et al. 1983):

$\dot{V}O_2$ (ml × kg⁻¹ × min⁻¹) = 8.2 + 0.08 (counts × min⁻¹)

EE (kcal × min⁻¹) = 5 × [[$\dot{V}O_2$ (ml × kg⁻¹ × min⁻¹) × body mass (kg)] / 1,000]

The estimated EE of the movement is continuously added to the resting EE value and summed across the specified observation period to yield a value of total EE. Because it cannot be programmed for interval-based time sampling, Caltrac provides only total daily "counts" or EE.

The Caltrac has been the most widely used accelerometer, and its reliability and validity has been frequently assessed (Bassett et al. 2000; Fogelholm et al. 1998; Jacobs et al. 1993; Montoye et al. 1983, 1996; Pambianco, Wing, and Robertson 1990; Richardson et al. 1995). Jacobs and colleagues (1993) reported 1-, 6-, and 13-month test-retest correlations of 0.69, 0.84, and 0.79, for Caltrac EE, and 0.34, 0.49, and 0.42 for Caltrac "counts." Montoye and colleagues (1983) reported strong correlations between Caltrac EE and measured $\dot{V}O_2$ (pooled $r = 0.74$, standard error of estimation [SEE] = 6.6 ml $\times$ kg^{-1} $\times$ min^{-1}) and test-retest correlations of 0.93 to 0.98 over two measurements. Melanson and Freedson (1995) reported a strong correlation between Caltrac and $\dot{V}O_2$ ($r = 0.89$) but no relation between Caltrac and treadmill grade ($r = 0.02$). The latter observation illustrates the inability of accelerometers to detect changes in the energy cost of activities due to increased resistance to movement (Freedson and Miller 2000; Haskell et al. 1993). The Caltrac overestimated EE by 9 to 13% during level treadmill walking with larger discrepancies among obese (>15% over ideal weight) individuals at slower speeds and among normal weight individuals (mean = 66 kg) at higher speeds (Pambianco, Wing, and Robertson 1990). Among free-living overweight (BMI = 27.7-37.0 kg/m^2) women, PA ratios (measured EE/resting metabolic rate [RMR]) were higher for Caltrac compared with doubly labeled water measures (Fogelholm et al. 1998). Bassett and colleagues (2000) recently observed a modest correlation (r_{pooled} = 0.58) and large variation in quantitative EE estimates between the Caltrac and $\dot{V}O_2$ under a variety of field and laboratory conditions.

MTI actigraph accelerometer. The MTI actigraph (Manufacturing Technology, Inc., Fort Walton Beach, FL [formerly called CSA Actigraph]) is one of the smallest accelerometers and has become increasingly popular for field studies of PA and EE. The acceleration signal is filtered and digitized, integrated over a specified sampling time, and stored for subsequent computer processing. MTI monitors can be single mode (counts only) or dual mode (counts and frequency of accelerations interpreted as "steps"). Unlike Caltrac, the MTI must be computer initialized and, depending on the sampling interval (e.g., seconds to minutes), can store data for up to 22 days. Data are presented as counts per unit sampling time (e.g., counts $\times$ minute^{-1} $\times$ day^{-1}). Regression equations have been developed to derive EE estimates from raw MTI count data (Freedson, Melanson, and Sirard 1998; Hendelman et al. 2000; Swartz et al. 2000). The majority of these equations were generated from controlled laboratory studies of treadmill exercise or limited simulations of lifestyle PA. The most common equations are those developed by Freedson and colleagues (Freedson, Melanson, and Sirard 1998):

$$EE \text{ (METs)} = 1.439008 + (0.000795 \times \text{counts} \times \text{min}^{-1})$$

$$EE \text{ (kcal} \times \text{min}^{-1}) = (0.00094 \times \text{counts} \times \text{min}^{-1}) + (0.1346 \times \text{mass in kg})$$

The precision of each equation was $R^2 = 0.82$ (SEE = 1.12 METs) for METs and $R^2 = 0.82$ (SEE = 1.4 kcal $\times$ min^{-1}) for kilocalories during treadmill exercise at 3, 4, and 6 mph (80, 106, and 162 m $\times$ min^{-1}).

Several recent studies have assessed the ability of the MTI to assess PA-related EE (Ainsworth, Bassett et al. 2000; Bassett et al. 2000; Hendelman et al. 2000; Masse et al. 1999; Melanson and Freedson 1995; Nichols et al. 2000; Swartz et al. 2000; Welk, Blair et al. 2000). Welk and colleagues (Welk, Blair et al. 2000) showed that MTI count data varied significantly with monitor placement at three different ipsilateral hip locations. Despite being correlated with $\dot{V}O_2$ during treadmill walking ($r = 0.82$), MTI counts $\times$ min^{-1} were unrelated to treadmill grade ($r = 0.03$) (Melanson and Freedson 1995). Nichols and colleagues (2000) showed that MTI counts $\times$ min^{-1} were sensitive to changes in velocity across three walking speeds ($p < 0.0001$), but that interinstrument reliability was substantially lower during slower (2 mph [53 m $\times$ min^{-1}], $R = 0.55$) versus faster (4 mph [107 m $\times$ min^{-1}], $R = 0.91$) speeds. Correlations between $\dot{V}O_2$ and MTI counts $\times$ min^{-1} have been stronger during controlled laboratory activity (e.g., $r = 0.80$ to 0.95) (Melanson and Freedson 1995; Welk, Blair et al. 2000) and weaker during simulated or actual field conditions of lifestyle activities (e.g., $r = 0.40$ to 0.60) (Bassett et al. 2000; Welk, Blair et al. 2000). Hendelman and colleagues (2000) showed differences between measured and predicted METs of 30 to 57% for a variety of daily lifestyle activities. MTI count $\times$ min^{-1} cutoff points for 3-, 6-, and 9-MET activities were considerably different when derived from equations based on walking only versus walking and lifestyle activities combined (Hendelman et al. 2000). Regression equations used to estimate EE have shown lower precision when derived from lifestyle activity ($R^2 = 0.32$-0.35, SEE = 0.96-1.2 METs) (Hendelman et al. 2000; Swartz et al. 2000) compared with laboratory activity ($R^2 = 0.82$-0.89, SEE = 1.1 METs) (Freedson, Melanson, and Sirard 1998; Nichols et al. 2000). Ainsworth and colleagues (Ainsworth, Bassett, et al. 2000) showed large discrepancies in time spent (e.g., min $\times$ day^{-1}) within defined EE categories under free-living conditions between detailed PA logs and MTI data using three sets of accelerometer count cutoff points (Freedson, Melanson, and Sirard 1998; Hendelman et al. 2000; Swartz et al. 2000).

Tritrac accelerometer. The Tritrac (Hemokinetics Inc., Madison, WI) has been the most frequently used triaxial accelerometer, although other types of triaxial devices have been developed (e.g., Tracmor; see Bouten et al. 1996). Typically these devices provide count data for each separate plane as well as an integrated vector magnitude (Vmag) of counts for all planes combined. Estimates of EE are available through equations that account for body mass and resting EE. A regression equation ($R^2 = 0.90$, SEE = 0.014 kcal $\times$ kg^{-1} $\times$ min^{-1}) has been developed during treadmill walking and running to estimate PA-related EE from Tritrac Vmag (Nichols et al. 1999):

$$EE \ (kcal \times kg^{-1} \times min^{-1}) = 0.018673 + (0.000029051 \times Vmag \times min^{-1})$$

It is curious that the preceding regression equation to predict EE using a triaxial monitor was developed during activity that results in acceleration in essentially one plane (e.g., vertical). Theoretically, measurement in three planes (vertical, horizontal, lateral) should

account for more sources of body movement and therefore provide a more precise estimate of PA-related EE, particularly under lifestyle conditions. This hypothesis, however, has not been universally supported. Some studies show that concurrent uniaxial and triaxial accelerometer measures provided similar information on PA patterns (Masse et al. 1999). Others have shown that triaxial devices have lower error in estimating EE under laboratory conditions and stronger correlations with both laboratory ($r_{triaxial} = 0.84$-0.93 versus $r_{uniaxial} = 0.76$-0.85) and lifestyle activity ($r_{triaxial} = 0.59$-0.62 versus $r_{uniaxial} = 0.48$-0.59) EE (Hendelman et al. 2000; Welk, Blair et al. 2000). Total daily EE estimated from doubly labeled water has been strongly correlated with triaxial accelerometer data ($r = 0.73$) (Bouten et al. 1996), whereas others report low correlations ($r \leq 0.26$) between doubly labeled water and several field PA measures, including an uniaxial accelerometer (Fogelholm et al. 1998).

Although data from accelerometers can be used to assess frequency, duration, and intensity of physical activity, the specific type of physical activity is unknown. Accelerometers tend to overestimate the EE of walking and underestimate the EE of lifestyle activities. Energy expenditure owed to activities involving the upper extremities or increased resistance to body movement (e.g., uphill walking) is not well accounted for. Large variability exists among laboratory-based accelerometer count cutoff points used to classify health-related levels of EE under free-living conditions. Population-specific equations may be required to categorize PA levels accurately among target populations (e.g., sedentary or overweight) that differ from the typical college-aged, active, Caucasian individuals commonly used to develop published regression equations. Device placement appears to be particularly important for the MTI accelerometer; however, whether increased central adiposity or increased ground reaction forces associated with large body mass also influence accelerometer measurements has yet to be empirically determined. Subject compliance issues, potentially altered physical activity patterns, and the cost of the more sophisticated instruments (uniaxial ~ $250, triaxial ~ $550 per unit) limit the practicality of using motion detectors to measure PA and EE in large studies of free-living individuals.

Summary of Direct Physical Activity Assessment Methods

PA records, logs, and recalls provide much detail on the type and pattern of PA and allow for easy computation of PA-related EE. However, issues related to individual recall ability, response bias (recall bias, social desirability bias), and the potential for altered physical activity patterns or poor compliance while completing the PA records or logs may limit their use in population-based studies or interventions. Motion sensors provide objective and reliable data on PA, especially walking behavior. However, methods for estimating EE from motion sensor data are only moderately precise, with particular limitations across the range of moderate-intensity lifestyle activities included in health-related PA recommendations.

Indirect Physical Activity Assessment Methods

Investigators use indirect assessment methods to acquire surrogate measures of PA among large populations of free-living individuals when direct methods would be cost prohibitive and impractical. Indirect PA measures are typically validated against objective direct measures of PA in controlled, small sample studies so that EE estimates can be reasonably precise. The most common indirect method is the self-report PA recall questionnaire.

PA Questionnaires

Self-report questionnaires are used most frequently to assess PA in public health surveillance systems, in large-scale epidemiological studies of health-related outcomes, and in some clinical research or intervention settings. Table 9.1 provides a list of questionnaires that have been used to estimate PA and EE expenditure in various studies. Based on their level of detail and subject burden, PA questionnaires are generally classified as global, recall, and quantitative history instruments (Ainsworth, Montoye, and Leon 1994; LaMonte and Ainsworth 2001; Montoye et al. 1996).

Global questionnaires. Global PA questionnaires are typically one- to four-item instruments that are used to estimate general levels of PA. Although they are short and easy to complete, global questionnaires provide little detail on specific types and patterns of PA, and allow for only simple PA classifications (e.g., active versus inactive) (Belloc and Breslow 1972; Siscovick et al. 1988). Global questionnaires have been used in large epidemiological studies (Salonen, Puska, and Tuomilehto 1982; Shapiro et al. 1965; Siscovick et al. 1988) that aim to identify information about health-related risk factors and disease cofactors. Global questionnaires are preferred in public health surveillance systems (Macera and Pratt 2000; Slater et al. 1987) where administrative time is limited and the PA assessment goal for PA is to track long-term population PA trends or to broadly determine whether or not respondents meet national PA recommendations (Macera and Pratt 2000).

The accuracy and reproducibility of these types of PA instruments has been acceptable (Ainsworth, Jacobs, and Leon 1993; Jacobs et al. 1993). Test-retest correlations of 0.90 and 0.81 for men and women, respectively, and an age- and sex-adjusted coefficient of determination between the PA question and maximal aerobic capacity of 0.29 was reported among respondents to the two-point Lipid Research Clinics PA question (Ainsworth, Jacobs, and Leon 1993; Siscovick et al. 1988). However, because of limited detail regarding the type, frequency, duration, and intensity of PA, global questionnaires are insufficient for estimating activity-related EE. Thus, global questionnaires have limited utility for assessing PA in weight loss settings or as a part of clinical intervention trials.

Recall questionnaires. Compared with the global survey, recall instruments are more complex (10 to 20 items) and more burdensome to complete. However, they allow for very specific assessment of frequency, duration, and types of PA during the past day, week, or month. Scoring systems differ among recall questionnaires, ranging from simple ordinal scales (e.g., 1-5 representing low to high levels of PA) (Baecke, Burema, and Frijters 1982; Magnus, Matroos, and Strackee 1979), to unitless summary indices (e.g., exercise units) (Mayer et al. 1991), to comprehensive scores of continuous data (e.g., kcal, kJ, or MET – min $\times$ day^{-1}) (Ainsworth, LaMonte et al. 2000; Blair et al. 1985; Paffenbarger et al. 1986). The advantage of the latter measure is the ability to evaluate dose-response relationships (Paffenbarger et al. 1986) between health outcomes

Table 9.1 Self-Report Methods and Cutoff Points Used to Quantify Levels of Physical Activity and Energy Expenditure in Free-Living Populations

Method or questionnaire[a]	Type of activity[b]	Recall time frame	Burden[c]	Expression of PA score[d,e]	Dose-response assessment[f]	Author (reference)
General recommendations:						
CDC-ACSM	JOB, EX, SP, LEIS, TRAN, HH			Light (<3 METs) Moderate (3-6 METs) Vigorous (>6 METs)		Pate et al. 1995
ACSM	EX, SP, LEIS			Very light (<20% HRR)* Light (20-39%) Moderate (40-59%) Hard (60-84%) Very hard (≥85%) Maximal (100%)		ACSM 1998
Surgeon General	JOB, EX, SP, LEIS, TRAN, HH			≥150 kcal × d⁻¹ or 1,000 kcal × wk⁻¹		U.S. Dept. of Health & Human Services 1996
Global questionnaires:						
NSPHPC	TOTAL (relative to peers)	General	Low	5-point qualitative scale 2-point qualitative scale	No No	Slater et al. 1987 Belloc et al. 1972
Lipid Research Clinics	JOB, EX JOB, NON-JOB, EX	Usual day	Low	2-point qualitative scale 4-point qualitative scale	No No	Siscovick et al. 1988 Ainsworth, Jacobs, & Leon 1993
HIP	JOB, NON-JOB, TRAN, TOTAL	General	Low	4-point ordinal scale 3-point qualitative scale	No	Shapiro et al. 1965
BRFSS	JOB, EX, SP, LEIS, HH, CARE	Usual day	Low	3-point qualitative scale	No	Macera et al. 2000
Recall questionnaires:						
Baecke	JOB, SP, LEIS	General	Moderate	5-point ordinal scale	No	Baecke et al. 1982
Magnus	EX, LEIS	Past year	Low	2- and 4-point ordinal scale	No	Magnus et al. 1979

San Luis Valley	JOB, EX, LEIS, HH	Past 7 days	Moderate	$kJ \times kg^{-1} \times wk^{-1}$ Ordinal scales	Yes	Mayer et al. 1991
Seven-Day Recall	EX, LEIS	Past 7 days	Moderate	$kcal \times kg^{-1} \times d^{-1}$	Yes	Blair et al. 1985
College Alumnus	EX, SP, LEIS	Past 7 days	Moderate	$kcal \times wk^{-1}$	Yes	Paffenbarger et al. 1986
Typical Week Survey	JOB, EX, SP, LEIS, TRAN, HH, YRD, CARE, VOL, TOTAL	Typical week during past month	Moderate	MET-min $\times d^{-1}$	Yes	Ainsworth, LaMonte, et al. 2000
Quantitative history questionnaires:						
MNLTPA	EX, SP, LEIS, HH	Past year	High	AMI $\times d^{-1}$	Yes	Taylor et al. 1978
Tecumseh OPA	JOB, TRAN	Past year	Moderate	MET-hr $\times wk^{-1}$	Yes	Montoye 1971
Parker LTPA	EX, SP, LEIS	Past year	High	Summary index in kcal $\times kg^{-1} \times wk^{-1}$	Yes	Parker et al. 1988
Historical PA	SP, LEIS	Lifetime	High	Ordinal scale in hr $\times wk^{-1}$ and kcal $\times wk^{-1}$	Yes	Kriska et al. 1988

[a] CDC = Centers for Disease Control; ACSM = American College of Sports Medicine; NSPHPC = National Survey of Personal Health Practices & Consequences; HIP = Health Insurance Plan of Greater New York Study of Coronary Heart Disease; BRFSS = Behavioral Risk Factor Surveillance System; San Luis Valley = San Luis Valley Diabetes Study; MNLTPA = Minnesota LTPA; Tecumseh OPA = Tecumseh, Michigan, Occupational PA Survey; LTPA = leisure-time physical activity.

[b] JOB = occupational; EX = exercise; SP = sport; TRAN = transportation; LEIS = leisure; HH = household; YRD = yard work; CARE = caregiving; VOL = volunteer; TOTAL = total physical activity.

[c] Administrative burden including cost, time to administer/respond, data management/processing time.

[d] MET = metabolic equivalent; AMI = Activity Metabolic Index; kcal = kilocalorie; kJ = kilojoule; kg = kilogram.

[e] Qualitative scale refers to categories such as "More Active versus Less Active" or "Sedentary versus Active." Ordinal scale refers to an ordered range of numbers (e.g., 1-5) used to rank activity status (e.g., low to high).

[f] It is possible to evaluate dose-response relationships with health-related outcomes using quantifiable units for the exposure (PA) variable that approximate the PA units used within the general public health recommendations

* HRR, heart rate reserve; ACSM (12,13) also presents intensity levels in terms of % maximal HR, % $\dot{V}O_2$ reserve, RPE, and by METs stratified on categories of age.

Reprinted, by permission, from "Quantifying energy expenditure and physical activity in the context of dose response," *Medicine and Science in Sports and Exercise* 33(6 Supl): S370-S378.

and levels of PA or estimated EE defined by published recommendations (Pate et al. 1995; U.S. Department of Health and Human Services 1996).

Recall surveys have demonstrated acceptable levels of accuracy and repeatability (Ainsworth, LaMonte et al. 2000; Ainsworth, Leon et al. 1993; Blair et al. 1985; Jacobs et al. 1993). One-month test-retest correlations for an EE index computed from self-reported walking, stair climbing, and sport activity (Paffenbarger et al. 1986) were 0.61 and 0.75 for men and women, respectively, who completed the College Alumnus questionnaire (Ainsworth, Leon et al. 1993). Among all participants, criterion validity correlations between the EE index and Caltrac accelerometer METs $\times$ day^{-1} and kcal $\times$ day^{-1} were 0.29 and 0.17, respectively. Most recall surveys do not adequately assess nonoccupational and nonleisure PA, which may be particularly relevant sources of health-related EE among women and minorities (Masse et al. 1998; Weller and Corey 1998). Ainsworth and colleagues (Ainsworth, LaMonte et al. 2000) reported test-retest correlations of 0.43 to 0.62, and criterion validity correlations of 0.45 to 0.47 between detailed PA logs and summary scores for total, light, moderate, and vigorous MET – min $\times$ day^{-1} from a comprehensive Typical Week PA Survey administered to minority women 40 and older.

Recall questionnaires are preferred for studies of PA and health. The administrative burden is relatively low, and summary scores can easily be computed for time spent in specific activities of interest (e.g., walking), or in units that equate with health-related levels of EE (Pate et al. 1995; U.S. Department of Health and Human Services 1996). PA recall instruments have three primary limitations. First, the PA estimate is subject to errors in recall that may result in under- or overestimating the actual PA performed (Durante and Ainsworth 1996; Lichtman et al. 1992). Second, the structure of the instrument may not include relevant population-specific sources of PA (LaMonte and Ainsworth 2001; Masse et al. 1998). Finally, interpretation of the wording of questionnaire items may vary considerably by sex, race/ethnicity, socioeconomic status, and cultural diversity (Warenecke et al. 1997).

Quantitative history questionnaires. The longest and most detailed of the PA questionnaires are quantitative histories, which generally have more than 20 items. Typically these instruments assess the frequency and duration of leisure time and/or occupational physical activities obtained in the past year (Taylor et al. 1978) or through a lifetime (Kriska et al. 1988). Activity scores are usually expressed as a continuous variable (e.g., kcal $\times$ kg^{-1} $\times$ wk^{-1}) (Jacobs et al. 1993; Kriska, Sandler et al. 1988; Parker, Leaf, and McAfee 1988), allowing for evaluation of total or activity-specific EE, or dose-response effects on health parameters using recommended EE cutoff points (e.g., $\geq$14 kcal $\times$ kg^{-1} $\times$ wk^{-1}) (U.S. Department of Health and Human Services 1996).

Two popular quantitative history questionnaires are the Minnesota Leisure Time Physical Activity Questionnaire (MNLTPA; Taylor et al. 1978) and the Tecumseh Self-Administered Occupational Questionnaire (TOQ; Montoye 1971). The MNLTPA uses a one-year recall frame to identify the frequency (events per year) and average duration (time per event) of 74 items. Activity items are clustered in categories for walking, conditioning, hunting and fishing, water, winter, sports, home repair, and household maintenance activities.

One-year test-retest correlations for total, light, moderate, and heavy MET-min $\times$ day^{-1} were 0.69, 0.60, 0.32, and 0.71, respectively, among adults responding to the MNLTPA (Richardson et al. 1994). Criterion validity correlations of 0.75, 0.72, 0.70, and 0.75 were reported between MNLTPA and four-week PA history summary scores of total, light, moderate, and heavy MET-min $\times$ day^{-1}. Additionally, the MNLTPA has been used by investigators to show an inverse association between PA and mortality among high-risk men enrolled in the Multiple Risk Factor Intervention Trial (Leon et al. 1987). The TOQ (Montoye 1971) also uses a one-year recall frame to identify time spent in 28 different job activities grouped according to the type and intensity of activity (e.g., light intensity, sitting, heavy manual labor). Ainsworth, Jacobs, and colleagues (1993) established the reliability and validity of this instrument. Because the MNLTPA and the TOQ use similar questionnaire formats, the summary scores can be added to create a score for the energy expended in leisure and occupational settings.

Similar to the "remote diet recall" used to assess past dietary habits (Willett 1998), quantitative PA histories are useful in settings in which investigators and practitioners are interested in identifying detailed PA patterns over a prolonged period. This level of PA assessment may be particularly important when relating activity exposure to chronic diseases with lengthy incubation periods, such as cancer and coronary artery disease, and perhaps progressive weight gain typical of middle-aged Americans. However, since quantitative history questionnaires can take 60 minutes or longer to complete, and because of the intensive recall required by the respondent, these instruments have limited use in most research and clinical settings.

Cardiorespiratory Fitness

Habitual PA levels are closely related to $\dot{V}O_2$ or "cardiorespiratory fitness" (*fitness*) (Blair, Mulder, and Kohl 1987; LaMonte, Durstine et al. 2001; Saltin and Rowell 1980; Stofan et al. 1998). While factors like age, sex, genetics, and health status contribute to individual differences in fitness, the major determinant of fitness is the degree to which a person is regularly active in moderate to vigorous intensity physical activity (Bouchard, Malina, and Perusse 1997; Saltin and Rowell 1980; Stofan et al. 1998). Therefore, submaximal and maximal exercise testing have been used to *estimate* fitness without the additional burden and cost of ventilatory gas analysis and indirect calorimetry procedures (American College of Sports Medicine 1995). Submaximal fitness is reported as the heart rate response at a standard submaximal work rate (Slattery and Jacobs 1988) or the rate of submaximal work achieved (e.g., $kg \times m^{-1} \times min^{-1}$) during a standard exercise protocol (Sobolski et al. 1987). Maximal fitness is typically reported as total work (e.g., $kg \times m^{-1} \times min^{-1}$) performed during cycle ergometry (Sandvick et al. 1993), or as METs derived from treadmill exercise time or the speed and grade of the final treadmill exercise stage (American College of Sports Medicine 1995; Bruce, Kusumi, and Hosmer 1973). Studies have shown strong favorable associations for cardiorespiratory fitness with disease risk factors (Blair et al. 1989; LaMonte et al. 2000), and with mortality from all causes and cardiovascular disease (Blair et al. 1989; Sandvick et al. 1993; Slattery and Jacobs 1988; Sobolski et al. 1987). Changes in fitness have been a strong predictor of long-term

weight status in several studies (DiPietro et al. 1998; Lewis et al. 1997). In the Aerobics Center Longitudinal Study (Blair et al. 1989), maximal fitness has been positively related to habitual PA (Stofan et al. 1998), attenuated weight gain (DiPietro et al. 1998), and lower risk of mortality even among men with BMI >30 (Wei, Kampert, Barlow et al. 1999). These observations do suggest that PA, per se, isn't a significant factor for weight loss and maintenance. Rather, it may be that PA of sufficient duration or intensity to achieve a certain level of fitness is required for successful management of body composition and related health risks.

Exercise testing is safe (Gibbons et al. 1989), precise (Blair et al. 1989; Bruce, Kusumi, and Hosmer 1973), and highly reproducible (Skinner et al. 1999; Wilmore et al. 1998) and can be performed among overweight and obese populations (Wei et al. 1999). Thus, it may be the most accurate assessment of sedentary or irregularly active lifestyles that are associated with habitually low levels of EE and resultant weight gain. An advantage of using cardiorespiratory fitness as an estimate of habitual PA is the ability to prescribe individualized PA interventions and verify changes in certain types of PA through changes in fitness (American College of Sports Medicine 1995; Yanowitz 1996). Although fitness is closely related to habitual PA, a fitness score (e.g., maximal METs) tells little about the type or pattern of lifestyle PA and EE that contributed to an individual's measured fitness level. This limits the use of fitness assessment as a quantitative measure of PA patterns in free-living individuals. Lack of agreement over the degree to which cardiorespiratory fitness, PA, and EE influence specific health parameters through shared or independent effects (Haskell 1994), as well as feasibility considerations, currently challenge the practicality of assessing fitness as the primary indirect measure of PA or EE in large-scale studies or interventions targeting specific PA behaviors (e.g., walking) and health outcomes (e.g., weight loss). Fitness assessment may be a useful adjuvant to other PA measures in research and clinical settings.

Summary of Indirect Physical Activity Assessment Methods

Questionnaires that elicit self-reports of PA are the most common method for assessing

PA in large epidemiological studies of free-living individuals. A variety of questionnaire structures have been used with adequate precision for broadly categorizing PA levels, assessing time spent in specific PA, and computing estimates of EE. Although concerns over the limitations of human recall and reporting biases are valid, self-report questionnaires provide a relatively easy, inexpensive, and nonreactive method of assessing PA and estimating EE in large free-living populations. Estimating cardiorespiratory fitness through clinical exercise testing provides an objective reproducible measure of recent PA that may be useful for differentiating sedentary and regularly active populations, or to verify changes in PA consequent to intervention. However, fitness measures tell little about individual or population patterns of free-living PA. Lack of a gold standard measure of PA in field settings complicates the choices of an appropriate instrument for assessing activity levels and the related EE in specific field, clinical, and intervention settings.

Measurement of Energy Expenditure

A large amount of heat energy results from the complex biochemical processes that provide the metabolic energy requirements to support skeletal muscle contraction during PA (Brooks, Fahey, and White 1996). Because the rate of heat production is directly proportional to the amount of energy expended, EE can be precisely assessed by directly measuring body heat at rest or during exercise (Montoye et al. 1996). The oxidation of food substrate is a primary source of energy production at rest and both during and following PA. Therefore, PA-related EE can be assessed indirectly by measuring the rate of oxygen consumption under various conditions of metabolic demand (Brooks, Fahey, and White 1996; Montoye et al. 1996). Following is an overview of direct and indirect methods (see figure 9.1) used to assess EE in a variety of research and clinical settings.

Direct Energy Expenditure Assessment Methods

Precise measures of free-living EE is extremely difficult, burdensome, and costly. The most accurate methods of direct EE assessment generally require sophisticated laboratory instrumentation, which further limits direct EE assessment in large free-living populations. However, direct methods of EE measurement are often used in small, controlled laboratory studies aimed at developing cost-effective field measures of PA-related EE.

Direct Calorimetry

The most precise measure of EE is direct calorimetry, which is the measurement of body heat production (Horton 1983; Montoye et al. 1996). Calorimetry is a laboratory-based measure performed with an individual in a small airtight chamber that contains insulated pipes used to circulate water through the calorimeter. By carefully measuring the temperature and flow rate of the water as well as all sources of heat loss from the chamber, a subject's heat production, and thereby EE, can be measured at rest to within 1 to 2% error (Horton 1983). Measurements are typically made over a 24-hour period and follow a 10- to 12-hour fast so that resting metabolic rate (RMR) can be accurately assessed. Because room calorimeters are small and confined, they are not practical for assessing the EE related to PA. Further, a lag time between body heat release during exercise and calorimeter measurement requires extended periods of observation to obtain precise EE measures during PA. To circumvent this issue, Webb, Annis, and Troutman (1980) used a mobile water-cooled suit to perform direct calorimetric measures of EE during controlled bouts of PA (e.g., cycle ergometry). Although this technique is more conducive to studies of PA-related EE, accuracy may be lower (EE within 3 to 23% of room calorimetry) (Webb, Annis, and Troutman 1980). Issues with dissipating perspiration may make moderate to vigorous PA intolerable and limit the types of PA that can be studied. Altered mechanical efficiency during exercise may bias the EE measure away from a true representation of free-living EE. Generally, cost and technical limitations make direct calorimetry infeasible for assessing PA-related EE in most settings.

Doubly Labeled Water (DLW)

The DLW method has been used to assess human energy expenditure under laboratory and field conditions (Black et al. 1996; Bouten et al. 1996; Conway et al. 1999; Lichtman et al. 1992; Livingstone et al. 1990; Ravussin et al. 1991; Seale 1995; Seale, Conway, and Canary 1993; Seale et al. 1990). Energy expenditure estimated from DLW is based on the rate of metabolic carbon dioxide production ($\dot{V}CO_2$) (Speakman 1998). DLW consists of the stable water isotopes ^2H_2O and $H_2^{18}O$, and is administered to subjects as a liquid dosed according to body size. Labeled hydrogen (^2H_2O) is excreted as water alone, while labeled oxygen ($H_2^{18}O$) is lost as water and CO_2 ($C^{18}O_2$) through the carbonic anhydrase system. The difference in isotope turnover rates provide an estimate of metabolic CO_2 production (Speakman 1998). Urinary isotope excretion is tracked with mass spectrometry over several days. Oxygen uptake ($\dot{V}O_2$) and EE are extrapolated from $\dot{V}CO_2$ and estimated respiratory quotient (RQ) derived from established equations.

DLW estimates of EE have been within 1 to 20% of those derived from measured oxygen uptake at rest and varied PA intensities (Conway et al. 1999; Seale et al. 1990; Westersterp et al. 1988). Apparent inaccuracies between DLW and indirect calorimetry may reflect the ability of DLW to capture a greater EE under free-living conditions than can be simulated and measured under controlled laboratory conditions. Although doubly labeled water provides precise estimates of free-living EE over prolonged periods (e.g., weeks), this technique is limited to studies of total energy expenditure and does not differentiate among the duration, frequency, or intensity of specific physical activities. Further, the isotope assays may be cost prohibitive for use in large population-based studies of PA and health outcomes.

Labeled Bicarbonate

The labeled bicarbonate ($NaH^{14}CO_3$) method is very similar to DLW and has been used in shorter study periods (e.g., days) of free-living EE (Elia et al. 1995). After the isotope is infused at a constant rate, it is diluted by the body's natural metabolic CO_2 production. After recovering the labeled carbons from expired air, blood, urine, or saliva, the extent of isotopic dilution is used to determine $\dot{V}CO_2$ from which EE can be calculated based on assumptions made about RQ. Recent studies under

controlled experimental conditions have reported EE estimates from this method within <6% of EE measured in a respiratory chamber (Elia, Fuller, and Murgatroyd 1992; Elia et al. 1995; el-Khoury et al. 1994).

Summary of Direct Energy Expenditure Assessment Methods

While direct measures provide the most precise assessment of EE, their expense and highly technical nature may preclude their use in population-based studies or interventions of PA and health outcomes. Field methods are limited to isotope studies that measure only total EE, which may have limited value for assessing and prescribing PA according to current health-related recommendations. The utility of direct measures of EE for clinical purposes and validating field techniques for assessing PA, however, should not be understated.

Indirect Energy Expenditure Assessment Methods

Several indirect methods have been used to assess PA-related EE outside the constraints of research or clinical laboratories. These procedures are typically validated against direct EE measures and provide more cost-effective options for assessing EE in free-living populations.

Oxygen Uptake ($\dot{V}O_2$)

Energy expenditure estimates derived from indirect calorimetry are based on assumed relations between $\dot{V}O_2$ and the caloric cost of substrate oxidation under various conditions (Brooks, Fahey, and White 1996; Ferrannini 1988; Montoye et al. 1996). Similar to the room calorimeter, the respiratory chamber is an airtight insulated temperature- and humidity-controlled room into which known concentrations of O_2 and CO_2 are introduced at a known flow rate and sampled as they leave the system (Jequier and Schutz 1983; Montoye et al. 1996; Rumpler et al. 1990). Based on the gas concentrations of expired air, rates of carbon dioxide production ($\dot{V}CO_2$) and oxygen uptake ($\dot{V}O_2$) can be determined. Together, $\dot{V}O_2$ and RQ ($\dot{V}CO_2/\dot{V}O_2$) can be used to estimate EE in kcal $\times$ min^{-1} according Weir's equation (Weir 1949):

$$EE \ (kcal \times min^{-1}) = \dot{V}O_2 \ (3.9 + 1.1 \ RQ)$$

Several factors can result in large differences between actual and estimated RQ, including differences in the caloric cost of specific substrate oxidation, bicarbonate buffering of metabolic CO_2 during exercise, and postexercise oxygen consumption kinetics. Therefore, obtaining a precise measure of RQ, which involves urinary nitrogen collection (Ferrannini 1988), is required for precise estimates of EE from indirect calorimetry.

Although respiratory chambers are expensive and require a large space and extensive upkeep, they have been used for studies of PA under a limited set of circumstances (Jequier and Schutz 1983; Schulz et al. 1991; Rumpler et al. 1990). Because free-living PA patterns are likely to be altered in a respiratory chamber, alternative methods for performing indirect calorimetry outside the chamber have been employed. These techniques are based on the same principles described previously and use an integrated measurement system comprised of an O_2 and CO_2 analyzer; a ventilation flow-volume meter; and a microcomputer that processes expired air collected through a fitted hood, face mask, or mouthpiece (Davis 1996; Voorrips et al. 1993). The development of small, portable indirect calorimeters (e.g., Cosmed K4 b²) have allowed for field assessment of $\dot{V}O_2$ (Bassett et al. 2000; Hausswirth, Bigard, and Le Chevalier 1997; King et al. 1999). However, issues pertaining to costs, the necessity of wearing cumbersome and obtrusive instrumentation, altered patterns of physical activity, and lack of well-established validity and reliability in a variety of field settings limit the usefulness of this approach to quantifying EE in free-living population studies of PA and health.

Heart Rate (HR)

One of the simplest measures related to EE is heart rate, for which several recording instruments exist (Montoye et al. 1996). Energy expenditure has been estimated from HR based on the assumption of a strong linear relation between HR and $\dot{V}O_2$ (Berggren and Christensen 1950; Consolazio et al. 1971; Wilmore and Haskell 1971). Individual HR–$\dot{V}O_2$ calibration curves (Haskell et al. 1993; Washburn and Montoye 1986) are recommended to overcome considerable between-person HR–$\dot{V}O_2$ variability. Variation in the HR–$\dot{V}O_2$ relationship during low-intensity PA (Christensen et

al. 1983) has led some researchers to recommend establishing a heart rate "threshold" prior to estimating EE from the HR–$\dot{V}O_2$ calibration curve (Livingstone et al. 1990). This threshold is referred to as the "FLEX HR" and is determined from metabolic studies at various work intensities. Resting EE is used to determine the energy cost of activities that elicit a HR below FLEX HR, while the individual HR–$\dot{V}O_2$ calibration curve is used to estimate EE for activities with an HR above FLEX HR. Other techniques that have been used to estimate EE from HR include time spent in specific HR intensity ranges (Fogelholm et al. 1998; Washburn and Montoye 1986) and activity HR minus sedentary HR (Andrews 1971).

Schulz, Westersterp, and Bruck (1989) reported correlations of 0.53 to 0.73 between EE estimated from DLW and HR using individual HR–$\dot{V}O_2$ calibration, while Livingstone and colleagues (1990) demonstrated a range of difference scores of –22% to +52% between EE estimates from DLW and FLEX HR. Two other studies reported differences of –11% to +20% in EE estimated with a respiratory chamber and with FLEX HR (Ceesay et al. 1989; Spurr et al. 1988). Strath and colleagues (2000) recently showed a strong correlation ($r = 0.87$, SEE = 0.76 METs) between EE estimated from HR reserve and EE estimated from indirect calorimetry among adults performing moderate-intensity lifestyle and laboratory activities. The authors emphasize the potential value of EE estimates based on relative versus absolute HR measures in reducing between-person sources of variation that may be related to age, sex, and fitness level. Recent evidence that the HR–$\dot{V}O_2$ relationship may differ among obese versus nonobese populations (Byrne and Hills 2002) emphasizes the need to develop HR monitoring methods of estimating free-living EE specific to obese individuals. Furthermore, some researchers have failed to demonstrate that estimating EE from HR is substantially more precise than estimating EE from detailed PA records (Acheson et al. 1980; Kwalkwarf et al. 1989).

Although the HR–$\dot{V}O_2$ relationship is linear over a wide range of PA intensities, this is frequently not the case during low and very high intensity activity (Christensen et al. 1983; Freedson and Miller 2000). Because many daily activities are low to moderate intensity (Ainsworth, Haskell et al. 2000), HR monitoring may not provide precise estimates of habitual daily EE among free-living individuals. Several factors influence HR without having substantial effects on oxygen uptake, which may result in imprecise estimates of PA-related EE. Such factors include body temperature, size of the active muscle mass (e.g., upper vs. lower body), type of exercise (static vs. dynamic), stress, and medication (Acheson et al. 1980; Freedson and Miller 2000; Montoye et al. 1996). Day-to-day HR variability is also likely to reduce the reliability of EE estimates (Christensen et al. 1983; Livingstone et al. 1990). Additionally, the need to develop individual HR–$\dot{V}O_2$ calibration curves (Haskell et al. 1993) and instrumentation costs ($\geq$\$150 per unit) make HR monitoring a less suitable surrogate of PA or EE in health-related research. Heart rate monitoring, however, may be useful as part of an integrated multisystem approach (e.g., combined HR-motion monitoring) to population-based PA or EE assessment (Haskell et al. 1993; Healey 2000).

Body Temperature and Ventilation

A close relationship between EE and core body temperature (Berggren and Christensen 1950) and ventilation (Consolazio et al. 1971) has been reported under laboratory conditions. Hence, continuous monitoring of these variables could provide a means of extrapolating EE under certain conditions. However, body temperature and ventilation measures of EE may be limited by time requirements, several confounding factors, and inconvenient measurement techniques (LaMonte and Ainsworth 2001). The utility of these measurements may be as part of an integrated monitoring system rather than as a single measure of EE among free-living individuals (Healey 2000).

Summary of Indirect Energy Expenditure Assessment Methods

Several indirect methods of estimating EE under field conditions are available for use by researchers and practitioners. Each method has limitations related to interindividual variation in the measured variable as well as ancillary factors that may confound each method's true association with EE. Portable indirect calorimeters may be the most accurate indirect method for assessing EE in the field; however, behavior would likely be altered using this technique. Development of small, nonobtrusive integrated systems that employ multiple indirect measures of EE may improve the accuracy and feasibility of estimating EE under field conditions or as part of PA interventions aimed at weight loss or related risk factor modification.

Physical Activity Assessment of Overweight Persons

Currently, no single technique is considered to be the gold standard for assessing PA or EE among free-living overweight or obese individuals. Methods that have been used to assess PA and estimate EE among overweight persons vary little from procedures used among persons with average body weight and adiposity. However, depending on the level of overweight, some measurement techniques may be less precise than expected.

Prediction equations used to estimate EE from direct and indirect measures of PA were generally developed among active and fit Caucasian men and women with average body mass and percent body fat (Freedson, Melanson, and Sirard 1998; Melanson and Freedson 1995; Nichols et al. 1999). Thus, the use of these equations to estimate the EE of movement among overweight and obese individuals may be inappropriate (Byrne and Hills 2002). Results of a recent study of weight-bearing PA among middle-aged lean and obese women suggest that MET intensities used to estimate the energy cost of human movement might lead to underestimation of true EE in overweight and obese individuals (Schmitz 1998). Race/ethnicity is another important modifying factor for both activity-related EE and levels of body fat (Hunter et al. 2000), and therefore must be considered when measuring and prescribing PA and weight loss among ethnically diverse populations. Because MET levels presented in the Compendium of Physical Activities (Ainsworth, Haskell et al. 2000) represent an absolute scale for assigning intensity levels to PA record, log, and questionnaire items, erroneous conclusions could be made about habitual levels of EE among obese individuals who may also be severely deconditioned (Howley 2001).

The pedometer and accelerometers are less accurate at slow walking speeds and fail to differentiate the energy cost of graded ambulation (Melanson and Freedson 1995; Nichols et al. 2000; Washburn, Chin, and Montoye 1980; Welk, Differding et al. 2000). Schmitz (1998) noted that the MET intensities used to estimate the energy cost of human movement may underestimate the true metabolic cost of PA-related EE in overweight and obese individuals. This researcher also showed that obese women self-select slower movement paces, and hence a lower rate of EE, compared with normal weight women when completing the same ambulatory task. This may result in underestimation of the actual movement and related EE obtained among overweight persons if the excessive body mass and adiposity limits walking to very slow speeds. Additionally, it is not currently known whether accelerometer and pedometer sensitivity to vertical forces of footstrike are different among obese individuals compared with normal weight individuals. The degree to which excessive abdominal or waist adipose tissue physically influences a motion sensor worn at the hip is also currently unknown.

Physical activity questionnaires are the most feasible method for measuring patterns of PA, inactivity, and related EE in large free-living populations of obese individuals. Unfortunately, no such instrument has been developed and validated for use in this population. Traditional PA questionnaires focusing mostly on moderate to vigorous occupational, sport, and leisure activities (Ainsworth, Montoye, and Leon 1994; LaMonte and Ainsworth 2001) may not be sensitive to activity patterns typical of obese individuals. Physical activity records or logs may be useful to establish usual patterns of PA and inactivity among several obese populations varying in geographical and cultural factors. Focus groups and individual debriefings could provide additional resolution to both the qualitative and quantitative aspects of information obtained for the records or logs. Such data would then be used to develop and validate PA recall questions that address PA patterns within the specific demographic and sociocultural characteristics of obese individuals. Concerns over minimizing recall bias (Durante and Ainsworth 1996) and whether to use absolute or relative activity-related energy costs to derive EE estimates from PA questionnaire response (Ainsworth, Haskell et al. 2000; Howley 2001) would need

to be addressed. Notwithstanding, development of a valid recall questionnaire for use in large populations of obese individuals would hopefully transfer to improved epidemiological surveillance of PA among the obese; more precise assessment of dose-response relationships between PA, EE, and obesity-related disease; and enhanced ability to target specific activities for successful weight loss intervention.

Summary

Physical activity is an important determinant of body weight and composition and is a requirement for successful programs aimed at achieving and maintaining weight loss (American College of Sports Medicine 2001). The exact amount of activity-related EE for weight loss and maintenance is currently unknown, partly because accurate assessment of free-living PA and EE is difficult (Grundy et al. 1999). Advantages and disadvantages exist for all of the currently available methods of assessing free-living PA and related EE. Motion sensors (e.g., the MTI accelerometer) can provide valid estimates of the time spent in sedentary activity, which may be a particularly important as sedentary and nonsedentary low-intensity leisure PA are considered separate domains with independent risks for obesity (Ching et al. 1996). Measures of fitness from clinical exercise testing provide a highly objective measure of the adverse cardiorespiratory effects of sedentary living, and can be used to individualize PA intervention and verify changes in specific types of PA. Use of PA logs and recall questionnaires are feasible for population-based assessment and provide both qualitative and quantitative information on patterns of PA and inactivity. The best measure of free-living activity-related EE among obese and nonobese populations may be an integrated method that provides both qualitative (PA log or recall questionnaire) and quantitative (accelerometer, DLW) information.

Research objectives to improve the aforementioned methods have been proposed (LaMonte and Ainsworth 2001). The degree to which these and other methodological issues in measuring PA and EE are realized will be an important impetus for advancing the current understanding of physical activity's role in the growing epidemic of obesity and will provide the correct referent point for prescribing additional levels of activity-related EE to promote weight loss, modify metabolic abnormalities associated with overweight or obesity, and prevent weight regain among the formerly obese.

References

Acheson, K.J., Campbell, I.T., Edholm, O.G., Miller, D.S., and Stock, M.J. 1980. The measurement of daily energy expenditure—An evaluation of some techniques. *American Journal of Clinical Nutrition* 33: 1155-1164.

Ainsworth, B.E., Bassett, D.R., Strath, S.J., Swartz, A.M., O'Brien, W.L., Thompson, R.W., Jones, D.A., Macera, C.A., and Kimsey, C.D. 2000. Comparison of three methods for measuring the time spent in physical activity. *Medicine and Science in Sports and Exercise* 32 (9 Suppl. l): S457-S464.

Ainsworth, B.E., Haskell, W.L., Whitt, M.C., Irwin, M.L., Swartz, A.M., Strath, S.J., O'Brien, W.L., Bassett, D.R., Schmitz, K.H., Emplaincourt, P.O., Jacobs, D.R., and Leon, A.S. 2000. Compendium of physical activities: An update of activity codes and MET intensities. *Medicine and Science in Sports and Exercise* 32 (9 Suppl.): S498-S516.

Ainsworth, B.E., Irwin, M.L., Addy, C.L., Whitt, M.C., and Stolarczyk, L.M. 1999. Moderate physical activity patterns of minority women: The Cross-Cultural Activity Participation Study. *Journal of Women's Health* 8: 805-813.

Ainsworth, B.E., Jacobs, D.R., and Leon, A.S. 1993. Validity and reliability of self-reported physical activity status: The Lipid-Research Clinics questionnaire. *Medicine and Science in Sports and Exercise* 25: 92-98.

Ainsworth, B.E., Jacobs, D.R., Leon, A.S., Richardson, M.T., and Montoye, H.J. 1993. Assessment of the accuracy of physical activity questionnaire occupational data. *Journal of Occupational Medicine* 35: 1017-1027.

Ainsworth, B.E., LaMonte, M.J., Drowatzky, K.L., Cooper, R.S., Thompson, R.W., Irwin, M.L., Whitt, M.C., and Gilman, M. 2000. Evaluation of the CAPS Typical Week Physical Activity Survey among minority women. In *Proceedings of the community prevention research in women's health conference*, 17. Bethesda, MD: National Institutes of Health.

Ainsworth, B.E., Leon, A.S., Richardson, M.T., Jacobs, D.R., and Paffenbarger, R.S. 1993. Accuracy of the College Alumnus Physical Activity Questionnaire. *Journal of Clinical Epidemiology* 46: 1403-1411.

Ainsworth, B.E., Montoye, H.J., and Leon, A.S. 1994. Methods of assessing physical activity during leisure and work. In *Physical activity, fitness, and health*, eds. C. Bouchard, R. Shephard, and T. Stephens, 146-159. Champaign, IL: Human Kinetics.

American Association for Active Lifestyles and Fitness. 2000. Proceedings from the 9th Measurement and Evaluation Symposium of the Movement and Evaluation Council of the American Association for Active Lifestyles and Fitness. *Research Quarterly for Exercise and Sport* 71 (2 Suppl.): 1-158.

American College of Sports Medicine. 1995. *Guidelines for exercise testing and prescription*, 5th ed. Baltimore: Williams & Wilkins.

American College of Sports Medicine. 1998. The recommended quantity and quality of exercise for developing and maintaining cardiorespiratory and muscular fitness, and flexibility in healthy adults. *Medicine and Science in Sports and Exercise* 30: 975-991.

American College of Sports Medicine. 2001. Appropriate intervention strategies for weight loss and prevention of weight regain for adults. *Medicine and Science in Sports and Exercise* 33: 2145-2156.

Andrews, R.B. 1971. Net heart rate as a substitute for respiratory calorimetry. *American Journal of Clinical Nutrition* 24: 1139-1147.

Baecke, J.A.H., Burema, J., and Frijters, J.E.R. 1982. A short questionnaire for the measurement of habitual physical activity in epidemiological studies. *American Journal of Clinical Nutrition* 36: 936-942.

Bassett, D.R., Ainsworth, B.E., Leggett, S.R., Mathien, C.A., Main, J.A., Hunter, D.C., and Duncan, G.E. 1996. Accuracy of five electronic pedometers for measuring distance walked. *Medicine and Science in Sports and Exercise* 28: 1071-1077.

Bassett, D.R., Ainsworth, B.E., Swartz, A.M., Strath, S.J., O'Brien, W.L., and King, G.A. 2000. Validity of four motion sensors in measuring moderate intensity physical activity. *Medicine and Science in Sports and Exercise* 32 (9 Suppl.): S471-S480.

Bassey, E.J., Dallosso, H.M., Fentem, P.H., Irving, J.M., and Patrick, J.M. 1987. Validation of a simple mechanical accelerometer (pedometer) for the estimation of walking activity. *European Journal of Applied Physiology* 56: 323-330.

Belloc, N.B., and Breslow, L. 1972. Relationship of physical health status and health practices. *Preventive Medicine* 1: 409-421.

Berggren, G., and Christensen, E.H. 1950. Heart rate and body temperature as indices of metabolic rate during work. *Arbeitsphysiologie* 14: 255-260.

Black, A.E., Coward, W.A., Cole, T.J., and Prentice, A.M. 1996. Human energy expenditure in affluent societies: An analysis of 574 doubly-labeled water measurements. *European Journal of Clinical Nutrition* 50: 72-92.

Blair, S.N. 1993. Evidence for success of exercise in weight loss and control. *Annals of Internal Medicine* 119: 702-706.

Blair, S.N., Haskell, W.L., Ho, P., Paffenbarger, R.S., Vranizan, K.M., Farquhar, J.W., and Wood, P.D. 1985. Assessment of habitual physical activity by a seven-day recall in a community survey and controlled experiments. *American Journal of Epidemiology* 122: 794-804.

Blair S.N., Kohl, H.W., Paffenbarger, R.S., Clark, D.G., Cooper, K.H., and Gibbons, L.W. 1989. Physical fitness and all-cause mortality. A prospective study of healthy men and women. *Journal of the American Medical Association* 262: 2395-2401.

Blair S.N., Mulder, R.T., and Kohl, H.W. 1987. Reaction to "secular trends in adult physical activity: Exercise boom or bust?" *Research Quarterly in Exercise and Sport* 58: 106-110.

Bouchard C., Malina, R.M., and Perusse, L. 1997. *Genetics of fitness and physical performance.* Champaign, IL: Human Kinetics.

Bouchard, C., Tremblay, A., Leblanc, C., Lortie, G., Savard, R., and Theriault, G. 1983. A method to assess energy expenditure in children and adults. *American Journal of Clinical Nutrition* 37: 461-467.

Bouten, C.V.C., Wilhelmine, P.H.G., De Venne, V., Westersterp, K.R., Verduin, M., and Janssen, J.D. 1996. Daily physical activity assessment: Comparison between movement registration and doubly labeled water. *Journal of Applied Physiology* 81: 1019-1026.

Brooks, G.A., Fahey, T.D., and White, T.P. 1996. *Exercise physiology. Human bioenergetics and its application,* 2nd ed. Mountain View, CA: Mayfield.

Bruce, R.A., Kusumi, F., and Hosmer, D. 1973. Maximal oxygen intake and nomographic assessment of functional aerobic impairment in cardiovascular disease. *American Heart Journal* 85: 546-562.

Byrne, N.M., and Hills, A.P. 2002. Relationships between HR and $\dot{V}O_2$ in the obese. *Medicine and Science in Sports and Exercise* 34: 1419-1427.

Ceesay, S.M., Prentice, A.M., Day, K.C., Murgatroyd, P.R., Goldberg, G.R., and Scott, W. 1989. The use of heart rate monitoring in the estimation of energy expenditure: A validation study using indirect whole-body calorimetry. *British Journal of Nutrition* 61: 175-186.

Ching, P.L.Y.H., Willett, W.C., Rimm, E.B., Colditz, G.A., Gortmaker, S.L., and Stampfer, M.J. 1996. Activity level and risk of overweight in male health professionals. *American Journal of Public Health* 86: 25-30.

Christensen, C.C., Frey, H.M.M., Foenstelien, E., Aadland, E., and Rafsum, H.E. 1983. A critical review of energy expenditure estimates based on individual O_2 consumption/heart rate curves and average daily heart rate. *American Journal of Clinical Nutrition* 37: 468-472.

Consolazio, C.F., Nelson, R.A., Daws, T.A., Krzywicki, H.J., Johnson, H.L., and Barnhart, R.A. 1971. Body weight, heart rate, and ventilatory volume relationships to oxygen uptake. *American Journal of Clinical Nutrition* 24: 1180-1185.

Conway, J.M., Seale, J.R., Irwin, M.L., Jacobs, D.R., and Ainsworth, B.E. 1999. Ability of 7-day physical activity diaries and recalls to estimate free-living energy expenditure. *Obesity Research* 7(Suppl. 1): 107S.

Davis, J.A. 1996. Direct determination of aerobic power. In *Physiological assessment of human fitness,* eds. P.J. Maud and C. Foster, 9-17. Champaign, IL: Human Kinetics.

DiPietro, L., Kohl, H.W., Barlow, C.E., and Blair, S.N. 1998. Improvements in cardiorespiratory fitness attenuate age-related weight gain in healthy men and women: The Aerobics Center Longitudinal Study. *International Journal of Obesity* 22: 55-62.

Durante, R., and Ainsworth, B.E. 1996. The recall of physical activity: Using a cognitive model of the question-answering process. *Medicine and Science in Sports and Exercise* 28: 1282-1291.

Elia, M., Fuller, N.J., and Murgatroyd, P.R. 1992. Measurement of bicarbonate turnover in humans: Applicability to estimation of energy expenditure. *American Journal of Physiology* 263: E676-E687.

Elia, M., Jones, M.G., Jennings, G., Poppitt, S.D., Fuller, N.J., Murgatroyd, P.R., and Jebb, S.A. 1995. Estimating energy expenditure from specific activity of urine urea during lengthy subcutaneous NaH14CO3 infusion. *American Journal of Applied Physiology* 269: E172-E182.

el-Khoury, A.E., Sanchez, M., Fukagawa, N.K., Gleason, R.E., and Young, V.R. 1994. Similar 24-h pattern and rate of carbon dioxide production, by indirect calorimetry vs. stable isotope dilution, in healthy adults under standardized metabolic conditions. *Journal of Nutrition* 124: 1615-1627.

Ferrannini, E. 1988. The theoretical bases of indirect calorimetry. *Metabolism* 37: 287-301.

Fogelholm, M., Hilloskorpi, H., Laukkanen, R., Oja, P., Van Marken Lichtenbelt, W., and Westersterp, K. 1998. Assessment of energy expenditure in overweight women. *Medicine and Science in Sports and Exercise* 30: 1191-1197.

Freedson, P.S., Melanson, E., and Sirard, J. 1998. Calibration of the Computer Science and Applications, Inc. accelerometer. *Medicine and Science and Sports and Exercise* 30: 777-781.

Freedson, P.S., and Miller, K. 2000. Objective monitoring of physical activity using motion sensors and heart rate. *Research Quarterly for Exercise and Sport* 71: 21-29.

Gayle, R., Montoye, H.J., and Philpot, J. 1977. Accuracy of pedometers for measuring distance walked. *Research Quarterly for Exercise and Sport* 48: 632-636.

Gibbons, L., Blair, S.N., Kohl, H.W., and Cooper, K. 1989. The safety of maximal exercise testing. *Circulation* 80: 846-852.

Grundy, S.M., Blackburn, G., Higgins, M., Lauer, R., Perri, M.G., and Ryan, D. 1999. Physical activity in the prevention and treatment of obesity and its co-morbidities: Evidence report of independent panel to assess the role of physical activity in the treatment of obesity and its comorbidities. *Medicine and Science in Sports and Exercise* 31 (11 Suppl.): S502-S508.

Haskell, W.L. 1994. Health consequences of physical activity: Understanding and challenges regarding dose-response. *Medicine and Science in Sports and Exercise* 26: 649-660.

Haskell, W.L., Yee, M.C., Evans, A., and Irby, P.J. 1993. Simultaneous measurement of heart rate and body motion to quantitate physical activity. *Medicine and Science in Sports and Exercise* 25: 109-115.

Hatano, Y. 1993. Use of pedometers for promoting daily walking exercise. *International Council for Health, Physical Education, and Recreation* 29: 4-8.

Hausswirth, C., Bigard, A.X., and Le Chevalier, J.M. 1997. The Cosmed K4 telemetry system as an accurate device for oxygen uptake measurements during exercise. *International Journal of Sports Medicine* 18: 449-453.

Healey, J. 2000. Future possibilities in electronic monitoring of physical activity. *Research Quarterly for Exercise and Sport* 71: 137-145.

Hendelman, D., Miller, K., Bagget, C., Debold, E., and Freedson, P. 2000. Validity of accelerometry for the assessment of moderate intensity physical activity in the field. *Medicine and Science in Sports and Exercise* 32 (9 Suppl.): S442-S449.

Henderson K.A., and Ainsworth, B.E. 2000. Sociocultural perspectives on physical activity on the lives of older African American and American Indian women: A Cross-Cultural Activity Participation Study. *Women & Health* 31: 1-20.

Hill, J.O., and Melanson, E.L. 1999. Overview of the determinants of overweight and obesity: Current evidence and research issues. *Medicine and Science in Sports and Exercise* 31: S515-S521.

Horton E.S. 1983. An overview of the assessment and regulation of energy balance in humans. *American Journal of Clinical Nutrition* 38: 972-977.

Howley, E.T. 2001. Type of activity: Resistance, aerobic, and leisure versus occupational physical activity. *Medicine and Science in Sports and Exercise* 33 (6 Suppl.): S364-S369.

Hunter, G.R., Weinsier, R.L., Darnell, B.E., Zuckerman, P.A., and Goran, M.I. 2000. Racial differences in energy expenditure and aerobic fitness in premenopausal women. *American Journal of Clinical Nutrition* 71: 500-506.

Irwin, M.L., Mayer-Davis, E.J., Addy, C.L., Pate, R.R., Durstine, J.L., Stolarczyk, L.M., and Ainsworth, B.E. 2000. Moderate-intensity physical activity and fasting insulin levels in women. *Diabetes Care* 23: 449-454.

Jacobs, D.R., Ainsworth, B.E., Hartman, T.J., and Leon, A.S. 1993. A simultaneous evaluation of 10 commonly used physical activity questionnaires. *Medicine and Science in Sports and Exercise* 25: 81-91.

Jequier, E. and Schutz, Y. 1983. Long-term measurements of energy expenditure in humans using a respiratory chamber. *American Journal of Clinical Nutrition* 38: 989-998.

Jones, D.A., Ainsworth, B.E., Croft, J.B., Macera, C.A., Lloyd, E.E., and Yusuf, H.R. 1998. Moderate leisure-time physical activity. Who is meeting the public health recommendations? A national cross-sectional study. *Archives of Internal Medicine* 7: 285-289.

King, G.A., McLaughlin, J.E., Howley, E.T., Bassett, D.R., and Ainsworth, B.E. 1999. Validation of Aerosport KB1-C portable metabolic system. *International Journal of Sports Medicine* 20: 304-308.

Klem, M.L., Wing, R.R., McGuire, M.T., Seagle, H.M., and Hill, J.O. 1997. A descriptive study of individuals successful at long-term maintenance of substantial weight loss. *American Journal of Clinical Nutrition* 66: 239-246.

Kriska, A.M., and Caspersen, C.J., eds. 1997. A collection of physical activity questionnaires for health-related research. *Medicine and Science in Sports and Exercise* 29 (6 Suppl.): S1-S205.

Kriska, A.M., Sandler, R.B., Cauley, J.A., LaPorte, R.E., Hom, D.L., and Pambianco, G. 1988. The assessment of historical physical activity and its relation to adult bone parameters. *American Journal of Epidemiology* 127: 1053-1063.

Kwalkwarf, H.J., Haas, J.D., Belko, A.Z., Roach, R.C., and Roe, D.A. 1989. Accuracy of heart-rate monitoring and activity diaries for estimating energy expenditure. *American Journal of Clinical Nutrition* 49: 37-43.

LaMonte, M.J., and Ainsworth, B.E. 2001. Quantification of energy expenditure and physical activity: Methods and issues in the context of dose response. *Medicine and Science in Sports and Exercise* 33 (6 Suppl.): S370-S378.

LaMonte, M.J., Durstine, J.L., Addy, C.L., Irwin, M.L., and Ainsworth, B.E. 2001. Physical activity, physical fitness, and Framingham 10-year risk score: The Cross-Cultural Activity Participation Study. *Journal of Cardiopulmonary Rehabilitation* 21: 63-70.

LaMonte, M.J., Eisenman, P.A., Adams, T.D., Shultz, B.B., Ainsworth, B.E., and Yanowitz, F.G. 2000. Cardiorespiratory fitness and coronary heart disease risk factors. The LDS Hospital Fitness Institute Cohort. *Circulation* 102: 1623-1628.

Leon, A.S., Connett, J., Jacobs, D.R., and Rauramaa, R. 1987. Leisure-time physical activity levels and risk of coronary heart disease and death. *Journal of the American Medical Association* 258: 2388-2395.

Levin, S., Jacobs, D.R., Ainsworth, B.E., Richardson, M.T., and Leon, A.S. 1999. Intra-individual variation and estimates of usual physical activity. *Annals of Epidemiology* 9: 481-488.

Lewis, C.E., Smith, D.E., Wallace, D.D., Williams, O.D., Bild, D.E., and Jacobs, D.R. 1997. Seven-year trends in body weight and associations with lifestyle and behavioral characteristics in black and white young adults: The CARDIA Study. *American Journal of Public Health* 87: 635-642.

Lichtman, S.W., Pisarska, K., Raynes Berman, E.R., Pestone, M., Dowling, H., Offenbacher, E., Weisel, H., Heshka, S., Matthews, D.E., and Heymsfield, S.B. 1992. Discrepancy between self-reported and actual caloric intake and exercise in obese subjects. *New England Journal of Medicine* 327: 1893-1888.

Livingstone, M.B., Prentice, A.M., Coward, W.A., Ceesay, S.M., Strain, J.J., McKenna, P.G., Nevin, G.B., Barker, M.E., and Hickey, R.J. 1990. Simultaneous measurement of free-living energy expenditure by the doubly labeled water method and heart-rate monitoring. *American Journal of Clinical Nutrition* 52: 59-65.

Macera, C.A., and Pratt, M. 2000. Public health surveillance of physical activity. *Research Quarterly for Exercise and Sport* 71: 97-103.

Magnus, K., Matroos, A., and Strackee, J. 1979. Walking, cycling, or gardening, with or without seasonal interruption, in relation to acute coronary events. *American Journal of Epidemiology* 110: 724-733.

Masse L.C., Ainsworth, B.E., Tortolero, S., Levin, S., Fulton, J.E., Henderson, K.A., and Mayo, K. 1998. Measuring physical activity in midlife, older, and minority women: Issues from an expert panel. *Journal of Women's Health* 7: 57-67.

Masse, L.C., Fulton, J.E., Watson, K.L., Heesch, K.C., Kohl, H.W., Blair, S.N., and Tortolero, S.R. 1999. Detecting bouts of physical activity in a field setting. *Research Quarterly for Exercise and Sport* 70: 212-219.

Matthews, C.E., DuBose, K.D., LaMonte, M.J., Tudor-Locke, C.E., and Ainsworth, B.E. 2002. Evaluation of a computerized 24-hour physical activity recall. *Medicine and Science in Sports and Exercise* 34 (5 Suppl.): S41.

Matthews, C.E., Freedson, P.S., Hebert, J.R., Stanek, E.J., Merriam, P.A., and Ockene, I.S. 2000. Comparing physical activity assessment methods in the Seasonal Variation of Blood Cholesterol Study. *Medicine and Science in Sports and Exercise* 32: 976-984.

Mayer, E.J., Alderman, B.W., Regensteiner, J.G., Marshall, J.A., Haskell, W.L., Baxter, J., and Hamman, R.F. 1991. Physical activity assessment measures compared in a biethnic rural population: The San Luis Valley Diabetes Study. *American Journal Clinical Nutrition* 53: 812-820.

McClung, C.D., Zahiri, C.A., Higa, J.K., Amstutz, H.C., and Schmalzried, T.P. 2000. Relationship between Body Mass Index and activity in hip or knee arthroplasty patients. *Journal of Orthopedic Research* 18: 35-39.

Melanson, E., and Freedson, P. 1995. Validity of the Computer Science and Applications, Inc. (CSA) activity monitor. *Medicine and Science in Sports and Exercise* 27: 934-940.

Montoye, H.J. 1971. Estimation of habitual physical activity by questionnaire and interview. *American Journal of Clinical Nutrition* 24: 1113-1118.

Montoye, H.J., Kemper, H.C.G., Saris, W.H.M., and Washburn, R.A. 1996. *Measuring physical activity and energy expenditure.* Champaign, IL: Human Kinetics.

Montoye, H.J., Washburn, R., Servais, S., Ertl, A., Webster, J.G., and Nagle, F.J. 1983. Estimation of energy expenditure by a portable accelerometer. *Medicine and Science in Sports and Exercise* 15: 403-407.

National Heart, Lung, and Blood Institute. 1998. *Clinical guidelines on the identification, evaluation, and treatment of overweight and obesity in adults: The evidence report.* Rockville, MD: National Institutes of Health; National Heart, Lung, and Blood Institute.

Nelson, T.E., Leenders, N.Y.J., and Sherman, W.M. 1998. Comparison of activity monitors worn during treadmill walking. *Medicine and Science in Sports and Exercise* 30 (5 Suppl.): S11.

Nichols, J.F., Morgan, C.G., Chabot, L.E., Sallis, J.F., and Calfas, K.J. 2000. Assessment of physical activity with the Computer Science and Applications, Inc., accelerometer: Laboratory versus field validation. *Research Quarterly for Exercise and Sport* 71: 36-43.

Nichols, J.F., Morgan, C.G., Sarkin, J.A., Sallis, J.F., and Calfas, K.J. 1999. Validity, reliability, and calibration of the Tritrac accelerometer as a measure of physical activity. *Medicine and Science in Sports and Exercise* 31: 908-912.

Paffenbarger, R.S., Hyde, R.T., Wing, A.L., and Hsieh, C.C. 1986. Physical activity, all-cause mortality, and longevity of college alumni. *New England Journal of Medicine* 314: 605-613.

Pambianco, G., Wing, R.R., and Robertson, R. 1990. Accuracy and reliability of the Caltrac accelerometer for estimating energy expenditure. *Medicine and Science in Sports and Exercise* 22: 858-862.

Parker, D.L., Leaf, D.A., and McAfee, S.R. 1988. Validation of a new questionnaire for the assessment of leisure time physical activity. *Annals of Sports Medicine* 4: 72-81.

Pate, R.R., Pratt, M., Blair, S.N., Haskell, W.L., Macera, C.A., Bouchard, C., Buchner, D., Ettinger, W., Heath, G.W., King, A.C., Kriska, A., Leon, A.S., Marcus, B.H., Morris, J., Paffenbarger, R.S., Patrick, K., Pollock, M.L., Rippe, J.M., Sallis, J., and Wilmore, J.H. 1995. Physical activity and public health. A recommendation from the Centers for Disease Control and Prevention and the American College of Sports Medicine. *Journal of the American Medical Association* 273: 402-407.

Ravussin, E., Harper, I.T., Rising, R., and Boagardus, C. 1991. Energy expenditure by doubly labeled water: Validation in lean and obese subjects. *American Journal of Physiology* 261: E402-E409.

Richardson, M.T., Leon, A.S., Jacobs, D.R., Ainsworth, B.E., and Serfass, R. 1994. Comprehensive evaluation of the Minnesota Leisure Time Physical Activity questionnaire. *Journal of Clinical Epidemiology* 47: 271-281.

Richardson, M.T., Leon, A.S., Jacobs, D.R., Ainsworth, B.E., and Serfass, R. 1995. Ability of the Caltrac accelerometer to assess daily physical activity levels. *Journal of Cardiopulmonary Rehabilitation* 15: 107-113.

Rowlands, A.V., Eston, R.G., and Ingledew, D.K. 1997. Measurement of physical activity in children with particular reference to the use of heart rate and pedometry. *Sports Medicine* 24: 258-272.

Rowlands, A.V., Eston, R.G., and Ingledew, D.K. 1999. Relationship between activity levels, aerobic fitness, and body fat in 8- to 10-yr-old children. *Journal of Applied Physiology* 86: 1428-1435.

Rumpler, W.V., Seale, J.L., Conway, J.M., and Moe, P.W. 1990. Repeatability of 24-h energy expenditure measurements in humans by indirect calorimetry. *American Journal of Clinical Nutrition* 51: 147-152.

Salonen, J.T., Puska, P., and Tuomilehto, J. 1982. Physical activity and risk of myocardial infarction, cerebral stroke and death. *American Journal of Epidemiology* 115: 526-537.

Saltin, B., and Rowell, L. 1980. Functional adaptations to physical activity and inactivity. *Federation Proceedings* 39: 1506-1513.

Sandvick, L., Erikssen, J., Thaulow, E., Erikssen, G., Mundal, R., and Rodahl, K. 1993. Physical fitness as a predictor of mortality among healthy, middle-aged Norwegian men. *New England Journal of Medicine* 328: 533-537.

Schmitz, M.K.H. 1998. The interactive and independent associations of physical activity, body weight, and blood lipid levels. Unpublished Ph.D. dissertation, University of Minnesota, Minneapolis, MN.

Schmitz, M.K.H., Jacobs, D.R., Leon, A.S., Schreiner, P.J., and Sternfeld, B. 1998. Physical activity and weight: Ten year follow-up in the CARDIA study. *Medicine and Science in Sports and Exercise* 30(5 Supl): S127.

Schulz, L.O., Nyomba, B.L., Alger, S., Anderson, T.E., and Ravussin, E. 1991. Effects of endurance training on sedentary energy expenditure measured in a respiratory chamber. *Journal of Applied Physiology* 260: E257-E261.

Schulz, S., Westersterp, K.R., and Bruck, K. 1989. Comparison of energy expenditure by the doubly labeled water technique with energy intake, heart rate, and activity recording in man. *American Journal of Clinical Nutrition* 49: 1146-1154.

Seale, J.L. 1995. Energy expenditure measurements in relation to energy requirements. *American Journal of Clinical Nutrition* 62: 1042S-1046S.

Seale, J.L., Conway, J.M., and Canary, J.J. 1993. Seven-day validation of doubly labeled water method using indirect calorimetry. *Journal of Applied Physiology* 74: 402-409.

Seale, J.L., Rumpler, W.V., Conway, J.M., and Miles, C.W. 1990. Comparison of double labeled water, intake balance, and direct- and indirect-calorimetry methods for measuring energy expenditure in adult men. *American Journal of Clinical Nutrition* 52: 66-71.

Shapiro, S, Weinblatt, E., Frank, C.W., and Sager, R.V. 1965. The H.I.P. Study of incidence and prognosis of coronary heart disease. Preliminary findings on incidence of myocardial infarction and angina. *Journal of Chronic Disease* 18: 527-558.

Shepherd, E.F., Toloza, E., McClung, C.D., and Schmalzried, T.P. 1999. Step activity monitor: Increased accuracy in quantifying ambulatory activity. *Journal of Orthopedic Research* 17: 703-708.

Siscovick, D.S., Ekelund, L.G., Hyde, J.S., Johnson, J.L., Gordon, D.J., and LaRosa, J.C. 1988. Physical activity and coronary heart disease among asymptomatic hypercholesterolemic men. *American Journal of Public Health* 78: 1428-1431.

Skinner, J.S., Wilmore, K.M., Jaskolska, A., Jaskolski, A., Daw, E., Rice, T., Gagnon, J., Leon, A.S., Wilmore, J.H., Rao, D.C., and Bouchard, C. 1999. Reproducibility of maximal exercise test data in the Heritage Family Study. *Medicine and Science in Sports and Exercise* 31: 1623-1628.

Slater, C.H., Green, L.W., Vernon, S.W., and Keith, V.M. 1987. Problems in estimating the prevalence of physical activity from national surveys. *Preventive Medicine* 16: 107-118.

Slattery M.L., and Jacobs, D.R., 1988. Physical fitness and cardiovascular disease mortality: The U.S. Railroad study. *American Journal of Epidemiology* 127: 571-580.

Sobolski, J., Kornitzer, M., De Backer, G., Dramaix, M., Abramowicz, M., Degre, S., and Denolin, H. 1987. Protection against ischemic heart disease in the Belgian Physical Fitness Study: Physical fitness rather than physical activity? *American Journal of Epidemiology* 125: 601-610.

Speakman, J.R. 1998. The history and theory of the doubly labeled water technique. *American Journal of Clinical Nutrition* 68: 932S-938S.

Spurr, G.B., Prentice, A.M., Murgatroyd, P.R., Goldberg, G.R., Reina, J.C., and Christman, N.T. 1988. Energy expenditure from minute-by-minute heart rate recording: Comparison with indirect calorimetry. *American Journal of Clinical Nutrition* 48: 552-559.

Stofan, J.R., DiPiettro, L., Davis, D., Kohl, H.W., and Blair, S.N. 1998. Physical activity patterns associated with cardiorespiratory fitness and reduced mortality: The Aerobics Center Longitudinal Study. *American Journal of Public Health* 88: 1807-1813.

Strath, S.J., Swartz, A.M., Bassett, D.R., O'Brien, W.L., King, G.A., and Ainsworth, B.E. 2000. Evaluation of heart rate as a method for assessing moderate intensity physical activity. *Medicine and Science in Sports and Exercise* 32 (9 Suppl.): S465-S470.

Swartz, A.M., Strath, S.J., Bassett, D.R., O'Brien, W.L., King, G.A., and Ainsworth, B.E. 2000. Estimation of energy expenditure using CSA accelerometers at hip and waist sites. *Medicine and Science in Sports and Exercise* 32 (9 Suppl.): S450-S456.

Taylor, H.L., Jacobs, D.R., Jr., Schucker, B., Knudsen, J., Leon, A.S., and De Backer, G. 1978. A questionnaire for the assessment of leisure time physical activities. *Journal of Chronic Disease* 31: 741-744.

Tudor-Locke, C.E., Ainsworth, B.E., Whitt, M.C., Thompson, R.W., Addy, C.L., and Jones, D.A. 2001. The relationship between Digiwalker-determined physical activity and body composition variables. *International Journal of Obesity and Related Metabolic Disorders* 25: 1571-1578.

Tudor-Locke, C.E., Bell, R.C., Myers, A.M., Harris, S.B., Mitek, N., and Rodger, N.M. 2002. Pedometer-determined ambulatory activity in individuals with type 2 diabetes. *Diabetes Research and Clinical Practice* 55: 191-199.

Tudor-Locke, C.E., and Myers, A.M. 2001. Methodological considerations for researchers and practitioners using pedometers to measure physical (ambulatory) activity. *Research Quarterly for Exercise and Sport* 71: 1-12.

U.S. Department of Health and Human Services. 1996. Physical Activity and Health: A Report of the Surgeon General. Atlanta, GA: U.S. Department of Health and Human Services, Centers for Disease Control and Prevention, National Center for Chronic Disease Prevention and Health Promotion.

Voorrips, L.E., van Acker, T.M-C.J., Deurenberg, P., and Staveren, W.A. 1993. Energy expenditure at rest and during standardized activities: a comparison between elderly and middle-aged women. *American Journal of Clinical Nutrition* 58: 15-20.

Warencke, R.B., Johnson, T.P., Chavez, N., Sudman, S., O'Rourke, D.P., Lacey, L., and Horm, J. 1997. Improving question wording in surveys of culturally diverse populations. *Annals of Epidemiology* 7: 334-342.

Washburn, R.A., Chin, M.K., and Montoye, H.J. 1980. Accuracy of pedometer in walking and running. *Research Quarterly in Exercise and Sport* 51: 695-702.

Washburn, R.A., and Montoye, H.J. 1986. Validity of heart rate as a measure of daily energy expenditure. *Exercise Physiology* 2: 161-172.

Webb, P., Annis, J.F., and Troutman, S.J. 1980. Energy balance in man measured by direct and indirect calorimetry. *American Journal of Clinical Nutrition* 33: 1287-1298.

Wei, M., Kampert, J.B., Barlow, C.E., Nichaman, M.Z., Gibbons, L.W., Paffenbarger, R.S., and Blair, S.N. 1999. Relationship between low cardiorespiratory fitness and mortality in normal-weight, overweight, and obese men. *Journal of the American Medical Association* 282: 1547-1553.

Weir, J.B. 1949. New methods for calculating metabolic rate with special reference to protein metabolism. *Journal of Physiology* 109: 1-9.

Welk, G.J., Blair, S.N., Wood, K., Jones, S., and Thompson, R.W. 2000. A comparative evaluation of three accelerometry-based physical activity monitors. *Medicine and Science in Sports and Exercise* 32 (9 Suppl.): S489-S497.

Welk, G.J., Differding, J.A., Thompson, R.W., Blair, S.N., Dziura, J., and Hart, P. 2000. The utility of the Digi-Walker step counter to assess daily physical activity patterns. *Medicine and Science in Sports and Exercise* 32 (9 Suppl.): S481-S488.

Weller I., and Corey, P. 1998. The impact of excluding non-leisure energy expenditure on the relation between physical activity and mortality in women. *Epidemiology* 9: 632-635.

Westersterp, K.R., Brouns, F., Saris, W.H.M., and Ten Hoor, F. 1988. Comparison of doubly labeled water with respirometry at low- and high-activity levels. *Journal of Applied Physiology* 65: 53-56.

Wilcox, S., Irwin, M.L., Addy, C.L., Ainsworth, B.E., Stolarczyk, L., Whitt, M.C., and Tudor-Locke, C.E. 2001. Agreement between participant-rated and compendium-coded intensity of daily activities in a triethnic sample of women ages 40 years and older. *Annals of Behavioral Medicine* 23: 253-262.

Willett, W.C. 1998. *Nutritional epidemiology,* 2nd ed. New York: Oxford Press.

Wilmore, J.H., and Haskell, W.L. 1971. Use of the heart rate-energy expenditure relationship in the individualized prescription of exercise. *American Journal of Clinical Nutrition* 24: 1186-1192.

Wilmore, J.H., Stanforth, P.R., Turley, K.R., Gagnon, J., Daw, E., Leon, A.S., Rao, D.C., Skinner, J.S., and Bouchard, C. 1998. Reproducibility of cardiovascular, respiratory, and metabolic responses to submaximal exercise: The HERITAGE Family Study. *Medicine and Science in Sports and Exercise* 30: 259-265.

Yamanouchi, K., Shinozaki, T., Chikada, K., Toshihiko, N., Katsunori, I., Shimizu, S., and Sato, Y. 1995. Daily walking combined with diet therapy is a useful means for obese NIDDM patients not only to reduce body weight but also to improve insulin sensitivity. *Diabetes Care* 18: 775-778.

Yanowitz, F.G. 1996. Exercise prescription and cardiovascular fitness screening. In *Office sports medicine,* 2nd ed., ed. M.B. Mellion, 12-21. Philadelphia: Hanley and Belfus.

PART III

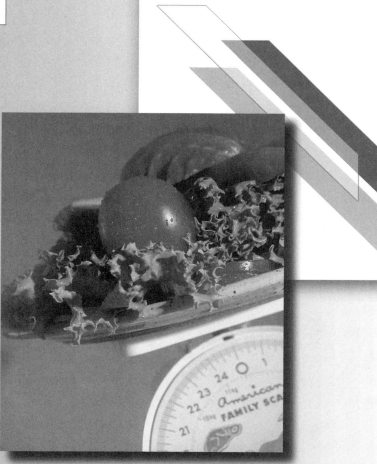

Treatment and Prevention

Chapter 10

The Importance of Body Weight Maintenance in Successful Aging

James Dziura, PhD, MPH
Loretta DiPietro, PhD, MPH
Yale University School of Medicine

Aging is associated with marked alterations in body composition. Of greater importance than obesity with regard to health and function in older age is the maintenance of body weight—specifically, the preservation of lean mass. Past the seventh decade of life, a decline in body weight occurs, which is at least partially explained by a loss of muscle mass or *sarcopenia*. Evidence suggests that muscle mass decreases 3 to 6% per decade (Flynn et al. 1989). Not totally distinct from sarcopenia is the increase in the proportion of total body fat that occurs with aging. As people age, body fat is redistributed within the body, with a preferential deposition to central and visceral, rather than subcutaneous, fat depots. As a result of these shifts in body composition, older individuals are at an increased risk for a number of functional (i.e., metabolic as well as physical) disorders.

This chapter will describe aging-related trends in body weight and the importance of these changes to the decline in metabolic and physical reserve. It will also discuss *disuse* and the importance of physical activity in the preservation of body weight and function in older people. Finally, the chapter will describe a number of determinants of physical activity in older populations and strategies for increasing physical activity among older sectors of the community.

Age-Related Changes in Body Weight

Body weight tends to increase throughout middle age, followed by a period of weight stabilization and then a decline in older age (>65 years) (Najjar and Rowland 1987) (see figure 10.1). More recent data from NHANES III report that mean body mass index (BMI = kg/m^2) steadily increases in men and women from ~ 24.9 and 24.0 kg/m^2, respectively, during ages 20 to 29 to ~ 27.5 and 28.5 kg/m^2 from ages 50 to 59 and then decreases to ~ 26.6 and 26.8 kg/m^2 by ages 70 to 74 (Flegal 1996). Several other cross-sectional studies corroborate this decline in body weight in later life (Butler et al. 1982; DiPietro et al. 1992; Shimokata, Andres et al. 1989; Shimokata, Tobin et al. 1989; Vaughan, Zurlo, and Ravussin 1991).

Although these observed cross-sectional age differences in body weight could be the result of selective survival, whereby lighter individuals have survived the putative factors associated with overweight in late middle age, Burr and Phillips (1984) argue

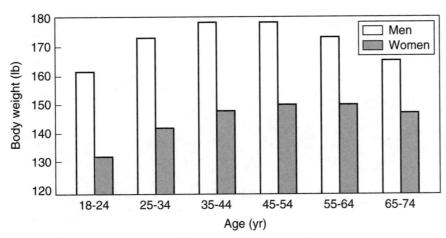

Figure 10.1 Age and body weight among U.S. men and women. From NHANES II, 1987.

that in older individuals mortality is associated with *underweight* rather than *overweight*. Furthermore, longitudinal studies confirm the decline in body weight with age, although the magnitude of this weight loss is variable (Dey et al. 1999; Shimokata, Andres et al. 1989; Steen, Lundgren, and Isaksson 1985; Stevens et al. 1991). Over the 25 years of follow-up in the Charleston Heart Study, Stevens and colleagues (1991) observed an increase in average body weight of 12 lb (5.4 kg) in those aged 37 to 46 at baseline and a *decline* of 6 lb (2.6 kg) in those aged 55 to 74 at baseline. Older men and women in the Yale Health and Aging Study lost an average of 1.3 lb (0.59 kg) *per year of aging* over the years between 1982 and 1994 (Dziura, Mendes de Leon, Kasl, and DiPietro, unpublished). Finally, Dey and colleagues (1999) reported a rate of weight loss among their cohort of older Swedish adults between 0.51 and 1.8 lb (0.23 and 0.80 kg) per year.

Aging-Related Changes in Body Composition

Possibly underlying the loss in body weight that occurs in older age is the dramatic shift in body composition. Most investigators agree that fat-free mass (FFM) declines with age while the proportion of body fat increases (Borkan et al. 1983; Evans 1995a, 1995b; Fiatarone-Singh 1998; Pollock et al. 1987; Steen 1988).

Lean Mass

Between the third and eighth decades of life FFM appears to decrease gradually by about 15% (Evans 1995a). A large part of the decline in FFM can be attributed to the loss of skeletal muscle tissue, as the maximal weight of human skeletal muscle achieved during early adulthood declines 40% by the age of 70 (Steen 1988). In comparison, losses of 18%, 11%, and 9% were observed for the liver, lungs, and kidney, respectively.

Using total body neutron activation methods, Cohn and colleagues (1980) verified cross-sectionally that declines in fat-free mass were primarily accounted for by losses in skeletal muscle. The muscle mass of older men (75 years) was observed to be 14% lower than that of younger men (21 years), and similarly, older women had 17% of the muscle mass of younger women. Measuring urinary creatinine excretion as a marker of total body muscle mass, Tzankoff and Norris (1977, 1978) also observed muscle mass to be 50% lower in the oldest men (~ 90 years) from the Baltimore Longitudinal Aging Study compared to the youngest men. In contrast, however, Flynn and colleagues (1989), using serial total body potassium analyses, observed slightly more modest declines in muscle mass of about 3 to 6% per decade in adult men and women.

Computed tomography (CT) scans comparing middle-aged (41 to 52 years) to older (59 to 76 years) men demonstrate that lean tissue areas were significantly smaller for cross-sections of the leg, abdomen, and upper arm in the older men, and that total lean body weight in older men was 88% of that of middle-aged men (Borkan et al. 1983). The term *sarcopenia*, derived from the Greek words *sarx* meaning "flesh" and *penia* meaning "loss," is now used to describe the age-related loss of muscle mass (Rosenberg 1997).

Body Fat

Not altogether distinct from sarcopenia is the aging-related increase in the proportion of body fat. Using total body potassium methods, Novak (1972) assessed cross-sectionally the amount of total body fat and fat-free mass in over 500 men and women between the ages of 18 and 85. Results showed that body fat was higher in older age groups than in younger age groups, ranging from 18 to 36% in young and old men, respectively, and from 33 to 45% in young and old women, respectively. The greater proportion of body fat with older age corresponded with a lower amount of fat-free mass, which dropped with age from 82 to 64% in men and from 67 to 55% in women. Similarly, the previously mentioned longitudinal study by Flynn and colleagues (1989) showed linear increases in the proportion of fat of between 3 and 5% per decade in men and women, respectively. Interestingly, among men the increase in the accumulation of body fat with time was accelerated in the oldest age group (i.e., >61 years).

Fat Distribution

Other investigators observed not only the increase in the proportion of fat mass with age but also the preferential redistribution of fat in the body (Borkan and Norris 1977; Carmelli, McElroy, and Rosenman 1991; Chien et al. 1975; Enzi et al. 1986). Current evidence suggests that regional differences in body fat distribution, particularly excess abdominal adiposity, are predictive of several chronic disorders including diabetes and cardiovascular diseases (Kissebah and Krakower 1994). Therefore, much attention has been given to the changes in fat patterning that occur with aging.

Shimokata and colleagues (1989a,b) observed that cross-sectional and five-year longitudinal measurements of waist and hip circumferences as well as waist-to-hip ratios (WHR) were higher with increasing age in both men and women aged 22 to 86 at baseline. Longitudinal data from the 23 years of follow-up of Caucasian men in the Western Collaborative Group Study showed that waist girth increased 6.2 cm and 3.5 cm (2.4 in. and

1.2 in.) in men aged 41 to 50 and 51 to 62 at baseline, respectively (Carmelli, McElroy, and Rosenman 1991). This corresponded to a similar aging-related increase in trunk-to-limb skinfold ratios observed in the same cohort. Further, regression analysis of the Charleston Heart Study cohort revealed a linear increase in abdominal girth, ranging from 2.8 to 7.5 cm (1 to 3 in.) over 25 years of follow-up, independent of changes in BMI (Stevens et al. 1991).

Measurement of subcutaneous versus visceral abdominal adipose tissue distribution using CT has revealed a distinct pattern with aging (Borkan et al. 1983; Borkan and Norris 1977; Enzi et al. 1986; Schwartz et al. 1991). Enzi and colleagues (1986) observed that subcutaneous-to-visceral fat ratios in both abdominal and thoracic compartments were inversely correlated with age, and that this correlation was primarily related to age-related increases in the visceral fat depot. Interestingly, despite relatively small differences in total body composition and circumference measures, Schwartz and colleagues (1991) reported that visceral fat depots were twofold greater in older men than in younger, whereas thigh subcutaneous fat was 48% lower in older men than in younger men. Similarly, in a comparison of middle-aged men to older men, Borkan and colleagues (1983) observed smaller areas of subcutaneous fat (206 cm^2 compared to 172 cm^2, respectively) and greater areas of visceral fat (126 cm^2 compared to 158 cm^2, respectively) in the older men. Furthermore, fat infiltration into and between muscles was significantly greater among the older men, a trend supported by a study of nursing home residents who had large deposits of intramuscular fat (Fiatarone et al. 1990).

In summary, it appears that the loss in body weight that accompanies older age is primarily the result of sarcopenia. Fat-free mass has been shown to decrease 15% between ages 30 and 90, with reductions in skeletal muscle mass accounting for the majority of this loss. Consequently, with the loss of lean tissue, the proportion of total body fat increases with age. While aging-related shifts in the storage of fat toward central and visceral depots are likely key components in the pathophysiology of metabolic disorders, the preservation of both the *quantity* and *quality* of skeletal muscle mass may also play an important role with regard to metabolic and functional resiliency.

Health Issues Related to Body Composition

Health issues related to excess body weight or adiposity may predominate in late middle age and early older age; however, in people over 75, anorexia, undernutrition, and consequent weight loss are concerns as well, as they often exist in combination with multiple chronic diseases. Andres and colleagues (1985) first reported the now well-recognized relationship between the extremes of body weight and mortality risk in aging. Indeed, this J- or U-shaped relationship between body weight and mortality suggests excess mortality risk among those who are overweight (due to cardiovascular disease and diabetes) and those who are underweight (due to cancer, pulmonary dysfunction, and infectious diseases). Although this pattern is observed across the age spectrum, generally it does not include persons considered the *oldest old* (i.e., ≥85 years) (Higgins et al. 1993). The lowest mortality associated with body weight for older people falls at a BMI of approximately 26 to 27 kg/m^2 (Andres et al. 1985), which is considerably higher than that observed for younger women (19 to 21 kg/m^2) (Willitt et al. 1995). Indeed, there is much controversy regarding the relative risks and benefits of small amounts of weight gain with aging (Fiatarone-Singh 1998).

The loss of lean mass with aging also poses a substantial threat to health in older people. Functional sequelae related specifically to the loss of muscle tissue include insulin resistance leading to type 2 diabetes (Pratley et al. 1995), as well as impairments in muscle strength (Nevitt et al. 1989), maximal aerobic capacity (Fleg and Lakatta 1988), resting metabolic rate (Tzankoff and Norris 1978), immune response (Morley, Glick, and Rubenstein 1995), and physical function and mobility (Fiatarone-Singh 1998). The loss of alpha motor neurons with aging contributes to this muscle atrophy (Fiatarone and Evans 1993), but increased sedentary behavior, catabolic illness, medications, and undernutrition play important roles as well (Fiatarone-Singh 1998).

Diabetes

Results from the National Health Interview Survey (NHIS) showed that the self-reported prevalence of physician-diagnosed diabetes was 1.3% in those aged 18 to 44 and >10% in those 65 years and older (National Center for Health Statistics 1992, 1994a, 1994b). Likewise, national estimates of type 2 diabetes incidence from the 1990-92 NHIS increased from 1.79 to 8.63 per 1,000 U.S. population for those aged 25 to 44 and 65 to 74, respectively (NCHS 1994b). Numerous community studies have also reported these age-related increases in both the incidence and prevalence of type 2 diabetes observed with national estimates (Barrett-Connor 1980; Bender et al. 1986; Butler et al. 1982; French et al. 1990; Hamman et al. 1989; Hanis et al. 1983).

Researchers have also studied the effect of age on the more functional outcomes of glucose tolerance and insulin sensitivity. The prevalence of impaired glucose tolerance in the United States follows a similar trend with age as seen with type 2 diabetes (Harris et al. 1987; Shimokata et al. 1991). Several smaller metabolic studies also offer supportive evidence for increased insulin resistance and poorer glucose tolerance with aging that can be explained primarily by aging-related impairments in peripheral tissue sensitivity (DeFronzo 1979; Fink et al. 1983; Rosenthal et al. 1982; Rowe et al. 1983).

Role of Lean Mass

Skeletal muscle is the primary tissue responsible for the clearance of a glucose load, and therefore a strong positive association exists between the loss of skeletal muscle mass and insulin resistance. Theoretically, sarcopenia has a profound effect on the ability of insulin to clear glucose from the bloodstream, as less muscle is available for glucose uptake and storage. Specifically, a preferential loss of type I muscle occurs (Saltin and Gollnick 1983), and the qualitative functional loss with regard to glucose homeostasis is exacerbated in the remaining muscle due to the reduction in fiber size, capillary density, and consequent lower diffusion capacity (Ivy, Zderic, and Fogt 1999). Data from strength training studies offer supportive evidence of a link between improvements in the quantity and quality of muscle mass and improved insulin sensitivity (Cüppers et al. 1982; Ivy, Zderic, and Fogt 1999). Unfortunately, epidemiological evidence relating sarcopenia in aging to insulin resistance or diabetes is lacking.

Role of Body Fat

Data from NHANES II and several prospective studies clearly show that being overweight (BMI ≥28) or overfat is associated with an increased risk of type 2 diabetes in younger people (Kriska, Blair, and Pereira 1994). On the other hand, the East Boston Seniors Project revealed a more modest relationship in overweight (BMI >26 kg/m²) men and women over the age of 65, who were 2.4 times more likely to develop diabetes when compared to their leaner peers (Gurwitz et al. 1994). Indeed, the *distribution* of body fat may be a more important determinant of diabetes risk than *overall* obesity in older people (Kissebah and Krakower 1994).

Several studies have identified central obesity as an important predictor of diabetes risk (Carey et al. 1997; Hartz et al. 1983; Kaye and Folsom 1991; Kohrt, Kirwan, and Staten 1993; Lundgren et al. 1989). For example, Kohrt, Kirwan, and Staten (1993) compared insulin-sensitive older subjects to insulin-resistant subjects of the same age and found that the major determinant of insulin resistance was the accumulation of abdominal fat. In fact, waist circumference accounted for over 40% of the variance in insulin action, while age explained only 2%. Other studies have shown visceral fat, as measured by scanning techniques, to be correlated with diabetes risk in older people (Bergstron et al. 1990; Brochu et al. 2000, 2001; Cefalu et al. 1995; Kelley et al. 2000; Matsuzawa, Shimomura, and Nakamura 1993).

Physical Function

The traditional view of aging has been one of inevitable decline in health and function. In reality, however, even though the absolute number of older people with physical disabilities increases with age, this number represents a relatively small proportion of the general older population (Haskell and Phillips 1995). Nonetheless, physical function is a key component of independence in older age, and the maintenance of both the quantity and the quality of muscle mass seems vital to increasing the "active life expectancy" of older adults (Katz et al. 1983).

The decline in strength with aging is well documented (Haskell and Phillips 1995; White 1995). Indeed, musculoskeletal weakness is cited as the most common determinant of frailty and disability in older people (Manton, Corder, and Stallard 1993); other determinants include cognitive and sensory deficits (Guralnik and Simonsick 1993). Fiatarone and colleagues (1994) provide strong evidence for the important role of improved muscle strength through resistance training in the oldest old. Data from this randomized, placebo-controlled trial on 100 older people between the ages of 72 and 98 show that this frail population achieved significant improvements in strength and muscle cross-sectional area. More important, however, these physiological improvements also translated into significant *functional improvements* in activities of daily living (ADLs). Indeed, gait speed increased by 9%, stair-climbing power by 34%, and overall physical activity by 50%.

Role of Physical Activity in Weight Maintenance

Central to any discussion of the loss in physiologic resiliency with older age is the distinction between *mandatory* and *facultative* aging (DiPietro and Seals 1995). Mandatory aging is that over which we have no control. In the absence of disease or injury, biological cells, tissues, systems, and organs undergo a process of irreversible senescence. The basis of mandatory aging has been debated for decades, and two simplified hypotheses for cell death (genetic programming and error buildup) are presented in figure 10.2. On the other hand, facultative aging refers to the age-related decline in function that is attributable to factors over which we do have control. One very important lifestyle factor in facultative aging is sedentary behavior—or disuse.

Disuse

Bortz (1982) was an early proponent of the hypothesis that disuse—or inactivity—causes many of the functional losses commonly attributed to aging at every level from cells and molecules to tissues and organs. He noted that many of the physiological changes ascribed to aging per se are similar to those induced by enforced inactivity, such as during bed rest or during prolonged spaceflight. Indeed,

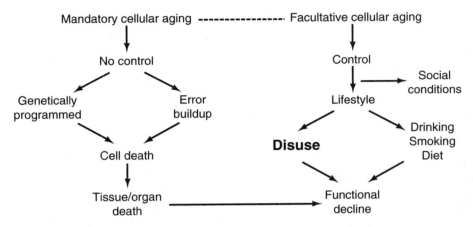

Figure 10.2 Hypothesized model of mandatory cellular and facultative cellular aging leading to functional decline.

hypogravity can serve as a useful model for studying the decline in functional reserve in aging—especially as the prevalence of physical inactivity increases steadily with increasing age and increasing reliance on automation in our society. Bortz further proposed that the decline in function can be attenuated, or even reversed, by exercise.

At least part of the reduced risk of metabolic and functional decline observed in physically active individuals is likely to be explained by the maintenance of body composition. Ample epidemiological and experimental data have demonstrated the inverse relationship between physical activity and overweight or obesity that persists even into early older age (DiPietro 1995). Perhaps of greater importance in older populations, however, is the relationship between physical activity and the preservation of muscle mass since, as discussed previously, sarcopenia has been linked to defects in carbohydrate metabolism as well as to physical frailty (Evans 1995b).

A cross-sectional study by Horber and colleagues (1996) indicated that physical activity may preserve lean body mass in old age. They used dual-energy X-ray absorptiometry (DXA) to compare lean mass in trained and untrained older men and untrained younger men. The lean mass in older untrained men was 3.5 kg (7.7 lb) lower than that in both trained older and untrained younger men—primarily the result of a lower skeletal muscle mass. No significant differences in lean or skeletal muscle mass were observed between older trained and younger untrained men. Forbes (1992) reviewed the results of several studies examining the relationship between physical activity and lean mass and concluded that exercise can preserve or even increase lean body mass, provided body weight is maintained. However, in the presence of weight loss, exercise cannot prevent a loss of lean mass. Unfortunately, Forbes never commented on the ability of physical activity to minimize the rate of decline in lean mass with aging.

Aerobic Exercise Training

Aerobic exercise training is often used to induce reductions in body fat in populations of any age. Two important studies of older people have observed significant improvements in central fat deposition that were independent of large changes in overall body weight or body composition (Kohrt, Obert, and Holloszy 1992; Schwartz et al. 1991). It is important to note, however, that these two studies used exercise intensities that were greater than 85% of peak heart rate reserve or peak aerobic capacity, with training frequencies of four to five times a week for durations of six months or longer. Indeed, the exercise stimulus used in these studies is greater than what the general older population can adhere to regularly. Nonetheless, this volume of exercise may be the necessary level of stimulus required to observe significant changes in the abdominal fat depot of otherwise healthy older people.

In general, however, aerobic exercise training without concurrent caloric restriction appears to have little effect on body composition in healthy older people. Numerous randomized controlled trials report the minimal impact of moderate- to higher-intensity training on body weight, body fat, fat deposition, and muscle mass (Fiatarone-Singh 1998). On the other hand, reasons to encourage this type of exercise in older people include increases in aerobic fitness and glucose tolerance that may occur independent of weight or body composition changes (DiPietro et al. 1998).

Resistance Training

Numerous studies have reported that high-intensity resistance training is associated with increases in FFM or muscle area, with minimal alterations in body weight (Fiatarone-Singh 1998). Typically, the largest changes are seen in cross-sectional areas of the trained muscles, whereas whole body measures of FFM or lean mass show more modest changes (Nelson et al. 1996). Two landmark studies by Frontera and colleagues (1988) and Fiatarone and colleagues (1990) reported the benefits of resistance training to improvements in muscle strength and function even in the oldest old.

Studies of resistance training also report favorable improvements in energy balance, again, even in the absence of weight change. Campbell and colleagues (1994) reported that total energy requirements for weight maintenance increased approximately 15% after 12 weeks of resistance training in healthy older men and women, presumably due to increases in the resting metabolic rate. This has important implications for very old people. If living arrangements change; if isolation and depression are present; or mobility is reduced as a result of fear, illness, or medication, older people may be at greater risk of sarcopenia from anorexia or disuse. Thus, resistance training, along with caloric supplementation in the very old, may be a successful strategy for maintaining muscle mass and body weight in this high-risk population.

Role of Lifestyle Activity

Because the accurate assessment of physical activity patterns over many years is difficult to achieve, estimates of the relative contribution of lifestyle activity to body composition changes over time vary widely among the population (Fiatarone-Singh 1998). At this time, we know of no published epidemiological data relating the benefits of habitual physical activity to body weight maintenance in older people. These longitudinal data are particularly important given that the fastest growing segment of the general population is those 85 years and older.

Most recently, Dziura and colleagues (Dziura, Mendes de Leon, Kasl, and DiPietro, unpublished) used mixed-effects longitudinal regression modeling to determine the impact of baseline physical activity on the trajectory of weight change (reported annually for 12 years) in men and women over 65 years in the Yale Health and Aging Project. In this older cohort, body weight significantly decreased as individuals aged, and although at baseline no cross-sectional association existed between reported physical activity and body weight, higher levels of baseline physical activity significantly *attenuated* the rate of weight loss in older individuals over time (see figure 10.3). After adjustment for multiple factors (including health status, functional ability, and pre-existing chronic conditions), each one-unit increase in baseline total physical activity score minimized the rate of aging-related weight loss by 0.11 lb (0.05 kg) per year. For instance, although initial weight tended to be 3.1 lb (1.4 kg) lower in women reporting a *moderate* total activity score of 4 (achieved by walking and gardening "often in the past month") compared to those women reporting no activity (a score of 0), after 12 years, weight loss was minimized by 5.3 lb (2.4 kg) in the more active women. This net savings in body weight that can be attributed to even moderate levels of habitual physical activity (and not to disease) translates into substantial health benefits for people in their later years.

In summary, evidence suggests that aging-related loss of muscle mass can be attenuated with regular exercise in older people. Although interventions of aerobic activity (e.g., brisk walking, aerobic dance, or swimming) have a minimal impact on changes in body composition in healthy, weight stable older people, the benefits of this type of activity to general health and function are not to be dismissed. The current data suggest that resistance training has a more specific impact on maintaining and even increasing muscle size and strength in older persons up to 100 years of age (Fiatarone et al. 1994; Fiatarone and Evans 1990). As discussed previously, the benefits of increased quantity, and perhaps quality, of muscle fiber are important to preserving both metabolic and physical resiliency.

As is the case with obesity among the more general population, however, *prevention* of sarcopenia and its metabolic and functional

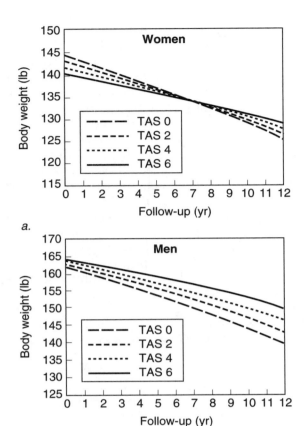

a.

b.

TAS = Total activity score

Figure 10.3 Physical activity attenuates the rate of aging-related weight loss in *(a)* women and *(b)* men: Yale Health and Aging Project, 1982-1994.

sequelae may be a more effective strategy for maintaining health and function. The few epidemiological data that exist suggest that regular (perhaps lifetime) patterns of physical activity, achieved from work or recreational activity, are important to minimizing the aging-related decline in body weight and muscle mass observed among the older population. The recent Surgeon General's Report (U.S. Department of Health and Human Services 1996) that recommended 30 minutes per day of accumulated activity of any type should be interpreted as a sufficient prescription for the *primary prevention* (i.e., delaying) of a wide array of health and functional decrements. As depicted in table 10.1, the amount of activity necessary to effectively alter more compromised function or already-existing disease is not clear and may be far greater. In any case, this modest amount of activity prescribed by the Surgeon General's Report is achievable by

most of the older segments of the population through lifestyle activities such as housework, yard work, use of the stairs, and most important, avoidance of labor-saving devices whenever possible. Although the absolute stimulus from a single episode of any of these activities is small, if these simple activities are performed regularly over years, the benefits will accumulate into a meaningful contribution to the maintenance of health and function.

Encouraging Physical Activity in Older People

Most important to the study of physical activity and exercise among older people are the determinants of regular participation or adherence to structured programs (King et al. 1992; Sallis et al. 1992). These determinants (e.g., physiological, psychosocial, or environmental), which may vary by age, sex, and socioeconomic status among the general population, must be clearly identified and subsequently managed before the public health potential of physical activity can be fulfilled.

Physiological attributes, such as strength, flexibility, and balance, may act as important incentives for exercise among older people as they will participate in activities at which they are more competent and feel safe. Exercise programs that promote perceptions of safety and efficacy among older people might include modifications to various structures that "equalize the playing field," such as hand railings, carpeted floors, lower steps, and built-in seating.

Information sharing about the health effects of exercise is an important contributor to adherence in any age group (Napolitano and Marcus 2002). Therefore, providing information updates via newsletters and individual progress reports that enlist the full cooperation of the client population in an exercise intervention will contribute substantially to both adherence and the sustainability of the program. Social influences on physical activity patterns appear to be strong throughout the life span (Sallis et al. 1992). Exercise programs that encourage social support via group activities within a structured time frame and randomized programs that allocate spouses to the same treatment group are key to the success of any program.

Table 10.1   *Public Health Strategy for the Prevention of Functional and Metabolic Decline*

Level of intervention	Health status	Amount of physical activity
Primary	Normal function	30 min or more of *moderate* intensity activity on most days
Secondary	Compromised function	?
Tertiary	Diseased state	??

Safety and accessibility are two important environmental factors associated with activity participation across the age span, and these two factors have only recently become public health funding priorities. Walking and running or bicycle paths and recreational areas, which are set away from traffic and are patrolled and well lighted, are very important for older people—especially those living in underserved urban environments where sidewalks are often in disrepair. Fear of crime is an important deterrent to physical activity in older populations. Also, among older adults, membership fees or lack of transportation often present insurmountable barriers to supervised programs in health clubs or recreational facilities. Thus, the provision of safe, supervised exercise programs and facilities may equalize access to physical activity across age, sex, and racial groups.

In summary, an array of physiological, psychological, and environmental factors may determine physical activity behavior throughout the life span, and these factors become even more important in older age. Many of these determinants, particularly some of the psychosocial and environmental factors, are particularly amenable to change and should be the focus of community intervention efforts. Strategies for increasing physical activity among the older sectors of the community include (1) increased public education about the health effects of moderate physical activity; (2) increased senior and community center programs that are supervised and provide social support and other incentives for exer-

cise; and (3) increased community availability and accessibility of safe physical activity and recreational facilities such as hiking, biking, and fitness trails; public swimming pools; and acres of park space.

Summary

Older people are not simply younger, untrained people. Therefore, determinants of health and function in older people differ substantially from those in younger or middle-aged people. Of significant importance to health and function in older age is the maintenance of body weight—specifically, the preservation of lean mass. Ample evidence demonstrates the relationship that aging-related decreases in muscle mass and increases in the relative proportion of abdominal adiposity have with regard to the loss of both metabolic and physical reserve.

Many of the physiological decrements commonly ascribed to aging per se may be related to disuse, as the prevalence of sedentary behavior increases steadily with age. Regular exercise and habitual physical activity can attenuate the aging-related loss of muscle mass. Although the current data suggest that resistance training has a more specific impact on maintaining and even increasing muscle size and strength, the health benefits of aerobic exercise should not be dismissed.

As is the case for obesity among the general population, the *prevention* of sarcopenia (along with its metabolic and physical sequelae) may actually be a more effective strategy than its reversal for maintaining health and function in aging. The few epidemiological data that do exist suggest that regular lifetime patterns are important in minimizing weight loss in older age.

References

Andres, R.A., Elahi, D., Tobin, J.D., and Muller, D.C. 1985. Impact of age on weight goals. *Annals of Internal Medicine* 103: 1030-1033.

Barrett-Connor, E. 1980. The prevalence of diabetes mellitus in an adult community as determined by history or fasting hyperglycemia. *American Journal of Epidemiology* 11: 705-712.

Bender, A.P., Sprafka, J.M., Jagger, H.G., Muckala, K.H., Martin, C.P., and Edwards, T.R. 1986. Incidence, prevalence, and mortality of diabetes mellitus in Wadena, Marshall, and Grand Rapids, Minnesota: The three-city study. *Diabetes Care* 9: 343-350.

Bergstron, R.W., Newell-Morris, L.L., Leonetti, D.L., Shuman, W.P., Wahl, P.W., and Fujimoto, W.Y. 1990. Association of elevated fasting C-peptide level and increased intra-abdominal fat distribution with development of NIDDM in Japanese-American men. *Diabetes* 39: 104-111.

Borkan, G.A., Hults, D.E., Gerzof, S.G., Robbins, A.H., and Silbert, C.K. 1983. Age changes in body composition revealed by computed tomography. *Journal of Gerontology* 38: 673-677.

Borkan, G.A., and Norris, A.H. 1977. Fat redistribution and the changing body dimensions of the adult male. *Human Biology* 49: 495-514.

Bortz, W.M. 1982. Disuse and aging. *Journal of the American Medical Association* 248: 1203-1208.

Brochu, M., Starling, R.D., Tchernof, A. et al. 2000. Visceral adipose tissue is an independent correlate of glucose disposal in older obese postmenopausal women. *Journal of Clinical Endocrinology and Metabolism* 85: 2378-2384.

Brochu, M., Tchernof, A., Dionne, I.J. et al. 2001. What are the physical characteristics associated with a normal metabolic profile despite a high level of obesity in postmenopausal women? *Journal of Clinical Endocrinology and Metabolism* 86: 1020-1025.

Burr, M.L., and Phillips, K.M. 1984. Anthropometric norms in the elderly. *British Journal of Nutrition* 51: 165-169.

Butler, W.J., Ostrander, L.D., Carman, W.J., and Lamphiear, D.E. 1982. Diabetes mellitus in Tecumseh, Michigan. *American Journal of Epidemiology* 116: 971-980.

Campbell, W.W., Crim, M.C., Young, V.R., and Evans, W.J. 1994. Increased energy requirements and changes in body composition with resistance training in older adults. *American Journal of Clinical Nutrition* 60: 167-175.

Carey, V.J., Walters, E.E., Coditz, G.A., Solomon, C.G., Willet, W.C., Rosner, B.A., Speizer, F.E., and Manson, J.E. 1997. Body fat distribution and risk of non-insulin dependent diabetes mellitus in women: The Nurses' Health Study. *American Journal of Epidemiology* 145: 614-619.

Carmelli, D., McElroy, M.R., and Rosenman, R.H. 1991. Longitudinal changes in fat distribution in the Western Collaborative Group Study: A 23-year follow-up. *International Journal of Obesity* 15: 67-74.

Cefalu, W.T., Wang, Z.Q., Werbel, S., Bell-Farrow, A., Crouse, I.I.I., Jr., Hinson, W.H., Terry, J.G., and Anderson, R. 1995. Contribution of visceral fat mass to the insulin resistance of aging. *Metabolism* 44: 954-959.

Chien, S., Peng, M.T., Chen, K.P., Huang, T.F., Chang, C., and Fang, H.S. 1975. Longitudinal studies on adipose tissue and its distribution in human subjects. *Journal of Applied Physiology* 30: 825-830.

Cohn, S.H., Vartsky, D., Yasumura, S., Sawitsky, A., Zanzi, I., Vaswani, A., and Ellis, K.J. 1980. Compartmental body composition based on total-body nitrogen, potassium, and calcium. *American Journal of Physiology* 239: E524-530.

Cüppers, H.J., Erdmann, D., Schubert, H., Berchtold, P., and Berger, M. 1982. Glucose tolerance serum insulin, serum lipids in athletes. In *Diabetes and exercise*, eds. M. Berger, P. Christancopolous, and J. Wahren, 115-165. Bern: Han Huber.

DeFronzo, R.A. 1979. Glucose intolerance and aging: Evidence for tissue insensitivity to insulin. *Diabetes* 28: 1095-1101.

Dey, D.K., Rothenberg, E., Sundh, V., Bosaeus, I., and Steen, B. 1999. Height and body weight in the elderly. I. A 25-year longitudinal study of a population aged 70 to 95 years. *European Journal of Clinical Nutrition* 53: 905-914.

DiPietro, L. 1995. Physical activity, body weight, and adiposity: An epidemiologic perspective. *Exercise and Sports Science Reviews* 23: 275-303.

DiPietro, L., Anda, R.F., Williamson, D.F., and Stunkard, A.J. 1992. Depression and weight change in a national cohort of adults. *International Journal of Obesity* 16: 745-753.

DiPietro, L., and Seals, D.R. 1995. Introduction to exercise in older adults. In *Perspectives in exercise science and sports medicine, vol. 8: Exercise in older adults*, eds. D.R. Lamb, C.V. Gisolfi, and E. Nadel, 1-10. Carmel, IN: Cooper Publishing Group.

DiPietro, L., Seeman, T.E., Stachenfeld, N.S., Katz, L.D., and Nadel, E.R. 1998. Moderate-intensity aerobic training improves glucose responses in aging independent of abdominal adiposity. *Journal of the American Geriatrics Society* 46: 875-879.

Dziura, J., Mendes de Leon, C., Kasl S., and DiPietro L. Physical activity attenuates aging-related weight loss in older people: The Yale Health and Aging Study, 1982-1994. (unpublished).

Enzi, G., Gasparo, M., Biondetti, P.R., Fiore, D., Semisa, M., and Zurlo, F. 1986. Subcutaneous and visceral fat distribution according to sex, age, and overweight, evaluated by computed tomography. *American Journal of Clinical Nutrition* 44: 739-746.

Evans, W. 1995a. Exercise, nutrition and aging. *Clinical Geriatric Medicine* 11: 725-734.

Evans, W.J. 1995b. What is sarcopenia? *Journal of Gerontology A: Biological and Medical Science* 50: 5-8.

Fiatarone, M.A., and Evans, W.J. 1990. Exercise in the oldest old. *Topics in Geriatric Rehabilitation* 5: 63-77.

Fiatarone, M.A., and Evans, W.J. 1993. The etiology and reversibility of muscle dysfunction in the aged. *Journal of Gerontology*.48: 77-83.

Fiatorone, M.A., Marks, E.C., Ryan, N.D., Meredith, C.N., Lipsitz, L.A., and Evans, W.J. 1990. High-intensity strength training in nonagenarians. Effects on skeletal muscle. *Journal of the American Medical Association* 263: 3029-3034.

Fiatarone, M.A., O'Neill, E.F., Ryan, N.D., Clements, K.M., Solares, G.R., Nelson, M.E., Roberts, S.R., Kehayias, J.K., Lipsitz, L.A., and Evans, W.J. 1994. Exercise training and nutritional supplementation for physical frailty in very elderly people. *New England Journal of Medicine* 330: 1769-1775.

Fiatarone-Singh, M.A. 1998. Body composition and weight control in older adults. In *Perspectives in exercise science and sports medicine, vol. 11: Exercise, nutrition, and weight control,* eds. D.R. Lamb and R. Murray, 243-293. Carmel, IN: Cooper Publishing Co.

Fink, R.I., Kolterman, O.G., Griffin, J., and Olefsky, J.M. 1983. Mechanisms of insulin resistance in aging. *Journal of Clinical Investigation* 71: 1523-1535.

Fleg, J., and Lakatta, E. 1988. Role of muscle loss in age-associated reduction in $\dot{V}O_2$max. *Journal of Applied Physiology* 65: 1147-1151.

Flegal, K.M. 1996. Trends in body weight and overweight in the U.S. population. *Nutrition Reviews* 54: S97-100.

Flynn, M.A., Nolph, G.B., Baker, A.S., Martin, W.A., and Krause, G. 1989. Total body potassium in aging humans: A longitudinal study. *American Journal of Clinical Nutrition* 50: 713-717.

Forbes, G.B. 1992. Exercise and lean weight: The influence of body weight. *Nutrition Reviews* 50: 157-161.

French, L.R., Boen, J.R., Martinez, A.M., Bushhouse, S.A., Sprafka, J.M., and Goetz, F.C. 1990. Population-based study of impaired glucose tolerance and type II diabetes in Wadena, Minnesota. *American Journal of Epidemiology* 39: 1131-1137.

Frontera, W.R., Meredith, C.N., O'Reilly, K.P., Knuttgen, H.G., and Evans, W.J. 1988. Strength conditioning in older men: Skeletal muscle hypertrophy and improved function. *Journal of Applied Physiology* 64: 1038-1044.

Guralnik, J.M., and Simonsick, E.M. 1993. Physical disability in older Americans. *Journal of Gerontology* 48: 3-10.

Gurwitz, J.H., Field, T.S., Glynn, R.J., Manson, J.E., Avorn, J., Taylor, J.O., and Hennekens, C.H. 1994. Risk factors for non-insulin-dependent diabetes mellitus requiring treatment in the elderly. *Journal of the American Geriatrics Society* 42: 1235-1240.

Hamman, R.F., Marshall, J.A., Baxter, J., Kahn, L.B., Mayer, E.J., Orleans, M., Murphy, J.R., and Lezotte, D.C. 1989. Methods and prevalence of non-insulin dependent diabetes mellitus in a biethnic Colorado population: The San Luis Valley diabetes study. *American Journal of Epidemiology* 129: 295-311.

Hanis, C.L., Ferrell, R.E., Barton, S.A., Aguilar, L., Garza-Ibarra, A., Tulloch, B.R., Garcia, C.A., and Schull, W.J. 1983. Diabetes among Mexican Americans in Starr County, Texas. *American Journal of Epidemiology* 118: 659-672.

Harris, M.I., Hadden, W.C., Knowler, W.C., and Bennett, P.H. 1987. Prevalence of diabetes and impaired glucose tolerance and plasma glucose levels in the U.S. population aged 20-74 yr. *Diabetes* 36: 523-534.

Hartz, A.J., Rupley, D.C., Kalkhoff, R.K., and Rimm, A.A. 1983. Relationship of obesity to diabetes: Influence of obesity level and body fat distribution. *Preventative Medicine* 12: 351-357.

Haskell, W.L., and Phillips, W.T. 1995. Exercise training, fitness, health, and longevity. In *Perspectives in exercise science and sports medicine, vol. 8: Exercise in older adults,* eds. D.R. Lamb, C.V. Gisolfi, and E. Nadel, 11-52. Carmel, IN: Cooper Publishing Group.

Higgins, M., D'Agostino, R., Kannel, W., Cobb, J., and Pinsky, J. 1993. Benefits and adverse effects of weight loss. Observations from the Framingham Study. *Annals of Internal Medicine* 119: 758-763.

Horber, F.F., Kohler, S.A., Lippuner, K., and Jaeger, P. 1996. Effect of regular physical training on age-associated alteration of body composition in men. *European Journal of Clinical Investigation* 26: 279-285.

Ivy, J., Zderic, G.M., and Fogt, D.L. 1999. Prevention and treatment of non-insulin-dependent diabetes mellitus. *Exercise and Sports Sciences Reviews* 27: 1-36.

Katz, S., Branch, L.G., Branson, M.H., Papsidero, J.A., Beck, J.C., and Greer, D.S. 1983. Active life expectancy. *New England Journal of Medicine* 309: 1218-1223.

Kaye, S.A., and Folsom, A.R. 1991. Is serum cortisol associated with body fat distribution in post menopausal women? *International Journal of Obesity* 15: 437-439.

Kelley, D.E., Thaete, F.L., Troost, F., Huwe, T., and Goodpaster, B.H. 2000. Subdivisions of subcutaneous abdominal adipose tissue and insulin resistance. *American Journal of Physiology: Endocrinology and Metabolism* 278: E941-948.

King, A.C., Blair, S.N., Bild, D.E. et al. 1992. Determinants of physical activity and interventions in adults. *Medicine and Science in Sports and Exercise* 24: S221-S236.

Kissebah, A.H., and Krakower, G.R. 1994. Regional adiposity and morbidity. *Physiological Reviews* 74: 761-811.

Kohrt, W.M., Kirwan, J.P., and Staten, M.A. 1993. Insulin resistance in aging is related to abdominal obesity. *Diabetes* 42: 273-281.

Kohrt, W.M., Obert, K.A., and Holloszy, J.O. 1992. Exercise training improves fat distribution patterns in 60- to 70-year-old men and women. *Journal of Gerontology* 47: M99-M105.

Kriska, A.M., Blair, S.N., and Periera M.A. 1994. The potential role of physical activity in the prevention of non-insulin-dependent diabetes mellitus. *Exercise and Sports Sciences Reviews* 22: 121-143.

Lundgren, H., Bengtsson, C., Blohme, G., Isaksson, B., Lapidus, L., Lenner, R.A., Saaek, A., and Winther, E. 1989. Dietary habits and incidence of noninsulin-dependent diabetes mellitus in a population study of women in Gothenburg, Sweden. *American Journal of Clinical Nutrition* 49: 708-712.

Manton, K.G., Corder, L.S., and Stallard, E. 1993. Estimates of change in chronic disability and institutional incidence and prevalence rates in the U.S. elderly population from the 1982, 1984, and 1989 National Long-Term Care Study. *Journal of Gerontology: Social Sciences* 48: S15.

Matsuzawa, Y., Shimomura, I., and Nakamura, T. 1993. Pathophysiology and pathogenesis of visceral fat obesity. *Annals of the New York Academy of Sciences* 676: 270-278.

Morley, J.E., Glick, Z., and Rubenstein, L.Z. 1995. *Geriatric nutrition: A comprehensive review*, 2nd ed. New York: Lippincott-Raven.

Najjar, M.F., and Rowland, M. 1987. Anthropometric reference data and prevalence of overweight, United States, 1976-80. *Vital Health Statistics* 11: 1-73.

Napolitano, M.A., and Marcus, B.H. 2002. Targeting and tailoring physical activity information using print and information technologies. *Exercise and Sports Sciences Reviews* 30: 122-128.

National Center for Health Statistics. 1992. Current estimates from the National Health Interview Survey, 1991. *Vital and Health Statistics*, Series 10, no. 184.

National Center for Health Statistics. 1994a. Current estimates from the National Health Interview Survey, 1992. *Vital and Health Statistics*, Series 10, no. 189.

National Center for Health Statistics. 1994b. Current estimates from the National Health Interview Survey, 1993. *Vital and Health Statistics*, Series 10, no. 190.

Nelson, M., Fiatarone, M.A., Layne, J., Trice, I., Economos, C., Fielding, R., Ma, R., Pierson, R., and

Evans, W. 1996. Analysis of body composition techniques and models for detecting changes in soft tissue with strength training. *American Journal of Clinical Nutrition* 63: 678-686.

Nevitt, M.C., Cummings, S.R., Kidd, S., and Black, D. 1989. Risk factors for recurrent nonsyncopal falls: A prospective study. *Journal of the American Medical Association* 261: 2663-2668.

Novak, L.P. 1972. Aging, total body potassium, fat-free mass, and cell mass in males and females between ages 18 and 85 years. *Journal of Gerontology* 27: 438-643.

Pollock, M.L., Foster, C., Knapp, D., Rod, J.L., and Schmidt, D.H. 1987. Effect of age and training on aerobic capacity and body composition of master athletes. *Journal of Applied Physiology* 62: 725-731.

Pratley, R., Hagberg, J., Rogus, E., and Goldberg, A. 1995. Enhanced insulin sensitivity and lower waist-to-hip ratio in master athletes. *American Journal of Physiology* 268: E484-E490.

Rosenberg, I.H. 1997. Sarcopenia: Origins and clinical relevance. *Journal of Nutrition* 127: 990S-991S.

Rosenthal, M., Doberne, L., Greenfield, M., Widstrom, A., and Reaven, G.M. 1982. Effect of age on glucose tolerance, insulin secretion, and in vivo insulin action. *Journal of the American Geriatrics Society* 30: 562-567.

Rowe, J.W., Minaker, K.L., Pallotta, J.A., and Flier, J.S. 1983. Characterization of the insulin resistance of aging. *Journal of Clinical Investigation* 71: 1581-1587.

Sallis, J.F., Simons-Morton, B.G., Stone, E.J., et al. 1992. Determinants of physical activity and interventions in youth. *Medicine and Science in Sports and Exercise* 24: S248-S257.

Saltin, B., and Gollnick, P.D. 1983. Skeletal muscle adaptability: Significance for metabolism and performance. In *Handbook of physiology. Skeletal muscle*, 551-563. Bethesda, MD: American Physiological Society.

Schwartz, R.S., Shuman, W.P., Larson, V., Cain, K.C., Fellingham, G.W., Beard, J.C., Kahn, S.E., Stratton, J.R., Cerqueira, M.D., and Abrass, I.B. 1991. The effect of intensive endurance exercise training on body fat distribution in young and older men. *Metabolism* 40: 545-551.

Shimokata, H., Andres, R., Coon, P.J., Elahi, D., Muller, D.C., and Tobin, J.D. 1989. Studies in the distribution of body fat. II. Longitudinal effects of change in weight. *International Journal of Obesity* 13: 455-464.

Shimokata, H., Muller, D.C., Fleg, J.L., Sorkin, J., Ziemba, A.W., and Andres, R. 1991. Age as independent determinant of glucose tolerance. *Diabetes* 40: 44-51.

Shimokata, H., Tobin, J.D., Muller, D.C., Elahi, D., Coon, P.J., and Andres, R. 1989. Studies in the distribution of body fat. I. Effects of age, sex, and obesity. *Journal of Gerontology* 44: M66-73.

Steen, B. 1988. Body composition and aging. *Nutrition Review* 46: 45-51.

Steen, B., Lundgren, B.K., Isaksson, B. 1985. Body composition at age 70, 75, 79, and 81 years: A longitudinal population study. In *Nutrition, immunity, and illness in the elderly*, ed. R.K. Chandra, 49-53. New York: Pergamon Press.

Stevens, J., Knapp, R., Keil, J., and Verdugo, R. 1991. Changes in body weight and girths in black and white adults studied over a 25 yr interval. *International Journal of Obesity* 15: 803-808.

Tzankoff, S.P., and Norris, A.H. 1977. Effect of muscle mass decrease on age-related BMR changes. *Journal of Applied Physiology* 43: 1001-1006.

Tzankoff, S.P., and Norris, A.H. 1978. Longitudinal changes in resting metabolic rate in man. *Journal of Applied Physiology* 33: 536-539.

U.S. Department of Health and Human Services. 1996. Physical activity and health: A report of the Surgeon General. U.S. Department of Health and Human Services, National Centers for Disease Control and Prevention, National Center for Chronic Disease Prevention.

Vaughan, L., Zurlo, F., and Ravussin, E. 1991. Aging and energy expenditure. *American Journal of Clinical Nutrition* 53: 821-885.

White, T.P. 1995. Skeletal muscle structure and function in older mammals. In *Perspectives in exercise science and sports medicine, vol. 8: Exercise in older adults*, eds. D.R. Lamb, C.V. Gisolfi, and E. Nadel, 115-174. Carmel, IN: Cooper Publishing Group.

Willitt, W., Manson, J., Stampfer, M., Colditz, G. et al. 1995. Weight, weight change, and coronary heart disease in women. *Journal of the American Medical Association* 273: 461-465.

Chapter 11

Treating and Preventing Pediatric Obesity

Marian Tanofsky-Kraff, MA

Unit on Growth and Obesity, Developmental
Endocrinology Branch, The National Institute
of Child Health and Human Development,
National Institutes of Health

Helen Hayden-Wade, PhD

Child and Adolescent Services Research Center,
Children's Hospital—San Diego

Paul A. Cavazos, BA

Center for Eating and Weight Disorders,
San Diego State University

Denise E. Wilfley, PhD

Departments of Psychiatry, Medicine, Pediatrics,
and Psychology, Washington University School
of Medicine, St. Louis

The prevalence of pediatric obesity has been increasing in recent decades both nationally (Troiano et al. 1995) and worldwide (Chinn and Rona 2001; Chunming 2000; de Onis and Blossner 2000; Troiano and Flegal 1998; World Health Organization 1998). Estimates in the United States indicate that 11 to 22% of children between the ages of 6 and 11, or one in five children, is presently overweight (Troiano et al. 1995). Moreover, the greatest increases in obesity are occurring among the heaviest children (Troiano et al. 1996). Such a rapid and steep increase is of serious concern, as obesity is associated with grim physiological and psychosocial ramifications in adulthood. Studies reveal that 24 to 44% of obese adults were obese children (Troiano et al. 1995). Since obese children are more likely to become obese adults (Serdula et al. 1993), particularly if one parent is obese (Whitaker et al. 1997), a focus on early intervention and prevention may be crucial in decreasing the development of adult obesity.

In this chapter, we will discuss the health and psychological risks associated with carrying excess weight early in life as well as the etiology of pediatric obesity. A focus of the chapter will be the specific treatment components that researchers have found to be promising when intervening with obese children for long-term positive outcomes. Given the limited empirical investigation of efficacious treatments for obese adolescents, this chapter will focus primarily on preadolescent obesity treatment, as early intervention increases the likelihood for prevention of adult obesity. Furthermore, we will emphasize the early intervention and prevention of adult obesity, and how it might be mobilized in school systems. We will discuss briefly the issue of eating disorder development and prevention, as well as the importance of sensitive consideration of differences when treating obese children of various ethnic and cultural groups.

Health and Psychosocial Risks Associated With Childhood Obesity

Aside from being associated with adult obesity, childhood obesity is itself a major health problem (Dietz 1995). Pediatric obesity, like adult obesity, is related to physical health problems such as increased blood pressure, dyslipidemia, increased risk of respiratory infections, and lowered physical fitness (Chu et al. 1998; Dietz 1995). In addition to the immediate negative effects on health, obesity in adolescence also increases the long-term (e.g., 50 years; Gunnell et al. 1998) risk of adult morbidity and mortality, independent of adult obesity status (Must et al. 1992). Research has shown that treatment of pediatric obesity is associated with significant health benefits including decreases in systolic and diastolic blood pressure and improved lipid profiles (for a review, see Epstein et al. 1998).

Obese children are frequently the target of discrimination and stigmatization (Dietz 1995) and suffer significant psychosocial consequences, such as being shamed, marginalized (Dietz 1995), and rejected (Goldfield and Chrisler 1995). Young children describe silhouettes of obese children as "lazy, dirty, stupid, cheats, and liars." They rank obese children as those they would least like to have as friends (Goldfield and Chrisler 1995; Staffieri 1967). Indeed, obese children report being more socially isolated than their non-overweight peers (Phillips and Hill 1997).

Consistent findings indicate that obese children are subjected to body- and weight-related teasing (Hayden et al. 1999; Shapiro, Baumeister, and Kessler 1991) and are also perceived negatively by their peers in both academic and social contexts (Bell and Morgan 2000). Shapiro, Baumeister, and Kessler (1991) found that among third- and fifth-graders, the most common content of teasing was related to appearance (39%), especially to being fat (13%). Overweight girls are especially vulnerable; they are more likely than their non-overweight peers to be teased about their weight, size, and overall appearance (Rieves and Cash 1996; Thompson et al. 1995). Teasing has also been correlated with a negative body image in overweight children. Indeed, obese children report more body image problems than non-overweight children (Hayden et al. 1999). Moreover, obese children report increased social isolation (Achenbach and Elderbrock 1991) and are at risk for social problems in comparison to their non-overweight peers (Epstein, Klein, and Wisniewski 1994).

Such negative social consequences typically continue into adolescence and adulthood. College completion rates for obese adolescents are lower than those for non-overweight adolescents of similar educational backgrounds (Gortmaker et al. 1993). Obese young adults are much less likely to marry than nonobese young adults (Gortmaker et al. 1993). When they do marry, obese women are far more likely than nonobese women to choose a partner in a lower socioeconomic class (Brownell 1995). Furthermore, obese individuals face discrimination from potential employers (Brownell 1995), and prospective evidence indicates that people who are obese as adolescents or young adults earn less money, have fewer years of schooling, and suffer higher rates of poverty than their nonobese peers. These findings remain even when controlling for IQ and parents' educational or income level (Gortmaker et al. 1993). Clearly, successful long-term treatment of pediatric obesity not only will help prevent children from becoming obese adults, but may also improve their physical, psychological, and social well-being.

Genetic and Environmental Influences

Beginning nearly 50 years ago, increasing evidence has shown that individuals within the same family are similar in terms of their degree of adiposity (Faith et al. 1997). In a pioneering study, Clark (1956) found degree of fatness to be more strongly correlated with monozygotic twins than dyzygotic twins. Moreover, adoption and twin studies have found that genetic influence is responsible for a substantial proportion of the variance accounting for body mass index (BMI) (MacDonald and Stunkard 1990; Sorensen et al. 1992; Stunkard et al. 1990). Results yielded from these and other studies led Faith and colleagues (1997) to posit that the genetic variation in BMI may be as high as 70% in industrialized nations. While few heritability studies have been conducted on children, by age 4 and older the degree of heritability is primarily stable throughout the lifetime (Cardon 1995), suggesting that a genetic influence is significant for many obese individuals.

Clinicians should remain cognizant of the strong influence genetics has in the development of obesity, particularly when treating children. In the past, obese individuals have been held responsible for their weight status, often by their treating physicians. Professional insensitivity has contributed to a standard of social discrimination and stigmatization that can have profound and lasting psychological effects (Dietz 1995). To reduce the larger societal attributional bias against obese individuals, medical and health professionals must gain an increased understanding of scientific information regarding the genetic mechanisms and biological processes involved in the etiology and maintenance of obesity.

Researchers have also demonstrated that environmental influences are associated with pediatric obesity. Obesity and the socioeconomic status of children living in industrialized societies may be related (Sobal and Stunkard 1989). Garn and Clark (1976) found that girls from lower-income backgrounds gained weight following adolescence, while girls from higher-income families tended to lose weight after adolescence.

Family dysfunction is an environmental influence that appears to be related to increased BMI among children and adolescents (Kinston, Loader, and Miller 1987; Mendelson, White, and Schliecker 1995). For instance, in a 10-year follow-up study, neglected children were significantly more likely (9.8 times) to become obese by age 14 than were children who were not neglected (Lissau and Sorensen 1994). The association between parental neglect and child obesity was stronger than other psychosocial risk associations (e.g., quality of dwelling) (Lissau and Sorensen 1994). The

authors speculate that a lack of supervision affects eating patterns in children. In particular, periods of unsupervised eating, especially after school, may likely be a time of high-caloric consumption.

Similar to making poor food choices when unsupervised, children tend to make poor choices when engaging in activities. It is more alluring for children to sit in front of the television, for example, than to be active. Parents may also feel more secure in the knowledge that their children are at home and not outside unsupervised. Recent national data indicate that children watch an average of more than 24 hours of television a week (Robinson 1999). Sedentary behavior such as television viewing has been found to be associated with increased BMI and a higher prevalence of overweight (Andersen et al. 1998; Muller et al. 1999). The relationship between higher BMI and increased sedentary behavior is likely because, for example, watching television and engaging in physical activity typically are not complementary (Vara and Epstein 1993). In fact, Robinson (1999) suggested three mechanisms that may link television viewing and obesity: (1) reduced energy expenditure by displacing physical activity; (2) increased energy intake through eating while viewing television, perhaps prompted by food advertising; and (3) decreased resting metabolic rate, which occurs while watching television. In sum, the genetic tendency toward a higher body weight coupled with environmental risk factors will likely result in the development of pediatric obesity.

Treatment of Pediatric Obesity

Compared to medical, educational, school-based, and individual behavioral treatments, behavioral family-based treatment programs have been the most studied intervention in pediatric obesity They have reliably produced the best-known short- and long-term treatment effects of any pediatric obesity treatment (Epstein et al. 1998; Jelalian and Saelens 1999). Indeed, the most effective family-based weight control programs show promising results even at 10-year follow-up for overweight children (Epstein, Valoski et al. 1995).

While the results presented in the pediatric treatment literature are variable, outcomes for nonpharmacological interventions for pediatric obesity are promising in the areas of improved blood pressure (Hoffman et al. 1995), physical fitness (Gutin et al. 1996), body fat mass (Gutin et al. 1996; Johnson et al. 1997; Wabitsch et al. 1996), cholesterol, triglycerides, lipoprotein levels (Gutin et al. 1996; Johnson et al. 1997), as well as insulin and fasting glucose (Gutin et al. 1996; Hoffman et al. 1995).

Of 21 published studies that assessed weight changes for at least one year, only three reported good maintenance in which participants maintained a 20% or greater decrease in percent overweight (Brownell, Kelman, and Stunkard 1983; Epstein, Wing, Penner, and Kress 1985; Epstein, Wing, Woodall et al. 1985). Of the more promising studies, Brownell and colleagues (1983) reported a 20.5% change in percent overweight at follow-up. Epstein and colleagues (1990) achieved an average of 20% decrease in percent overweight, which was maintained at the 10-year follow-up. Studies on pharmacotherapy and surgery are omitted because of the sparse empirical literature on children (for detailed descriptions of these studies, see Goldfield, Raynor, and Epstein 2002).

Promising long-term weight loss produced from comprehensive behavioral treatments for childhood obesity are in contrast to the less-than-encouraging findings from adult weight control interventions (Epstein, Valoski, Wing, and McCurley 1990, 1994; Epstein, Valoski et al. 1995). Moreover, in a review of 11 school-based programs, interventions focusing on younger children were more successful than those focusing on adolescents (Story 1999). The finding that younger individuals are more responsive to intervention than adolescents and adults is encouraging for pediatric obesity programs (Epstein, Valoski et al. 1995).

Obesity intervention aimed at younger individuals targets an ideal developmental time point during which individuals are more sensitive and receptive to instigating crucial life changes. In fact, preadolescent treatment can take advantage of growth and increases in lean body mass, as well as weight change (Epstein et al. 1998). Experts posit several reasons to explain why children show superior long-term outcomes as compared to adolescents and adults in obesity treatment (Epstein, Valoski et al. 1995; Wilson 1994). First, children require less self-motivation than adults to persist with weight loss programs and the behavior changes involved, as it is the parents who ensure their children's attendance at appointments and regulate the quantity and quality of the foods to which their children have access. Second, children have less ingrained, and therefore more malleable, physical activity and dietary habits than do obese adolescents and adults who present for treatment. Finally, children are generally more physically active than adults, which may be beneficial for long-term weight maintenance, as physical activity is associated with better long-term maintenance in adults (Klem et al. 1997).

Who Should Be Treated

Assessment is an important evaluative step to determine who should be treated for childhood overweight or obesity in primary care and other health professional settings. Presenting age, as well as severity of obesity, are important factors that relate to obesity persistence and should be considered when assessing a child for treatment.

A practical method of assessing children's severity of overweight or obesity is to use BMI. Recommendations by a committee of pediatric obesity experts (see Barlow and Dietz 1998) suggest that children with a BMI greater than or equal to the 85th percentile (with complications of obesity) or 95th percentile (with or without complications) should be evaluated and, based on that assessment, possibly treated for obesity. More recently, a workshop organized by the International Obesity Task Force recommended that adult BMI cutoff points in widest use (body mass index of 25 kg/m^2 for overweight; 30 kg/m^2 for obesity) can also be applied as cutoff points in the assessment of pediatric overweight and obesity status (Bellizzi and Dietz 1999; Cole et al. 2000; Dietz and Robinson 1998).

It should be emphasized that careful assessment of children is necessary; only those whose weight status puts them at risk for health complications should be treated (Barlow and Dietz 1998; Himes and Dietz 1994). In addition, a family history of cardiovascular disease, parental hypercholesterolemia, unknown family medical history (American Academy of Pediatrics 1992), a family history of diabetes mellitus, or an obese parent or parents also warrant intervention (Faith et al. 2001). In addition, high blood pressure (Second Task Force on Blood Pressure Control in Children 1987), elevated total cholesterol (National Cholesterol Education Program 1991), a recent larger-than-expected increase in BMI, and psychological or emotional displays and concerns about one's weight status (Barlow and Dietz 1998) are considered complications associated with pediatric obesity.

In sum, proper assessment is crucial in order to identify who is at risk and decide the level of treatment. Himes and Dietz (1994) provided the guidelines in figure 11.1 as a recommendation for the medical assessment of pediatric obesity.

Primary Treatment Components of Efficacious Intervention

Several components of treatment have been shown to increase the odds of a successful intervention (Epstein et al. 1998). The primary components of treatment—dietary change, increases in physical activity, and parental involvement—will be discussed in the ensu-

ing paragraphs. A recent comprehensive review of the child obesity treatment literature concluded that substantial work is needed to reduce the considerable relapse that occurs even in the most well-validated treatments for overweight children (Epstein et al. 1998). We will discuss the promising directions for extending the effects of weight loss treatment into long-term weight maintenance, as well as recommendations for improving long-term weight maintenance treatment outcomes.

Dietary Change

Researchers have demonstrated that changes in the types and quantity of food are crucial to weight loss in children (see Goldfield, Raynor, and Epstein 2002; Faith et al. 2000). Weight loss results when energy expenditure exceeds energy intake. This can be achieved by altering one's diet to reduce caloric and fat intake while increasing the nutritional value of food intake. Several studies have demonstrated the efficacy of dietary changes in obtaining weight loss in children (e.g., Amador et al. 1990; Epstein, Valoski et al. 1994; Epstein, Wing, Penner, and Kress 1985; Rocchini, Katch, and Anderson 1988). Two recent literature reviews (Epstein et al. 1998; Goldfield, Raynor, and Epstein 2002) described several

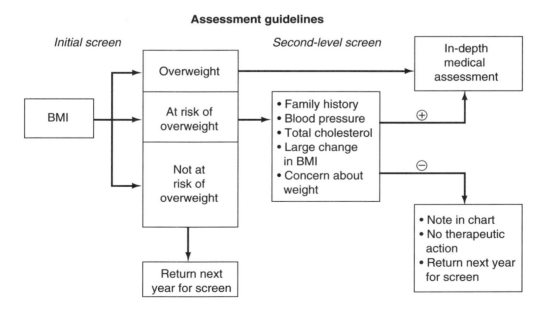

Figure 11.1 Recommended assessment.

Reprinted, by permission, from J.H. Himes and W.H. Dietz, 1994, "Guidelines for overweight in adolescent preventive services: Recommendations from an expert committee," *American Journal of Clinical Nutrition* 59: 307-316.

different dietary approaches to treating pediatric obesity, including moderate and more restrictive decreasing of caloric intake; protein-sparing modified fast (PSMF); and the stoplight diet (Epstein and Squires 1988), a behavioral approach designed for children that is easily understood and based on the USDA food guide pyramid guidelines (see chapter 12, page 181). Moderate caloric restriction and gradual reductions in unhealthy and high-fat food intake have been recommended when instituting a weight loss program for children (Faith et al. 2001).

Epstein and colleagues (1998) found that reductions in high-fat, nutrient-poor foods have been observed after treatment, a behavior change linked with weight loss or decrease in percent overweight. Furthermore, children treated with the stoplight diet also exhibited greater decreases in rated palatability for high-fat and high-sugar foods, with a concomitant greater increase in rated palatability for low-fat and low-sugar foods than their nontreated, lean counterparts (Epstein, Valoski et al. 1994).

Experts working with obese children have endorsed gradually decreasing caloric intake while striving to meet FDA recommended nutritional guidelines (Barlow and Dietz 1998). Behavioral approaches may be particularly useful in obesity treatment, as behavior modification techniques (i.e., behavioral contracting, stimulus control, and specific dietary planning) have been shown to be effective (Coates et al. 1982; Epstein et al. 1980; Johnson et al. 1997). Self-monitoring increases children's awareness of eating habits and is recommended as a first step. Moderate caloric restriction within the range of 1,100 to 1,400 kcal per day, a lessening of fat intake, and a gradual exchange of unhealthy foods for better choices can instigate a shift in negative energy balance. Epstein's stoplight diet (Epstein and Squires 1988) has proven useful in attaining these goals.

Less is known about using PSMF and very low calorie diets for mild to moderately obese children, although studies suggest that long-term outcome is similar to that induced by a more moderate program (Figueroa-Colon et al. 1993). For severely obese children, more restrictive diets are recommended, but only in combination with regular physician supervision (Stallings et al. 1988).

Physical Activity

Weight loss is best achieved through both dietary change and physical activity in concert (Epstein, Coleman, and Myers 1996). Although some studies have demonstrated the effectiveness of physical activity alone, the most successful weight loss treatments have included a physical activity component in addition to a dietary component (Epstein, Valoski et al. 1994). Exercise accelerates weight loss via increased caloric expenditure and increases the likelihood of maintaining lost weight (Brownell and Wadden 1991). In terms of specific activities, aerobic exercise has proven to be more efficacious than calisthenics (Epstein, McKenzie et al. 1994; Epstein et al. 1982).

Reducing sedentary behavior has also been found to increase physical activity (Epstein, Saelens, and Giancola O'Brian 1995) and to induce weight loss (Epstein, Valoski et al. 1995). Saelens and Epstein (1998) found that children for whom television watching was contingent on physical activity increased their physical activity and decreased their television viewing, even when other sedentary activities were available. Moreover, in a study directly comparing children who increased their physical activity to children decreasing sedentary behavior (all of whom were participating in a comprehensive weight loss treatment program), both groups experienced significant decreases in percent overweight and body fat and improved aerobic fitness (Epstein et al. 2000). Therefore, either behavioral intervention objective (i.e., decreasing sedentary behavior or increasing physical activity) can be efficacious in weight loss interventions. The essential component to be coupled with either of these activity-targeted intervention strategies, however, is a dietary intervention (Epstein et al. 1998).

For nonoverweight children, the U.S. Department of Health and Human Services (USDHHS) (1996) recommends that children two or more years of age engage in moderately intense physical activity for at least 30 minutes daily. While not proposing specific guidelines for obese children, the USDHHS has advised that children attempting weight loss increase the duration, frequency, and intensity of physical activity. Furthermore, the USDHHS report suggests that children self-monitor their physical activity, with the aim of becoming more aware of their sedentary behaviors. Helping children to identify and become more cognizant of their current activity as well as the physical activities available to them has been useful, as children are then more likely to initiate change. This is achieved by increasing cues for and providing access to physical activity.

While more research is needed, Epstein and colleagues (Epstein et al. 1982; Epstein, Wing, Koeske, and Valoski 1985; Epstein, Valoski et al. 1994) have found success with a lifestyle approach for pediatric treatment. Lifestyle exercise incorporates energy expenditure through activity into daily events (Epstein et al. 1998), such as taking the stairs instead of the elevator or riding one's bicycle to school (Faith et al. 1997). Moderate or lifestyle activities are encouraged prior to attempting more rigorous physical activities (Faith et al. 2001). In fact, Epstein, Valoski, and colleagues (1994) found that lifestyle activities may be superior to more structured activities (such as aerobics classes) and may be more easily maintained in the long term given that it can be worked into one's daily activity pattern.

Parental Involvement

Parental involvement is a necessary component of successful treatment of pediatric obesity (Brownell, Kelman, and Stunkard 1983; Epstein et al. 1981). Programs for children have varied with respect to degree of parental involvement, but most have found that it is clearly an important factor in helping children achieve weight loss (Goldfield, Raynor, and Epstein 2002). Various clinical studies have found success with interventions in which the parent and child participate together (Epstein, Valoski et al. 1995; Israel et al. 1994), while other settings included only the parents (Golan et al. 1998) or the child alone (e.g., Brownell, Kelman, and Stunkard 1983; Kirschenbaum, Harris, and Tomarken 1984). Although findings have varied regarding which combination is best, Epstein, Valoski, and colleagues (1995) found separate but simultaneous parental participation to be the strongest intervention. Thus, the involvement of parents in weight loss treatment, particularly with young children, is strongly recommended.

We emphasize the importance of parental assistance with the child's self-monitoring of diet and exercise. Involving the entire family in exercise in order to make physical activity more fun has also proven helpful. Similarly, parents can serve as a model to children by exercising along with their children. Other recommendations include following basic parenting skills (Barlow and Dietz 1998), such as finding reasons to praise and correct their child's behavior, restraining from using food as a reward, and establishing daily family meals and snack times (Barlow and Dietz 1998). Figure 11.2 outlines a more comprehensive list of the parenting skills especially valuable in the treatment of pediatric obesity.

Psychological Aspects of Treatment

Few treatments for pediatric obesity have outlined recommendations for coping with the psychological ramifications of obesity in order to facilitate weight loss. Wilfley and colleagues are conducting a study funded by the National Institute of Child Health and Human Development to test two different

- Find reasons to praise the child's behavior.
- Never use food as a reward.
- Offer "rewards" for childen in exchange for the changes in the children's behavior.
- Establish daily family meal and snack times.
- Determine what food is offered and when; let the child decide whether to eat.
- Offer only healthy options.
- Remove temptations.
- Be a role model.
- Be consistent.

Figure 11.2 Recommended parenting skills.
Reproduced with permission from *Pediatrics*, Vol. 102, pages 1-11, Table 5, Copyright 1998.

weight maintenance treatment approaches. The first approach is a behavioral-skills approach that focuses on, for example, the acquisition of coping strategies during high-risk situations for weight control, the use of cognitive restructuring in converting negative self-thoughts during high-risk situations into more appropriate positive self-thoughts, and continued use of parent-facilitated behavior change strategies and reinforcement techniques. Children are often in situations that may be considered high risk in terms of healthy eating, such as birthday parties, or face high peer influence to engage in sedentary behaviors, such as watching television or playing video games. Therefore, coping skills for weight maintenance are most likely important for children, as such skills (e.g., the ability to generate coping responses in hypothetical high-risk situations for weight control, the use of coping strategies during high-risk situations, and the frequent use of problem solving) have been demonstrated to be predictive of their successful maintenance of weight loss in adulthood (Drapkin, Wing, and Shiffman 1995; Grilo, Shiffman, and Wing 1989; Kayman, Bruvold, and Stern 1990; Perri et al. 1989, 1984).

The second weight maintenance approach involves the examination of peer interaction in relation to weight maintenance behaviors. For example, parents and children work together to make the peer environment more supportive of healthful eating and physical activity (Stein, Saelens, and Wilfley 2000). Parents can research and explore community programs that provide physical activity opportunities with other children and can also arrange with other parents for get-togethers where healthy food options are served and physical activity is encouraged (Stein, Saelens, and Wilfley 2000). Working with parents and children in order to teach them to draw on peer support and peer interaction may increase the likelihood that children will be successful in the long-term achievement of healthy weight ranges.

In addition, overweight children report self-consciousness about and reluctance to show their bodies when engaging in physical activity. The social facilitation approach helps promote parent awareness of media influence on one's evaluation of self-worth, the self-exploration of dysfunctional beliefs about

physical appearance, and ways to model positive body acceptance by eliminating negative self-statements and appearance-related comments. Children also learn to critique media images and the promotion of homogeneous body types; focus on the functional, positive aspects of their bodies; and determine multiple ways to feel good about themselves.

Finally, our social facilitation weight maintenance intervention teaches children skills to more effectively cope with negative feelings stemming from societal stigmatization and discrimination (Epstein et al. 2001; Faith et al. 2001; Wilfley et al. 2000). For example, coping with weight-related teasing from peers is taught and role-played with both parents and children in order to help facilitate more appropriate in vivo implementation of these skills. It is hypothesized that such skills, along with other social facilitation components (e.g., promotion of healthy body image, peer support for physical activity and healthy eating, facilitating an educated-consumer approach to a variety of media images) will assist in the long-term maintenance of weight loss. Preliminary findings suggest that addressing psychological and social aspects of obesity in treatment may prove significant in helping children lose weight and maintain a healthy weight.

Challenges to Treatment

When treating obese children, certain barriers to treatment can make treatment progression particularly challenging for child, parent, and therapist alike. Figure 11.3 summarizes the numerous clinical challenges encountered

- Failure to self-monitor
- Motivation
- Sabotage within the family
- Decreased use of positive reinforcement
- Multiple caregivers
- Time constraints
- Poor-quality school lunches
- Festive occasions

Figure 11.3 Challenges to treatment.

throughout the implementation of our pediatric obesity treatment program.

Failure to Self-Monitor

An important component of the weight loss and weight maintenance process is monitoring one's progress and behavior in light of certain treatment goals, such as limiting one's daily calories to a certain number or increasing one's physical activity participation from 30 minutes to 45 minutes per day. It is critical that parents involved in treatment take an active role in their child's monitoring process by providing a structured, consistent schedule for them to complete their monitoring forms. Self-monitoring can be burdensome and time-consuming to the child and parent (Goldfield, Raynor, and Epstein 2002). Therapists must work creatively with the parent and child to find a way to fit recording into busy schedules.

In addition to the time burden, children may also resist self-monitoring due to the discomfort it may induce. Some children report that recording at lunch makes them feel different from the other children in their school cafeteria, for example. However, since recording is most accurate when most immediate to the event, therapists must again work creatively with the children in finding a way that they can record comfortably in a variety of situations (Goldfield, Raynor, and Epstein 2002). In sum, self-monitoring is crucial to weight loss and weight maintenance and must be continued despite the challenges involved.

Motivation

Motivation to continue with treatment can wane over time, especially if the weight loss is less than desired or expected. Children may also feel frustrated with regard to the necessary permanence of the behavior change. Parents must maintain continued, regular positive reinforcement of the child's healthy eating and physical activity behavior changes. Parents must also work with children to accept the new behaviors and habits as a lifestyle change (i.e., behaviors that will remain automatic and permanent).

When children become discouraged, they may express a sense of unfairness in that they feel different from their peers who do not seem as conscientious with regard to their

eating. In this situation, the therapist can help children reframe feeling different in a more positive way, such as considering their family as a family that eats healthfully. The therapist can then model for the parent ways to express support and reinforce learning, thereby motivating their child to persist with the healthy eating and physical activity behavior changes they have worked hard to attain. In sum, because motivation may wane over time, behavioral changes need to be reinforced by both therapist and parent.

Sabotage Within the Family

Even when both child and participating parent are progressing well in treatment, other family members may introduce barriers or challenges to treatment. Specifically, we have encountered situations in which older siblings bring their own high-fat, calorie-dense foods into the house. Participating parents' spouses may also express disagreement with the treatment protocol, thus undermining the child's motivation.

Nonparticipating parents may see the child's weight as a nonissue and disagree with the need for treatment. In this situation, the therapist should encourage the entire family to join in the therapy sessions to emphasize the importance of a supportive environment so that the treatment will have a positive effect. It is also important that the family not single out the overweight child as "the problem" or "a nuisance." In fact, family involvement and support is essential for the child's behavior changes made during treatment to persist in the long term (Goldfield, Raynor, and Epstein 2002) and to avoid sabotage from individual family members.

Decreased Use of Positive Reinforcement

Across the length of treatment, parents may decrease their use of positive reinforcement of the child's healthy eating and physical activity behavior changes (Goldfield, Raynor, and Epstein 2002). Parents are more likely to criticize mistakes or "slips" than to praise positive changes. Some parents may feel that positive reinforcement is not necessary, emphasizing that children should be intrinsically motivated to lose weight and maintain weight changes. Therapists must consistently remind parents to provide regular positive reinforcement for their children, emphasizing that even small rewards create the needed motivation to maintain health behavior change. It has also proven helpful to brainstorm with parents regarding inexpensive reinforcers, especially for those families who cannot afford to provide more expensive reinforcers for their children each month.

Multiple Caregivers

In contemporary society, multiple caregivers are common as a result of the widespread phenomenon of divorced as well as blended families (Hunter et al. 1998). This family structure provides a particularly challenging situation for treatment in that the therapist must work hard to involve all caregivers so that they might better understand the program objectives and lend increased support and sensitivity to the child in treatment. Some divorced parents may actually sabotage treatment in order to win the affection of the child by giving the child foods that the other parent has been eliminating from the child's environment. Again, it is essential that the therapist involve all caregivers in order to clarify the importance of the changes being made and to explain how vital the parents' support is for that behavior change to occur.

Time Constraints

Given the time commitment involved in a weekly behavioral weight loss treatment program, many parents and children find that they lack the time to follow through with the weekly assignments and monitoring involved. This may be because the child is involved in too many extracurricular activities or the parents' schedules are prohibitive. Single-parent homes are especially challenging in this regard. The therapist's task involves meeting with the family to take an intensive look at the many activities they are involved in at the time and to encourage them to reconsider their schedules in light of long- and short-term goals. In short, the therapist must work with the family to focus on short-term goals (i.e., the weight loss program) in order to achieve healthy long-term goals (i.e., long-term healthy weight maintenance). In

this regard, the therapist should recommend that other activities impeding progress (e.g., softball practices and games) be reconsidered so as to better focus on the specific weight loss goals at hand.

Poor-Quality School Lunches

Unfortunately, in the United States, poor-quality school lunches are a deplorable reality (Osganian et al. 1995). The low nutritional value of school lunches as well as the introduction of fast-food chains into some school cafeterias is reprehensible. For many families, packing lunch each morning is viewed as time consuming. Therapists must take a creative approach to school lunches and encourage children to choose the healthiest possible option or to pack healthy snacks to supplement the lunch choice. On the broader societal level, health professionals must work together to challenge school districts on the healthy school lunch issue.

Festive Occasions

Holidays, parties, and family functions create challenges to healthy eating for children. Many families view food as a necessary part of the celebration, and often these foods are of the high-calorie, high-fat variety. Children may express the fear of insulting or offending relatives when refusing homemade foods and may find themselves under social pressure to participate in the festivities by consuming that food. The family can be taught coping skills and appropriate behaviors for such situations. The therapist should challenge the notion that food must be an inherent part of the entertainment. Engaging the family in role-plays so that coping skills can be strategized, practiced, and later implemented in vivo can also be helpful.

Prevention

Given that adult obesity is so resistant to treatment, we must shift our focus toward obesity prevention (National Institutes of Health 1998) through both broad, population-based intervention as well as explicit, early intervention. Specifically, the Institute of Medicine (1995) described three types of prevention: primary, secondary, and tertiary.

Primary prevention best encompasses the idea of obesity *prevention* in that its aim is to intervene with children *before* the excess weight has been gained, with the goal of thwarting adult obesity. This will be discussed as those prevention efforts that target all children in a school program regardless of current weight status. Robinson (1999) has found promising results in this regard.

Secondary prevention seeks to treat obesity shortly after it has emerged. While it is not as immediate as primary prevention, the goal is to intervene before the problem becomes more severe and steadfast. Given the strong link between childhood obesity and adult obesity, successful long-term treatment for pediatric obesity is one of the most promising directions in the prevention of adult obesity (Institute of Medicine 1995; World Health Organization 1998), as it reduces the risk of obese children tracking obesity into adulthood. This form of secondary prevention has also been referred to as "indicated prevention" (Institute of Medicine 1995) or "targeted prevention" (World Health Organization 1998).

The last form of prevention is tertiary prevention, which refers to the treatment of obesity after the condition has existed for a period of time (Faith et al. 1997). This chapter will focus on primary and secondary forms of prevention.

Empirical Literature on Prevention

Of the prevention programs specifically geared toward reduction of fat and energy intake in children, only three studies have proven effective in reducing adiposity. One primary prevention study that reported efficacious findings employed nutrition education versus a conventional diet with the parents of 80 neonates (Piscano et al. 1978). Study findings revealed that a significantly greater percentage of the infants in the comparison group were overweight as compared to the those in the intervention group.

A second study involving tenth-graders (Killen and Robinson 1989) was based on the conceptual perspectives of social cognitive theory (Bandura 1986) and social inoculation theory (McGuire 1964). This 20-session curriculum produced significant reductions in adiposity at two-month follow-up in comparison to controls (Killen et al. 1988).

The third empirically efficacious study, which was aimed at reducing television viewing, has demonstrated promising results (Robinson 1999). The intervention consisted of eighteen 30- to 50-minute lessons across the first six months of the school year (September through April). In this curriculum, lessons emphasized self-monitoring of television, videotape, and video game use. Classes also taught children to be selective viewers and to act as advocates for reducing media consumption. Students participated in a television turnoff for 10 days and were encouraged to follow a seven-hour-per-week budget. Each family was also given a television monitor to effectively budget the use of television viewing.

After completion of the intervention (six months beyond baseline measurement), the children in the intervention group experienced significant decreases in BMI, triceps skinfold thickness, waist circumference, and waist-to-hip ratio in comparison to the control group. Moreover, the intervention children reported less television viewing and less food consumption while watching television. Although there were no differences in high-fat food consumption, physical activity, or cardiorespiratory fitness (Robinson 1999), this curriculum may offer a potentially beneficial component to a school-based prevention program. Perhaps combined with health education, a dietary component, and physical activity, the results might be even more robust.

Recommendations for Prevention

The ensuing sections will discuss several areas to focus on when implementing prevention efforts.

Timing of Prevention

Researchers disagree on the age at which prevention is best undertaken. Some believe that optimal results are achieved during critical periods. Dietz (1994) proposed three critical periods for prevention: the first and second trimesters of pregnancy, between 5 and 7 years of age, and adolescence. Preadolescence is also a particularly sensitive time due to crucial physiological changes occurring during puberty that can cause excess weight to track from childhood and adolescence into adulthood (Robinson and Killen 2001).

Furthermore, thwarting the maintenance of pediatric obesity into adolescence and adulthood may help prevent some of the excess morbidity and mortality associated with adult obesity (Robinson and Killen 2001). As such, early intervention is likely most effective for more positive, longer-lasting health behavior changes (Wilson 1994). Thus, it is recommended that prevention programs be aimed at elementary school children.

Primary and Secondary Prevention in the School

Positive effects have been observed for school-based prevention programs using health education, physical education, health services, and school food services to target health behaviors (e.g., smoking, fitness, diet; see Story 1999). Schools are a promising forum for child-targeted prevention efforts for several reasons. School staff have ongoing contact with 95% of American children between the ages of 5 and 17 (Resnicow 1993). Furthermore, school programs are made available to children of low-income families who might not otherwise be able to afford treatment. Ideally, school cafeterias can provide healthier meals while offering children an opportunity to learn about healthy food choices through informational posters and flyers. Optimally, physical activity is promoted through physical education classes at school, with appropriate equipment made frequently available. School nurses can also provide screening, counseling, and other medical supervision (Story 1999).

However, those involved in school-based obesity prevention efforts have encountered a variety of obstacles. Clinical researchers are deterred by results such as those from a recent meta-analysis that found school-based interventions significantly less efficacious than non-school-based programs (Haddock et al. 1994). Moreover, school prevention programs have not typically achieved significant reductions in adiposity (Resnicow and Robinson 1997).

Researchers may also lack enthusiasm for initiating obesity prevention efforts because of the sensitive nature of such programs. While school systems may be a prime environment for intervention, if not conducted carefully, harmful effects such as labeling, coercion, and stigmatization may occur (Parcel, Greene, and Beetes 1988). In interviewing overweight children from inner-city public schools, Neumark-Sztainer and colleagues (1997) confirmed that a concern about involvement in a school-based program did include the possibility of being teased and stigmatized. Many children requested that a program be undertaken in a supportive and respectful manner, include sensitive leaders who understand the difficulty of being overweight, not be labeled a "weight control" program, and ensure that participation remain anonymous (Neumark-Sztainer et al. 1997).

Despite obstacles encountered, more obesity prevention studies have recently been undertaken in the schools. These interventions have been successful at broadening student knowledge and improving attitudes about being healthy, while instigating positive behavioral changes. However, they are not typically successful at inducing weight loss (Resnicow 1993; Resnicow and Robinson 1997).

Nevertheless, two ongoing studies may prove both promising and informative. The Stanford Obesity Prevention for Pre-Adolescents (OPPrA) Trial (Robinson and Killen 2001) is a multitiered intervention focusing on the primary and secondary prevention of obesity. This three-year program intervenes at school and home with high-risk children from grades 3 through 5 and is based on social cognitive theory. The OPPrA school component includes a classroom curriculum, a physical education intervention, and a school lunch intervention. The home component involves sending newsletters and videos to parents. Children at high risk for developing adult obesity are eligible to participate with a parent in a more intense treatment-oriented program (Robinson and Killen 2001). OPPrA uses state-of-the-art prevention programs for children and may set the standard for multitiered population-based obesity prevention interventions.

Another multicenter, ongoing study called Pathways (Caballero et al. 1998; Davis, Going et al. 1999; Davis, Hunsberger et al. 1999) employs physical activity, food service, classroom curriculum, and family involvement to treat approximately two thousand third-grade Native American children. These children are considered to be at high risk for the development of adult obesity due to their ethnic background (Kumanyika 1993). The study promises to provide rich information regarding the efficacy of school-based programs in ethnically diverse children (Story 1999).

While shortcomings are clearly inherent in school-based programs, given the amount of time children spend in school, it is critical to involve the school in prevention programs in order to infiltrate all aspects of children's daily lives. Such programs may benefit from having interventions tailored to specific behavior changes as they are more likely to establish and promote lasting behavioral changes.

Physical Education

Physical education (PE) classes can assist with increased energy expenditure, and physical education teachers can advise students to engage in regular and frequent activity (Parcel, Green, and Beetes 1988). Specifically, the U.S. Department of Health and Human Services (USDHHS) (1997) recommends that children engage in moderately intense physical activity for at least 30 minutes daily. Moreover, the USDHHS recommends that children from kindergarten through grade 12 be involved in a comprehensive physical education program.

Physical education, particularly as a part of a prevention program, needs to offer enjoyable moderate to vigorous activities for children in school and provide children with the skills to perform similar activities outside of school (Robinson and Killen 2001). CATCH PE (NHLBI) and SPARK PE (Sallis, Chen, and Castro 1995) are two state-of-the-art physical education programs that may prove to be promising obesity prevention programs (Robinson and Killen 2001). These interventions encourage maximum student participation during class time by making more equipment available to children and decreasing inactive physical education time.

Health Education

Health education within an obesity prevention program has two primary aims: teaching children to adopt healthy eating habits and encouraging regular physical activity (Story 1999). Moreover, health education curriculum should focus on the short- and long-term consequences of healthy eating, increasing physical activity, and decreasing sedentary behavior while helping children develop a positive attitude toward more healthful behaviors. The curriculum should encourage the development of healthy food preferences, skills for necessary behavior change, and skills to influence the environment (Robinson and Killen 2001). Similar to obesity treatment, a reduction of calorie-dense foods is a focus of health education (Dietz 1999). Key learning concepts include portion size estimation; safe, healthy, individualized weight management; physical activity techniques; social and emotional influences of positive health; behavioral skills (e.g., monitoring, goal setting); and the initiation and maintenance of change (Parcel et al. 1988; Story 1999). These goals are taught under the premise of making permanent lifestyle changes that promote healthier living and help in protecting against excess weight gain.

School Food Service

The vast majority of school systems in the United States provide foods that are high in fat and sugar and low in nutrition. Particularly in junior and senior high schools, foods that are easily accessible (e.g., cafeteria, vending machines) tend to be unhealthy (Story 1999; Story, Hayes, and Kalina 1996). While the government has taken preliminary steps to require nutritious school meals that follow the Dietary Guidelines for Americans (U.S. Department of Agriculture and Health and Human Services 1995), no widespread legislation has been enacted to enforce such standards. Moreover, many schools use vendor-prepared meals that are delivered prepackaged to schools. As such, prevention programs may have difficulty restructuring food services (Robinson and Killen 2001). Nevertheless, children can be taught to choose healthier options; in fact, the promotion of nutrient-dense foods may enhance healthier taste preferences (Robinson and Killen 2001).

Teacher and Parent Involvement

Teacher training is a key program component to increase classroom emphasis on nutrition education (Story 1999). Instructors must attain proficiency in didactic methods such as discovery learning, cross-age and peer teaching, personal commitment to change, and goal setting, while providing opportunities to increase self-efficacy in modifying health behaviors (Seffrin 1992).

Parents should also serve as collaborators with school instructors and provide much of the same support that has been found to be efficacious in pediatric treatment modalities. To be involved appropriately, parents need to be taught basic skills, such as how to monitor their child's behavior, use contingencies, negotiate, set limits, and praise. Furthermore, parents need to be taught how to provide a low-fat, healthful diet for their family and how to promote the development of healthy food preferences in their child. Finally, they need to be trained to assist their child in reducing sedentary behavior and to build activity into their family routine (Robinson and Killen 2001).

Future Directions for Prevention Research

The prevention of adult obesity is a daunting and complicated endeavor. Continued genetic research will likely ease the difficulty of whom to target (Faith et al. 1997) in prevention efforts. In the meantime, a stepwise program, in which all children are targeted for prevention while those at risk are involved in a more rigorous intervention, may offer a potential compromise.

Manipulating the environment necessitates widespread change, such as taxing fattening foods (Jeffery 1998) or implementing community programs focused on increasing parental involvement (Epstein, Valoski et al. 1994). Furthermore, a potent prevention program is one that includes both individual and environmental approaches. Multilevel or multitiered approaches to prevention hold promise (e.g., Robinson and Killen 2001) in that they target the child both as an individual and in the context of the family, the school, and the broader community. Robinson and Killen (2001) posited that more specificity for behavior change (e.g., altering food preferences; reducing television, videotape, and video game use; and invoking children as health advocates) in the implementation of multilevel prevention efforts is likely to lead to better outcome and may thereby influence healthy eating and physical activity.

Special Concerns of Obesity Intervention and Prevention Programs

Eating disorders, culture and ethnicity, and weight discrimination are important concerns when implementing obesity intervention and prevention programs. They are discussed in the following sections.

Eating Disorders

When working with overweight and obese children, clinicians must be sensitive to the issue of eating disorders. Overweight children and adolescents, particularly girls, are at increased risk for pathology specifically related to eating, shape, and weight (Friedman et al. 1995; Striegel-Moore et al. 1995). Given overweight children's increased risk for an eating disorder, treatment must be considered in terms of how the child will respond to a dietary intervention.

Two recent childhood weight control study findings indicate that weight loss treatment employing moderate caloric restriction may reduce, rather than increase, the risk of overweight children developing eating disorders. Braet and Bettens (1998) as well as Epstein and colleagues (2001) found that eating disorder symptomatology decreased or did not change at follow-up among children receiving weight loss treatment. Furthermore, these rates were lower at follow-up than in overweight children who had not entered weight loss treatment (Braet and Bettens 1998).

The positive benefits of treatment for overweight children are best realized by emphasizing moderate, gradual change by helping children, for example, establish realistic weight goals, increase lifestyle activity (taking the stairs, walking to school), choose activities based on their own preferences, choose from a variety of healthy foods (to increase the likelihood that one or a few of the options will be acceptable to the child), understand the importance of eating three meals per day, and learn to eat healthfully without food restriction. These are just a few examples of ways in which treatment goals can be implemented gradually and reasonably without encouraging pathological eating habits. Similar aims should likewise be incorporated within the prevention context.

Cultural and Ethnicity Issues

The prevalence of obesity in children and adolescents differs significantly by ethnic group (Rosner et al. 1998; Troiano et al. 1995). Data from the largest set of normative height and weight for ethnically diverse children (aged 5 to 11) and adolescents (aged 12 to 17) in the

United States (Rosner et al. 1998) indicate that among females aged 5 to 17, blacks and Hispanics have the highest BMIs. These rates are substantially higher than those of white and Asian females, and differences are especially apparent after age 9. Differences by race among males aged 5 to 17 are less distinct, but Hispanic boys have significantly higher BMIs than boys in the other groups. Native Americans as a whole consistently have high rates of obesity (Kumanyika 1993).

The high rates of obesity in certain ethnic groups as well as in specific subgroups can be explained by the interaction of several culturally and biologically based risk factors. Specific factors that have been examined include socioeconomic status (Sobal and Stunkard 1989); reduced energy expenditure resulting from decreased physical activity (Andersen et al. 1998; Striegel-Moore, Tucker, and Hsu 1990); increased dietary fat intake and higher fast-food consumption (Williams, Achterberg, and Sylvester 1993), especially while watching television (Robinson and Killen 1995); genetic differences in resting metabolic rate (Foster, Wadden, and Vogt 1997; Yanovski et al. 1997); and racial differences in physical maturation and sexual development (Doswell et al. 1998).

Addressing the importance of differences among ethnicities can help improve approaches in treatment. Indeed, Shintani and colleagues (1991) found that weight loss research using an intervention designed to match participants' cultures resulted in enhanced treatment adherence, as well as increased cultural pride. For collectivistically oriented cultures (e.g., Hispanic, Native American, Asian) (Triandis 1995), experts recommend that treatment target the larger family system rather than just the individual (Dounchis, Hayden, and Wilfley 2001).

Education to Reduce Discrimination

Given the emotional toll on obese children and adults, a component focusing on increasing awareness as well as decreasing discrimination and stigmatization is an important facet of prevention programs. Classes should disseminate counterstereotypical information (such as the finding that some overweight people eat healthfully and exercise) to modify biases against obese persons (Faith et al. 2001; Wilder, Simon, and Faith 1996). Faith and colleagues (2000) suggest having obese and non-obese children interact on superordinate goals to increase understanding and compassion. This activity may be particularly appropriate in a school setting where teachers can monitor the interaction.

Moreover, children should be taught to understand that their weight status is largely the result of genetic influences, which are not under their own control, as opposed to controllable factors such as willpower (Allison, Basile, and Yuker 1991; Bell and Morgan 2000; Faith et al. 2000; Weiss 1980). Indeed, findings reveal that an emphasis on external, uncontrollable factors as opposed to internal, controllable factors tends to generate less negative attitudes toward obese individuals (Allison et al. 1991; Weiss 1980). Thus, teaching children in a sensitive manner about the external factors of obesity might help them to realize that people are largely not responsible for their weight status (Faith, Fontaine et al. 2000). While educating children regarding the stereotypical myths of obesity may not prevent excess weight gain, it may help to reduce the psychosocial problems with which obese individuals struggle.

Summary

Pediatric obesity is a rising and significant concern in contemporary society. While treatment has demonstrated to be promising, novel approaches for long-term weight maintenance work need to be applied creatively. The development and empirical assessment of prevention programs need be a priority of researchers and clinicians. Experts advise that part of this effort include continued research to determine which children are at greatest risk for the development of adult obesity. Treatment protocols as well as multilevel prevention programs with a certain level of specificity appear to hold promise as they serve to better guide the intervention. Moreover, both treatment and prevention interventions are best conducted in a way that is sensitive to risk factors for eating and shape-related psychopathology, as well as cultural and ethnic differences among children and their families.

References

Achenbach, T.M., and Elderbrock, C. 1991. *Manual for the Child Behavior Checklist and Revised Child Behavior*

Profile. Burlington, VT: University of Vermont Department of Psychiatry.

Allison, D.B., Basile, V.C., and Yuker, H.E. 1991. The measurement of attitudes toward and beliefs about obese persons. *International Journal of Eating Disorders* 10: 599-607.

Amador, M., Ramos, L.T., Morono, M., and Hermelo, M.P. 1990. Growth rate reduction during energy restriction in obese adolescents. *Experimental & Clinical Endocrinology* 96: 73-82.

American Academy of Pediatrics. 1992. Statement on cholesterol. *Pediatrics* 90: 469-473.

Andersen, R.E., Crespo, C., Bartlett, S.J., Cheskin, L., and Pratt, M. 1998. Relationship of physical activity and television watching with body weight and level of fatness among children. *Journal of the American Medical Association* 279: 938-942.

Bandura, A. 1986. *Social foundations of thought and action.* Englewood Cliffs, NJ: Prentice Hall.

Barlow, S.E., and Dietz, W.H. 1998. Obesity evaluation and treatment: Expert committee recommendations. *Pediatrics* 102: 1-11.

Bell, S.K., and Morgan, S.B. 2000. Children's attitudes and behavioral intentions toward a peer presented as obese: Does a medical explanation for the obesity make a difference? *Journal of Pediatric Psychology* 25: 137-145.

Bellizzi, M.C., and Dietz, W.H. 1999. Workshop on childhood obesity: Summary of the discussion. *American Journal of Clinical Nutrition* 70: 173-175S.

Braet, C., and Bettens, C. 1998. *Overweight in childhood: A risk factor for the development of eating disorders in adolescence?* Unpublished raw data.

Brownell, K.D. 1995. Psychosocial consequences of obesity. In *Eating disorders and obesity: A comprehensive handbook,* eds. K. D. Brownell & C. G. Fairburn, 417-421. New York: Guilford Press.

Brownell, K.D., Kelman, J.H., and Stunkard, A.J. 1983. Treatment of obese children with and without their mothers: Changes in weight and blood pressure. *Pediatrics* 71: 515-523.

Brownell, K.D., and Wadden, T.A. 1991. The heterogeneity of obesity: Fitting treatments to individuals. *Behavior Therapy* 22: 153-177.

Caballero, B., Davis, S., Davis, C.E., Ethelbah, B., Evans, M., Lohman, T., Stephenson, L., Story, M., and White, J. 1998. Pathways: A school-based program for the primary prevention of obesity in American Indian children. *Journal of Nutrition and Biochemistry* 9: 535-543.

Cardon, L.R. 1995. Genetic influences on body mass index in early childhood. In *Behavior genetic approaches in behavioral medicine,* eds. J. R. Turner, L. R. Cardon, and J. K. Hewitt, 133-143. New York: Plenum.

Chinn, S. and Rona, R.J. 2001. Prevalence and trends in overweight and obesity in three cross sectional studies of British children, 1974-1994. *British Medical Journal* 322: 24-26.

Chu, N., Rimm, E.B., Wang, D., Liou, H., and Shieh, S. 1998. Clustering of cardiovascular disease risk factors among obese schoolchildren: The Taipei Children Heart Study. *American Journal of Clinical Nutrition* 67: 1141-1146.

Chunming, C. 2000. Fat intake and nutritional status of children in China. *American Journal of Clinical Nutrition* 72: 1368S-1372S.

Clark, P.J. 1956. The heritability of certain anthropometric characters as ascertained from measurements of twins. *American Journal of Human Genetics* 8: 49-54.

Coates, T.J., Jeffery, R.W., Slinkard, L.A., Killen, J.D., and Danaher, B.G. 1982. Frequency of contact and monetary reward in weight loss, lipid change, and blood pressure reduction with adolescents. *Behavior Therapy* 13: 175-185.

Cole, T.J., Bellizzi, M.C., Flegal, K.M., and Dietz, W.H. 2000. Establishing a standard definition for child overweight and obesity worldwide: International survey. *British Medical Journal* 320: 1240-1253.

Davis, S., Hunsberger, S., Murray, D., Fabsitz, R., Himes, J.H., Stephenson, L.K., Cabellero, B., and Skipper, B. 1999. Design and statistical analysis for Pathways. *American Journal of Clinical Nutrition* 69 (4 Suppl.): 760-763.

Davis, S.M., Going, S., Heliker, D., Tuefel, N., Snyder, P., Gittelsohn, J., Metcalfe, L., Arviso, V., Evans, M., Smyth, M., Brice, R., and Altaha, J. 1999. Pathways: A culturally appropriate obesity-prevention program for American Indian school children. *American Journal of Clinical Nutrition* 69 (4 Suppl.): 796-802.

De Onis, M., and Blossner, M. 2000. Prevalence and trends of overweight among preschool children in developing countries. *American Journal of Clinical Nutrition* 72: 1032-1039.

Dietz, W.H. 1994. Critical periods in childhood for the development of obesity. *American Journal of Clinical Nutrition* 59: 955-959.

Dietz, W.H. 1995. Childhood obesity: Prevalence and effects. In *Eating disorders and obesity,* eds. K.D. Brownell and C.G. Fairburn. 438-440. New York: Guilford Press.

Dietz, W.H. 1999. How to tackle the problem early? The role of education in the prevention of obesity. *International Journal of Obesity and Related Metabolic Disorders* 23 (Suppl. 4): S7-S9.

Dietz, W.H., and Robinson, T.N. 1998. Use of the body mass index (BMI) as a measure of overweight in children and adolescents. *Journal of Pediatrics* 132: 191-193.

Doswell, W.M., Millor, G.K., Thompson, H., and Braxter, B. 1998. Self-image and self-esteem in African-American preteen girls: Implications for mental health. *Issues in Mental Health Nursing* 19: 71-94.

Dounchis, J.Z., Hayden, H.A., and Wilfley, D.E. 2001. Obesity, body image, and eating disorders in ethnically diverse children and adolescents. In *Body image, eating disorders, and obesity in children and adolescents: Theory, assessment, treatment, and prevention,* eds. J. K. Thompson and L. Smolak, 67-98. Washington, DC: American Psychological Association.

Drapkin, R.G., Wing, R.R., and Shiffman, S. 1995. Responses to hypothetical high risk situations: Do they predict weight loss in a behavioral treatment program or the context of dietary lapses? *Health Psychology* 14: 427-434.

Epstein, L.H., Coleman, K.J., and Myers, M.D. 1996. Exercise in treating obesity in children and adolescents. *Medicine and Science in Sports and Exercise* 28: 428-435.

Epstein, L. H., Klein, K.R., and Wisniewski, L. 1994. Child and parent factors that influence psychological problems in obese children. *International Journal of Eating Disorders* 15: 151-158.

Epstein, L.H., McKenzie, S.J., Valoski, A.M., Klein, K.R., and Wing, R.R. 1994. Effects of mastery criteria and contingent reinforcement for family-based child weight control. *Addictive Behaviors* 19: 135-145.

Epstein, L.H., Myers, M.D., Raynor, H.A., and Saelens, B.E. 1998. Treatment of pediatric obesity. *Pediatrics* 101: 554-570.

Epstein, L.H., Paluch, R.A., Gordy, C.C., and Dorn, J. 2000. Decreasing sedentary behaviors in treating pediatric obesity. *Archives of Pediatric & Adolescent Medicine* 154: 220-226.

Epstein, L.H., Paluch, R.A., Saelens, B.E., Ernst, M.M., and Wilfley, D.E. 2001. Changes in eating disorder symptoms with pediatric obesity treatment. *Journal of Pediatrics* 139: 58-65.

Epstein, L.H., Saelens, B.E., and Giancola O'Brien, J. 1995. Effects of reinforcing increases in active behavior versus decreases in sedentary behavior for obese children. *International Journal of Behavioral Medicine* 2: 41-50.

Epstein, L.H., and Squires, S. 1988. *The stoplight diet for children: An eight-week program for parents and children.* Boston: Little, Brown.

Epstein, L.H., Valoski, A.M., Kalarchian, M.A., and McCurley, J.J. 1995. Do children lose and maintain weight easier than adults: A comparison of child and parent weight changes from six months to ten years. *Obesity Research* 3: 411-417.

Epstein, L.H., Valoski, A.M., Wing, R.R., and McCurley, J.J. 1990. Ten-year follow-up of behavioral family-based treatment for obese children. *Journal of the American Medical Association* 264: 2519-2523.

Epstein, L.H., Valoski, A.M., Wing, R.R., and McCurley, J.J. 1994. Ten-year outcomes of behavioral family-based treatment of childhood obesity. *Health Psychology* 13: 573-583.

Epstein, L.H., Wing, R.R., Koeske, R., Andrasik, F., and Ossip D.J. 1981. Child and parent weight loss in family-based behavior modification programs. *Journal of Consulting and Clinical Psychology* 49: 674-685.

Epstein, L.H., Wing, R.R., Koeske, R., Ossip, D., and Beck, S. 1982. A comparison of lifestyle change and programmed exercise on weight and fitness changes in obese children. *Behavior Therapy* 13: 651-665.

Epstein, L.H., Wing, R.R., Koeske, R., and Valoski, A.M. 1985. A comparison of lifestyle exercise, aerobic exercise, and calisthenics on weight loss in obese children. *Behavior Therapy* 16: 345-356.

Epstein, L.H., Wing, R.R., Penner, B.C., and Kress, M.J. 1985. Effects of diet and controlled exercise on weight loss in obese children. *Journal of Pediatrics* 107: 358-361.

Epstein, L.H., Wing, R.R., Steranchak, L., Dickson, B., and Michelson, J. 1980. Comparison of family-based behavior modification and nutrition education for childhood obesity. *Journal of Pediatric Psychology* 5: 25-36.

Epstein, L.H., Wing, R.R., Woodall, K., Penner, B.C., Kress, M.J., and Koeske, R. 1985. Effects of family-based behavioral treatment on obese 5- to-8-year-old children. *Behavior Therapy* 16: 205-212.

Faith, M.S., Fontaine, K.R., Cheskin, L.R., and Allison, D.B. 2000. Behavioral approaches to the problems of obesity. *Behavior Modification* 24: 459-493.

Faith, M.S., Pietrobelli, A., Allison, D.B., and Heymsfield, S.B. 1997. Prevention of pediatric obesity: Examining the issues and forecasting research directions. In *Preventive Nutrition: The Comprehensive Guide for Health Professionals* (1st ed.), eds. A. Bendich and R.J. Deckelbaum 471-486. Totowa, NJ: Humana Press.

Faith, M.S., Saelens, B.E., Wilfley, D.E., and Allison, D.B. 2001. Behavioral treatment of childhood and adolescent obesity: Current status, challenges, and future directions. In *Body image, eating disorders, and obesity in children and adolescents: Theory, assessment, treatment, and prevention,* eds. J. K. Thompson and L. Smolak, 313-340. Washington, DC: American Psychological Association.

Figueroa-Colon, R., von Almen, T.K., Franklin, F.A., Schuftan, C., and Suskind, R.M. 1993. Comparison of two hypocaloric diets in obese children. *American Journal of Diseases of Children* 147: 160-166.

Foster, G.D., Wadden, T.A., and Vogt, R.A. 1997. Resting energy expenditure in obese African American and Caucasian women. *Obesity Research* 5: 1-8.

Friedman, M.A., Wilfley, D.E., Pike, K.M., Striegel-Moore, R.H., and Rodin, J. 1995. The relationship between weight and psychological functioning among adolescent girls. *Obesity Research* 3: 57-62.

Garn, S.M., and Clark, D.C. 1976. Trends in fatness and the origins of obesity. *Pediatrics* 57: 443-456.

Golan, M., Weizman, A., Apter, A., and Fainaru, M. 1998. Parent as the exclusive agents of change in the treatment of childhood obesity. *American Journal of Clinical Nutrition* 67: 1135.

Goldfield, A., and Chrisler, J. C. 1995. Body stereotyping and stigmatization of obese persons by first graders. *Perceptual & Motor Skills* 81: 909-910.

Goldfield, G.S., Raynor, H.A., and Epstein, L.H. 2002. Treatment of pediatric obesity. In *Handbook of obesity treatment*, eds. A. J. Stunkard and T. Wadden, 532-555. New York: Guildford Press.

Gortmaker, S.L., Must, A., Perrin, J.M., Sobol, A.M., and Dietz, W.H. 1993. Social and economic consequences of overweight in adolescence and young adulthood. *The New England Journal of Medicine* 329: 1008-1012.

Grilo, C.M., Shiffman, S., and Wing, R.R. 1989. Relapse crises and coping among dieters. *Journal of Consulting & Clinical Psychology* 57: 488-495.

Gunnell, D.J., Frankel, S.J., Nanchahal, K., Peters, T.J., and Smith, G.D. 1998. Childhood obesity and adult cardiovascular mortality: A 57-year follow-up study based on the Boyd Orr cohort. *American Journal of Clinical Nutrition* 67: 1111-1118.

Gutin, B., Cucuzzo, N., Islam, S., Smith, C., and Stachura, M.E. 1996. Physical training, lifestyle education, and coronary risk factors in obese girls. *Medicine and Science in Sports and Exercise* 28: 19-23.

Haddock, K.C., Shadish, W.R., Klesges, R.C., and Stein, R.J. 1994. Treatments for childhood and adolescent obesity. *Annals of Behavioral Medicine* 16: 235-244.

Hayden, H.A., Stein, R.I., Zabinski, M.F., Saelens, B.E., Dounchis, J.Z., and Wilfley, D.E. 1999, April. Effects of teasing experiences among obese children versus normal-weight peers. Fourth London International Conference on Eating Disorders, London, England.

Himes, J.H., and Dietz, W.H. 1994. Guidelines for overweight in adolescent preventive services: Recommendations from an expert committee. *American Journal of Clinical Nutrition* 59: 307-316.

Hoffman, R.P., Stumbo, P.J., Janz, K.F., and Nielsen, D.H. 1995. Altered insulin resistance is associated with increased dietary weight loss in obese children. *Hormone Research* 44: 17-22.

Hunter, A.G., Pearson, J.L., Ialongo, N.S., and Kellam, S.G. 1998. Parenting alone to multiple caregivers: Child care and parenting arrangements in Black and White urban families. *Family Relations: Interdisciplinary Journal of Applied Family Studies* 47 (4): 343-353.

Institute of Medicine. 1995. *Weighing the options: Criteria for evaluating weight management programs*. Washington, DC: National Academy Press.

Israel, A.C., Guile, C.A., Baker, J.E., and Silverman, W.K. 1994. An evaluation of enhanced self-regulation training in the treatment of childhood obesity. *Journal of Pediatric Psychology* 19: 737-749.

Jeffery, R.W. 1998. Prevention of obesity. In *Handbook of obesity*, eds. G.A. Bray, C. Bouchard, and W.P.T. James, 819-830. New York: Marcel Dekker.

Jelalian, E., and Saelens, B.E. 1999. Empirically supported treatments in pediatric psychology: Pediatric obesity. *Journal of Pediatric Psychology* 24 (3): 223-248.

Johnson, W.G., Hinkel, L.K., Carr, R.E., Anderson, D.A., Lemmon, C.R., Engler, L.B., and Bergeron, K.C. 1997. Dietary and exercise interventions for juvenile obesity: Long-term effects of behavioral and public health models. *Obesity Research* 5: 257-261.

Kayman, S., Bruvold, W., and Stern, J.S. 1990. Maintenance and relapse after weight loss in women: Behavioral aspects. *American Journal of Clinical Nutrition* 52: 800-807.

Killen, J.D., and Robinson, T.N. 1989. School-based research on health behavior change: The Stanford adolescent heart health program as a model for cardiovascular disease risk reduction. In *Review of research in education*, ed. E. Rothkopf, 171-200. Washington, DC: American Educational Research Association.

Killen, J.D., Telch, M.J., Robinson, T.N., Maccoby, N., Taylor, C.B., and Farquhar, J.W. 1988. Cardiovascular disease risk reduction for tenth-graders: A multiple-factor school-based approach. *Journal of the American Medical Association* 260(12), 1728-1733.

Kinston, W., Loader, P., and Miller, L. 1987. Emotional health of families and their members where a child is obese. *Journal of Psychosomatic Research* 31: 583-599.

Kirschenbaum, D.S., Harris, E.S., and Tomarken, A.J. 1984. Effects of parental involvement in behavioral weight loss therapy for preadolescents. *Behavior Therapy* 15: 485-500.

Klem, M.L., Wing, R.R., McGuire, M.T., Seagle, H.M., and Hill, J.O. 1997. A descriptive study of individuals successful at long-term maintenance of substantial weight loss. *American Journal of Clinical Nutrition* 66: 239-246.

Kumanyika, S. 1993. Ethnicity and obesity development in children. Prevention and treatment of childhood obesity. *Annals of the New York Academy of Sciences* 699: 81-92.

Lissau, I. and Sorensen, T.I. 1994.. Parental neglect during childhood and increased risk of obesity in young adulthood. *Lancet* 343: 324-327.

MacDonald, A., and Stunkard, A.J. 1990. Body-mass index of British separated twins. *New England Journal of Medicine* 332: 1483-1487.

McGuire, W. 1964. Inducing resistance to persuasion. In *Advances in experimental social psychology*, ed. L. Berkowitz, 191-229. New York: Academic Press.

Mendelson, B.K., White, D.R., and Schliecker, E. 1995. Adolescents' weight, sex, and family functioning. *International Journal of Eating Disorders* 17: 73-79.

Muller, M.J., Koertringer, I., Mast, M., Languix, K., and Frunch, A. 1999. Physical activity and diet in 7- to 11-year-old children. *Public Health Nutrition* 2: 443-444.

Must, A., Jacques, P.S., Dallal, G.E., Bajema, C.J., and Dietz, W.H. 1992. Long-term morbidity and mortality of overweight adolescents. *New England Journal of Medicine* 327: 1350-1355.

National Cholesterol Education Program. 1991. *Report of the Expert Panel on Blood Cholesterol Levels in Children and Adolescents* (Publication No. 91-2732). Washington, DC: U.S. Government Printing Office.

National Institutes of Health; National Heart, Lung, and Blood Institute. 1998. Clinical guidelines on the identification, evaluation, and treatment of overweight and obesity in adults— The evidence report. *Obesity Research* 6 (Suppl. 2): 51S-209S.

Neumark-Sztainer, D., Story, M., French, S.A., and Resnick, M.D. 1997. Psychosocial correlates of health compromising behaviors among adolescents. *Health Education Research* 12: 37-52.

Osganian, S.K., Nicklas, T., Stone, E., Nichaman, M., Ebzery, M.K., Lytle, L., and Nader, P.R. (1995). Perspectives on the School Nutrition Dietary Assessment Study from the Child and Adolescent Trial for Cardiovascular Health. *American Journal of Clinical Nutrition* 61 (Suppl. 1): 241S-244S.

Parcel, G.S., Green, L.W., and Beetes, B.A. 1988. School-based programs to prevent or reduce obesity. In *Childhood obesity: A biobehavioural perspective*, eds. N. A. Krasnegor, G. D. Grave, and N. Kretchmer, 143-157. Caldwell, NJ: Jedfor Press.

Perri, M.G., Nezu, A.M., Patti, E.T., and McCann, K.L. 1989. Effect of length of treatment on weight loss. *Journal of Consulting & Clinical Psychology* 57: 450-452.

Perri, M.G., Shapiro, R. M., Ludwig, W.W., Twentyman, C.T., and McAdoo, W.G. 1984. Maintenance strategies for the treatment of obesity: An evaluation of relapse prevention training and post-treatment contact by mail and telephone. *Journal of Consulting & Clinical Psychology* 52: 404-413.

Phillips, R.G. and Hill, A. 1997, April. Friendless, fat, and dieting: Peer popularity and weight control in 9-year-old girls. Third London International Conference on Eating Disorders, London, England.

Piscano, J.C., Lichter, H., Ritter, J., and Siegal, A.P. 1978. An attempt at prevention of obesity in infancy. *Pediatrics* 61: 360-364.

Resnicow, K. 1993. School-based obesity prevention: Population versus high-risk interventions. In *Prevention and treatment of childhood obesity*, eds. C.L. Williams and S.Y.S. Kimm, 154-166). New York: New York Academy of Sciences.

Resnicow, K., and Robinson, T.N. 1997. School-based cardiovascular disease prevention studies: Review and synthesis. *Annals of Epidemiology* (Suppl. 7): S14-S31.

Rieves, L., and Cash, T.F. 1996. Social developmental factors and women's body image attitudes. *Journal of Social Behavior and Personality* 11: 63-78.

Robinson, T.N. 1999. Behavioural treatment of childhood and adolescent obesity. *International Journal of Obesity* 23 (Suppl. 2): S52-S57.

Robinson, T.N., and Killen, J.D. 1995. Ethnic and gender differences in the relationships between television viewing and obesity, physical activity, and dietary fat intake. *Journal of Health Education* 26 (Suppl. 2): S94-S98.

Robinson, T.N., and Killen, J.D. 2001. Obesity prevention for children and adolescents. In *Body image, eating disorders, and obesity in children and adolescents: Theory, assessment, treatment, and prevention*, eds. J. K. Thompson and L. Smolak, 261-292. Washington, DC: American Psychological Association.

Rocchini, A.P., Katch, V., and Anderson, J. 1988. Blood pressure in obese adolescents: Effect of weight loss. *Pediatrics* 82: 16-23.

Rosner, B., Prineas, R., Loggie, J., and Daniels, S.R. 1998. Percentiles for body mass index in U.S. children 5 to 7 years of age. *Journal of Pediatrics* 132: 211-222.

Saelens, B.E., and Epstein, L.H. 1998. Behavioral engineering of activity choice in obese children. *International Journal of Obesity and Related Metabolic Disorders* 22: 275-277.

Sallis, J.F., Chen, A.H., and Castro, C.M. 1995. School-based interventions for childhood obesity. In *Child health, nutrition and physical activity*, eds. L.W.Y. Cheung and J.B. Richmond, 179-204. Champaign, IL: Human Kinetics.

Second Task Force on Blood Pressure Control in Children. 1987. Report on the Second Task Force on Blood Pressure Control in Children. *Pediatrics* 79: 1-25.

Seffrin, J. 1992. Why school health education? In *Principles and practices of student health*, eds. H.M. Wallace,

K. Patrick, G. Parcel, and J.B. Igbe, 393-422. Oakland: Third Party Publishing.

Serdula, M.K., Ivery, D., Coates, R.J., Freedman, D.S., Williamson, D.F., and Byers, T. 1993. Do obese children become obese adults? A review of the literature. *Preventive Medicine* 22: 167-177.

Shapiro, J.P., Baumeister, R.F., and Kessler, J.W. 1991. A three-component model of children's teasing: Aggression, humor, and ambiguity. *Journal of Social and Clinical Psychology* 10: 459-472.

Shintani, T.T., Hughes, C.K., Beckham, S., and O'Connor, H.K. 1991. Obesity and cardiovascular risk intervention through the ad libitum feeling of traditional Hawaiian diet. *American Journal of Clinical Nutrition* 53: 1647S-1651S.

Sobal, J., and Stunkard, A.J. 1989. Socioeconomic status and obesity: A review of the literature. *Psychological Bulletin* 105: 260-275.

Sorensen, T.A., Holst, C., Stunkard, A.J., and Skovgaard, L.T. 1992. Correlations of body mass index of adult adoptees and the biological and adoptive relatives. *International Journal of Obesity* 16: 227-236.

Staffieri, J.R. 1967. A study of social stereotype of body image in children. *Journal of Personality and Social Psychology* 7: 101-104.

Stallings, V.A., Archibald, E.H., Pencharz, P.B., Harrison, J.E., and Bell, J.E. 1988. One-year follow-up of weight, total body potassium, and total body nitrogen in obese adolescents treated with the protein-sparing modified fast. *American Journal of Clinical Nutrition* 48: 91-94.

Stein, R.I., Saelens, B.E., and Wilfley, D.E. 2000. Peer influences on children's body weight: Getting a little help from friends. *The Weight Control Digest* 10: 891, 894-897, 906.

Story, M. 1999. School-based approaches for preventing and treating obesity. *International Journal of Obesity* 23 (Suppl. 2): S43-S51

Story, M., Hayes, M., and Kalina, B. 1996. Availability of foods in high schools: Is there cause for concern? *Journal of American Dietetic Association* 96: 123-126.

Striegel-Moore, R.H., Schreiber, G.B., Pike, K. M., Wilfley, D.E., and Rodin, J. 1995. Drive for thinness in black and white preadolescent girls. *International Journal of Eating Disorders* 18: 59-69.

Striegel-Moore, R.H., Tucker, N., and Hsu, J. 1990. Body image dissatisfaction and disordered eating in lesbian college students. *International Journal of Eating Disorders* 9: 493-500.

Stunkard, A.J., Harris, J.R., Pedersen, N.L., and McClearn, G.E. 1990. The body-mass index of twins who have been reared apart. *New England Journal of Medicine* 21: 1483-1487.

Thompson, J.K., Coovert, M.D., Richards, K.J., and Johnson, S. 1995. Development of body image, eating disturbance, and general psychological functioning in female adolescents: Covariance structure modeling and longitudinal investigations. *International Journal of Eating Disorders* 18: 221-236.

Triandis, H.C. 1995. *Individualism and collectivism.* Boulder, CO: Westview Press.

Troiano, R.P., and Flegal, K.M. 1998. Overweight children and adolescents: Description, epidemiology, and demographics. *Pediatrics* 101: 497-504.

Troiano, R.P., Flegal, K.M., Kuczmarski, R.J., Campbell, S.M., and Johnson, C.L. 1995. Overweight prevalence and trends for children and adolescents. *Archives of Pediatric Adolescent Medicine* 149: 1085-1091.

Troiano, R.P., Frongillo, E.A. Jr., Sobal, J., and Levitski, D.A. 1996. The relationship between body weight and mortality: A quantitative analysis of combined information from existing studies. *International Journal of Obesity and Related Metabolic Disorders* 20: 63-75.

U.S. Department of Agriculture and Health and Human Services. 1995. *Nutrition and your health: Dietary guidelines for Americans,* 4th ed. Washington, DC: U.S. Court Printing Office.

U.S. Department of Health and Human Services. 1996. *Physical activity and health: A report of the surgeon general.* Atlanta, GA: U.S. Department of Health and Human Services, Centers for Disease Control and Prevention, National Center for Chronic Disease Prevention and Health Promotion.

U.S. Department of Health and Human Sciences. 1997. *Guidelines for school community programs to promote lifelong physical activity among young people.* Atlanta, GA: U.S. Department of Health and Human Services, Centers for Disease Control and Prevention, National Center for Chronic Disease Prevention and Health Promotion.

Vara, L.S., and Epstein, L.H. 1993. Laboratory assessment of choice between exercise or sedentary behavior. *Research Quarterly for Exercise and Sport* 64: 356-360.

Wabitsch, M., Braun, U., Heinze, E., Muche, R., Mayer, H., Teller, W., and Fusch, C. 1996. Body composition in 5-18-y-old obese children and adolescents before and after weight reduction as assessed by deuterium dilution and bioelectrical impedance analysis. *American Journal of Clinical Nutrition* 64: 1-6.

Weiss, E. 1980. Perceived self-infliction and evaluation of obese and handicapped persons. *Perceptual & Motor Skills* 50: 1268-1271.

Whitaker, R.C., Wright, J.A., Pepe, M.S., Seidel, K.D., and Dietz, W.H. 1997. Predicting obesity in young adulthood from childhood and parental obesity. *New England Journal of Medicine* 337: 869-873.

Wilder, D.A., Simon, A.F., and Faith, M. 1996. Enhancing the impact of counterstereotypic information: Dispositional attributions for deviance. *Journal of Personality and Social Psychology* 71: 276-287.

Wilfley, D.E., Stein, R.I., Saelens, B.E., and Epstein, L.E. 2000. Models of weight regain and weight loss maintenance in overweight children. Manuscript in preparation.

Williams, J.D., Achterberg, C., and Sylvester, G.P. 1993. Target marketing of food products to ethnic minority youth. In *Prevention and treatment of childhood obesity,* eds. C. L. Williams and S. Y. Kimm, 107-114. New York: New York Academy of Sciences.

Wilson, G.T. 1994. Behavioral treatment of obesity: Thirty years and counting. *Advances in Behaviour Research & Therapy* 16: 31-75.

World Health Organization. 1998. *Obesity: Preventing and managing the global epidemic* (Publication No. xv-276). Geneva: World Health Organization.

Yanovski, S.Z., Reynolds, J.C., Boyle, A.J., and Yanovski, J.A. 1997. Resting metabolic rate in African-American and Caucasian girls. *Obesity Research* 5: 321-525.

Chapter 12

Medical Nutrition Therapy Application

Laure Sullivan, RD
Johns Hopkins School of Medicine

Maintaining a healthy weight throughout one's lifetime, and avoiding the "yo-yo" dieting syndrome, can reduce the risk of many health problems. Eating to control weight and eating for good health should be viewed as the same goal rather than as two separate goals. A registered dietitian or other qualified nutrition expert can provide patients with an individualized plan and nutrition education aimed at making lifestyle changes to promote a lifetime of healthy weight management.

Determining Caloric Deficit to Promote Weight Loss

To lose weight, individuals must expend more calories (kcals) than they consume. Several methods can be used to determine the estimated caloric deficit necessary to promote a healthy weight loss. Mathematically, a 500-kcal-per-day deficit will produce a weight loss of approximately 1 lb (0.45 kg) per week. This may be discouraging to a patient who needs to lose in excess of 100 lb (45 kg). However, the amount of the initial weight loss seen in the first few weeks can be motivating, as larger patients tend to lose weight faster initially. It is not unusual to see a loss of 4 lb (1.8 kg) or more the first week

of a restricted diet. This may be due in part to diuresis.

Estimating Basal Metabolic Rate (BMR)

To determine an individualized calorie deficit, the clinician must first have an idea of the patient's resting and nonresting energy requirements. The most accurate way of measuring this is using a respiratory calorimeter or a metabolic cart. This equipment is typically available in university and hospital settings. In the absence of such equipment, the equations used most frequently by registered dietitians in a clinical setting are the Harris-Benedict equations (Harris and Benedict 1919; Blackburn et al. 1977; Consultant Dieticians in Health Care Facilities 2001). These formulas estimate basal energy expenditure (BEE) based on height in centimeters, weight in kilograms, gender, and age. The BEE is then multiplied by an activity factor and, if appropriate, a stress factor.

The basal metabolic rate can be thought of as the minimum amount of energy needed to keep the body in energy balance in the waking state. The terms *basal metabolic rate* and *resting metabolic rate* are often used interchangeably. Following are the gender-specific

Harris-Benedict equations (Harris and Benedict 1919):

Male: Basal energy expenditure (kcal/day) = 66 + (13.7 × weight [kg]) + (5 × height [cm]) − (6.8 × age)

Female: Basal energy expenditure (kcal/day) = 655 + (9.6 × weight [kg]) + (1.8 × height [cm]) − (4.7 × age)

Factors That Affect Energy Expenditure

For most people, food has a stimulating effect on metabolism because of the metabolic cost of digestion and absorption and the excretion of consumed food. This is often called the thermic effect of feeding (TEF) and tends to reach its peak about one hour after a meal is consumed. The TEF tends to represent about 10% of the daily energy expenditure in most healthy adults.

Physical activity stimulates energy expenditure most intensely. Most healthy adults can increase their resting energy requirements by 8 to 10 times above their resting levels during sustained aerobic exercise, such as jogging, cycling, swimming, and aerobic dance. Individuals who do manual labor also tend to expend far more calories than their sedentary counterparts. Thus, to estimate total daily energy expenditure, clinicians must estimate a patient's activity level. After querying about leisure-time and work-related energy expenditure, the following activity factors should be recorded:

Activity Factors (AF)

Confined to bed	1.1
Confined to bed or chair	1.2
Light	1.3
Moderate	1.4
Active	1.5
Very active	2.0

Many medical factors are known to affect a person's rate of energy metabolism. If appropriate, the following stress or medical factors should be used to help estimate daily energy requirements:

Stress Factors (SF)

Postoperative

(No complications)	1.00 – 1.05
Peritonitis	1.05 – 1.25
Minor surgery	1.2
Cancer	1.10 – 1.45
Long bone fracture	1.15 – 1.30

Decubitus ulcers

Stage I	1.0 – 1.1
Stage II	1.3 – 1.4
Stage III	1.3 – 1.4
Stage IV	1.5 – 1.6

Fever, per each degree

Fahrenheit above 98.6	1.07

Wound healing	1.2 – 1.6
Blunt trauma	1.25 – 1.5
Skeletal trauma	1.35
Severe infection/ multiple trauma	1.3 – 1.5
Multiple trauma/ on ventilator	1.5 – 1.7
Trauma with steroid sepsis	1.75 – 1.85

Thermal burns (% of total body surface)

0-20%	1.0 – 1.5
20-40%	1.5 – 1.8
40-100%	1.8 – 2.1

Estimating Daily Nutrient Needs

To estimate the total daily calories (ETDC) needed, multiply the BMR times the activity factor (AF) times the stress factor (SF), if appropriate.

ETDC = (BMR) × (AF) × (SF)

Establishing a Healthy Caloric Deficit

Most experts agree that a weight loss of approximately 1 to 2 lb (0.45 to 0.9 kg) per week is safest. A 500-kcal-per-day deficit will result in a loss of approximately 1 lb (0.45 kg) per week, whereas a 1,000-kcal-per-day reduction will be associated with a 2-lb (0.9 kg) loss.

Therefore, to estimate what daily requirements should be for an individual, clinicians can subtract 500 to 1,000 kcal from the estimated total daily calories calculated earlier.

A woman is considered obese if she is ≥120% of her IBW. A man is considered obese at 125% or greater than his IBW. IBW is based on sex and height. The calculations are as follows:

> Men: IBW = 106 lb (48.2 kg) for the first 5 ft (60 in. or 152.4 cm). Add to that 6 lb (2.7 kg) for each additional inch above 5 ft.
>
> Women: IBW = 100 lb (45.5 kg) for the first 5 ft. Add to that 5 lb (2.3 kg) for each additional inch above 5 ft.
>
> (For anyone below 5 ft tall, subtract 2 lb [0.9 kg] for each inch below 5 ft.)

(In the case of any amputated limbs, there is an additional adjustment factor which I will not go into here.)

For example, following is a calculation for an overweight 42-year-old female who stands 5 ft, 2 in. tall (157.5 cm) and weighs 150 lb (68 kg). Assuming she has a relatively sedentary lifestyle and is otherwise healthy, her ideal body weight (IBW), metabolically active weight (MAW), and her energy needs for weight maintenance and weight loss would be calculated as follows:

> IBW = 110 lb [100 lb + (2 in. × 5 lb)]
>
> % IBW = 136% [150 lb ÷ 110 lb (actual body weight ÷ IBW)]
>
> Because by definition she is considered obese, we would use her MAW in the calculation for BEE.
>
> MAW = [0.25 × (ABW − IBW) + IBW
>
> = 0.25 × (150 − 110) +110
>
> = 120 lb (54.5 kg)
>
> BEE = 655 + (9.6 × 54.5 kg) = 1,178
>
> + (1.8 × 157.5 cm) = 283.5
>
> - (4.7 × 42 yr) = 197.4
>
> = (1,178 + 283.5) − 197.4
>
> = 1,265 kcal

> Multiply by the appropriate activity factor, but no stress factor since she is healthy:
>
> ETDC = BEE × 1.3 (light activity)
>
> = 1,265 × 1.3
>
> = 1,645
>
> Subtract 500 kcal to create a deficit predicting 1 lb of weight loss per week:
>
> = 1,645 kcal − 500
>
> = 1,145 kcal/day needed for weight loss

Knowing that most people underestimate their intake, clinicians would be wise to have them aim for approximately 1,200 kcal, knowing that they will likely overshoot this and may consume 1,400 to 1,500 kcal. The more nutrition education patients receive, the more accurate they will be in estimating their intake. This is where a registered dietitian can be very helpful to a health care professional without formal training in the food sciences. For example, I have a patient who was referred to me by her physician. Her doctor gave her a sheet of paper with an example of a 1,200-kcal diet and had instructed her to lose weight. This frustrated patient came to me stating that she had been following this 1,200-kcal diet and had lost a total of only 6 lb (2.7 kg) over four months and then had hit a plateau and had been weight stable for seven weeks. Upon interviewing this patient, I discovered that she was actually consuming approximately 2,200 kcal per day. At 215 lb (97 kg), 2,200 calories was what her caloric needs for weight maintenance would be, based on the rule of thumb that obese patients need 10 kcal/lb (22 kcal/kg) to maintain their current level of obesity (Bray 1998). The main reason for this patient's lack of success was that she was not properly educated on measuring or estimating portion sizes of foods. In fact, she was underestimating her intake by approximately 1,000 kcal per day.

Unfortunately, this is not an uncommon scenario. Many of my patients enter treatment consuming 2,000 to 3,000 kcal per day while expecting to lose weight. When patients receive ongoing nutrition education in conjunction with behavior modification, they learn to make lower-fat, lower-calorie, and higher-fiber food choices. These changes may allow them to eat a greater quantity of food than their typical high-fat, calorie-dense choices, while maintaining a caloric deficit. A patient that is not physically hungry is much more likely to comply with a reduced calorie diet and weight management program.

Adjusting for Physical Activity and Increased Energy Expenditure

Patients who dramatically increase their physical activity levels may need to gradually increase their calorie levels. The previously referenced patient, for example, began walking just 10 minutes per day, aiming for most days of the week, and built up to 30 minutes per day, five days per week. At that level, and walking at a moderate intensity of 4 mph, she was burning off an additional 150 kcal per day, or 750 kcal per week (*Practical guide* 2000). In her case, the prescribed caloric deficit was decreased by approximately 107 kcal per day (750 calories per week divided by seven days). In other words, she was able to consume an additional 750 kcal per week and still maintain an average rate of 1 to 2 lb (0.45 to 0.9 kg) weight loss per week.

Generally, patients should not restrict kcal below 1,200 per day, with the exception of a protein-sparing modified fast in which a physician follows the patient closely and monitors blood work frequently (Flynn and Walsh 1993; National Task Force on the Prevention and Treatment of Obesity 1993). Patients should always increase physical activity as tolerated in addition to restricting calories. In addition to its obvious health benefits, exercise can help to offset the decrease in the resting metabolic rate associated with caloric restriction. Many patients seek professional guidance after an initial weight loss success followed by a frustrating plateau. Often they have not maintained any form of physical activity, and as soon as they increase their levels of activity, whether in the form of walking, weight training, jogging, lifestyle activities, or some combination, they generally break through the plateau and resume losing weight.

Macronutrient Distribution

In general, clinicians should encourage most patients to reduce saturated fat intake and the amount of protein they consume. Furthermore, they should also encourage patients to eat more complex carbohydrates and to consume mostly unsaturated fats (Food and Nutrition Board, Institute of Medicine 2002). The recommended intake of carbohydrate, protein, and fat is as follows:

45-65% of kcal from carbohydrate (CHO),* mainly from whole grains, fruits, and vegetables

10-35% of kcal from protein

20-35% of kcal from fat

(No more than 10% of total kcal should be from saturated fatty acids.)

   * A patient with diabetes may benefit from a smaller percentage of CHO, perhaps 45 to 55%.

A registered dietitian can calculate an individual's calorie requirements and distribute the calories appropriately, taking into consideration the patient's medical status, food preferences, and micronutrient needs. Calories are distributed using the following information and formulas:

Source of energy	kcal/g
Carbohydrate	4
Protein	4
Fat	9
Alcohol	7

Establishing a meal plan

Step 1. Multiply total kcal by each percentage used to arrive at the kcal needed of each nutrient—for example, 0.65 for CHO, 0.10 for protein, and 0.25 for fat. (Alcohol provides "empty" calories and is included for reference.)

Step 2. Divide each figure obtained in step 1 by the kcal/g of that nutrient, which is the grams of that nutrient to be distributed through the day.

The patient in the previous example had been prescribed a 1,200-kcal diet. To provide 65% of her kcal as CHO, 10% as protein, and 25% as fat, we perform the following calculations:

$$1{,}200 \text{ kcal} \times 0.65 = 780 \text{ kcal from CHO}$$
$$780 \div 4 = 195 \text{ g CHO}$$

$$1{,}200 \text{ kcal} \times 0.10 = 120 \text{ kcal from protein}$$
$$120 \div 4 = 30 \text{ g protein}$$

$$1{,}200 \text{ kcal} \times 0.25 = 300 \text{ kcal from fat}$$
$$300 \div 9 = 33 \text{ g fat}$$

Using the grams of each nutrient, we then use an exchange list, such as the Exchange Lists for Weight Management, available from the American Diabetes Association. This booklet can be ordered by visiting their Web site at www.diabetes.org, or by calling 800-Diabetes (800-342-2383).

Ideally, calories should be divided among three meals and two to three snacks, or six smaller meals. This promotes a healthy me-tabolism and takes advantage of the thermic effect of foods. A meal plan of 1,200 kcal, however, is usually divided up into three meals and one snack. Bray (1976) reported that individuals who consume only one or two meals a day are more likely to be obese than those who consume three or more smaller meals per day.

Without an exchange list, many patients find the food guide pyramid (see figure 12.1) a helpful tool. The food guide pyramid (FGP) was developed by the U.S. Department of Agriculture (USDA) and the U.S. Department of Health and Human Services (USDHHS) and is based on the *Dietary Guidelines for Americans*. The most recent set of *Dietary Guidelines for Americans* was released in May 2000. Every five years, current research on the guidelines is reviewed by a committee of invited experts who may make changes to the guidelines and release a new FGP to the public.

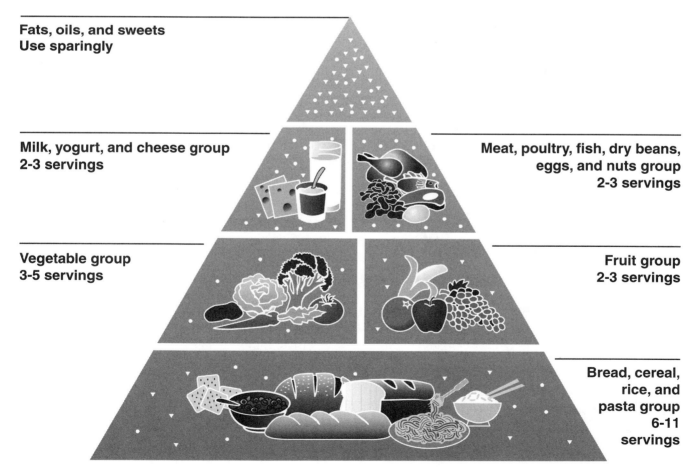

**Fats, oils, and sweets
Use sparingly**

**Milk, yogurt, and cheese group
2-3 servings**

**Meat, poultry, fish, dry beans,
eggs, and nuts group
2-3 servings**

**Vegetable group
3-5 servings**

**Fruit group
2-3 servings**

**Bread, cereal,
rice, and
pasta group
6-11
servings**

Figure 12.1 U.S. Department of Agriculture food guide pyramid.

The pyramid is a tool designed to help people choose a balanced diet while eating a variety of foods. If they choose the low end of the serving range for all five food groups, they will consume approximately 1,600 kcal. This means they would choose six servings from the bread, cereal, rice, and pasta group; two servings from the fruit group; three servings from the vegetable group; two servings from the milk, yogurt, and cheese group; and two servings from the meat, poultry, fish, dry beans, eggs, and nuts group. The midrange of servings would provide about 2,200 kcal, and the upper end would provide about 2,800 kcal. Everyone should choose sparingly from the group located at the tip of the pyramid—fats, oils, and sweets.

When using the food guide pyramid to help patients with weight management, dieticians should emphasize low-fat, low-calorie choices, as the Pyramid itself does not differentiate. For example, whole milk is equivalent to fat-free milk when following the Pyramid. However, whole milk has approximately 150 kcal and 8 g of fat per serving, while fat-free milk contains about 90 kcal and 0 g of fat per serving.

Limiting Dietary Fat to Reduce Caloric Intake

Counting fat grams is also a useful tool in cutting calories and planning a healthy diet. Table 12.1 provides the upper limit of fat (30% of calories) for several calorie levels. Patients should keep a daily food diary that tracks calories consumed, fat intake, and physical activity. Research has consistently demonstrated that systematically recording food and exercise is one of the strongest predictors of weight management success (Bray 1998; Duyff 1998; National Task Force on the Prevention and Treatment of Obesity 1993; *Practical guide* 2000). Many clients find that when they are writing down everything they eat, they tend to make leaner, healthier food choices.

When referring to the food guide pyramid, patients should understand what constitutes a single food serving. Table 12.2 illustrates examples of typical single food servings (*Food Guide Pyramid* 1992). Six breads may sound like a great deal of food until you realize that one cup of oatmeal would use up two bread servings, one sandwich is equivalent to another two servings, and one cup of cooked pasta is two more servings for a total of six servings.

Lowering Dietary Fat Intake

By making small changes, patients can cut down on calories without drastically sacrificing taste or satiety value. For example, by choosing a 3.5-oz serving of roasted tenderloin instead of a 3.5-oz portion of a braised chuck blade roast, calories would be reduced by 182, and fat intake by 21 g (Bowes, Church, and Church 1994). Keeping in mind that it takes a 500-kcal-per-day reduction (3,500 kcal per week) to lose 1 lb (0.45 kg), this is a good start.

Following are some suggestions for preparing meals and choosing lower-fat foods:

Protein foods

- Choose fish, chicken, turkey, and lean red meats most often.
- When buying beef and pork, remember that the leanest cuts of meat contain the words *round* or *loin*—for example, ground round, round steak, tenderloin, loin chop, and sirloin.
- Remember that the white meat of chicken and turkey contains considerably less fat than the dark meat.
- Trim meats of all visible fat before cooking.
- Remove chicken and turkey skin before cooking.

Table 12.1 Maximum Fat Intake per Calorie Level

Daily caloric intake	Daily fat intake (upper limit)
1,200	40 grams
1,500	50 grams
1,600	53 grams
1,800	60 grams
2,000	66 grams
2,200	73 grams
2,400	80 grams

Table 12.2 — *Single Food Pyramid Servings*

Bread, Cereal, Rice, and Pasta

1 slice of bread

1 oz of ready-to-eat cereal

1/2 c of cooked cereal, rice, or pasta

Vegetable

1 c raw, leafy vegetables

1/2 c other vegetables, cooked or chopped raw

3/4 c vegetable juice

Fruit

1 medium apple, banana, or orange

1/2 c chopped, cooked, or canned fruit

3/4 c fruit juice

Milk, Yogurt, and Cheese

1 c milk or yogurt

1 1/2 oz of natural cheese

2 oz of processed cheese

Meat, Poultry, Fish, Dry Beans, Eggs, and Nuts

2-3 oz cooked lean meat, poultry, or fish

1/2 c cooked dry beans, 1 egg, or 2 tbsp peanut butter count as 1 oz of lean meat

- Use low-fat cooking methods (see following).
- Prepare soups and stews containing meats the day before. Refrigerate so that the fat congeals on top. Skim off the fat and reheat.

Milk and dairy products

- Use fat-free milk. Wean down from whole milk to reduced fat to 1% to fat free.
- Use fat-free or low-fat yogurt instead of regular yogurt.
- Try low-fat sour cream or use yogurt instead of sour cream in dips.
- Try fat-free frozen yogurt or sherbet or sorbet instead of ice cream.
- Reduce the use of whole eggs. Use two egg whites in place of one whole egg in cooking.

Vegetables

- Stir-fry using a vegetable spray such as Pam™.
- Omit or limit the use of butter, margarine, and oils when preparing vegetables. Experiment with seasonings.

Snack foods

- Watch out for hidden fats in crackers, cookies, and snack foods.
- Many low-fat and fat-free snack foods are also higher in sugar and calories. Read the nutrition facts label.
- Cut the fat in baked goods. Start by reducing the fat in recipes by one-third.
- Limit pastries and rich baked goods. Avoid croissants.

General

- Limit the use of butter, margarine, oils, gravies, and sauces.
- Whiten coffee with evaporated skim milk or fat-free half-and-half.

Table 12.3 provides additional suggestions to further reduce caloric and fat intake when preparing food. As an example, by substituting 1 tbsp cocoa powder for a 1 oz square of unsweetened baking chocolate, one would eliminate approximately 128 kcal and 15 g of fat (Bowes, Church, and Church 1994).

Choosing a Responsible, Safe Weight Loss Program

Weight control must be considered a lifelong effort. Most people can and have lost weight, but unfortunately, most fail to keep the weight off. A knowledgeable consumer should look for a program with the following features (*Choosing a Safe* 1993):

- The weight loss diet should be safe. It should meet the Recommended Dietary Allowance (RDA) of all vitamins and minerals. The diet should be low in calories

Table 12.3 *Recipe Modifications for Reducing Fat and Calories*

Recipe calls for:	Substitute:
1 c fat (oil, butter, margarine)	1/2 c fruit puree (apple sauce, banana, prune)
1 whole egg	2 egg whites
1 whole egg	1/4 c egg substitute
1 oz cream cheese	1 oz fat-free cream cheese
1 oz cream cheese	1 oz Neufchatel cheese
1 c whole milk	1 c skim milk
1 tbsp butter	1 tbsp extra light margarine
1 c ricotta cheese	1 c 1% ricotta cheese
1 c ricotta cheese	1 c fat-free ricotta cheese
1 oz cheddar cheese	1 oz light cheddar cheese
1 oz cheddar cheese	1 oz fat-free cheddar cheese
1 tbsp heavy cream	1 tbsp half & half
1 tbsp heavy cream	1 tbsp evaporated skim milk
1 tbsp mayonnaise	1 tbsp light mayonnaise
1 tbsp mayonnaise	1 tbsp fat-free mayonnaise
1 c sour cream	1 c nonfat yogurt
1 c sour cream	1 c nonfat sour cream
1 tbsp fudge sauce	1 tbsp chocolate syrup
1 oz baking chocolate	1 tbsp cocoa powder
1 c ice cream	1 c fat-free ice cream
1 c ice cream	1 c fat-free yogurt
1 c ice cream	1 c ice milk

only; it should not eliminate or severely restrict any one or more food groups, such as carbohydrates (fruits and starches).

▫ The diet should promote a healthy, steady weight loss of 1 to 2 lb (0.45 to 0.9 kg) per week following the first week or two.

▫ The diet should include a variety of foods from the food guide pyramid.

▫ No foods should be "forbidden." Any food may fit into a healthy eating plan. The key is moderation.

▫ The diet should combine nutrition education and behavior modification to help patients maintain weight loss. It should also promote or encourage increasing physical activity rather than relying solely on caloric restriction.

▫ A commercial weight loss program should be upfront in providing detailed information of all fees and additional costs such as food products and dietary supplements.

Selecting a Qualified Nutrition Professional

A registered dietitian (RD) or *qualified* nutritionist can provide the nutrition counseling and education necessary for successful weight loss and maintenance. A word of caution is in order here: The term *nutritionist* is not regulated. This means that anyone can claim to be a nutritionist without having any education, training, or credentials. With the growing popularity of commercial weight loss programs and natural remedies, there are more self-proclaimed nutrition experts now than ever before. They are often employed in health clubs or health food and vitamin shops, or leading many of the popular weight loss programs and support groups. Many have authored nutrition and weight loss books that promote methods that have little or no scientific backing and can often pose a danger to the consumer. When considering a nutritionist, ask for credentials. A qualified nutritionist should have a four-year college degree in nutrition science or dietetics, and many have advanced degrees and are often practicing in research settings.

A registered dietitian (RD) is a food and nutrition expert with a minimum of a bachelor's degree in nutrition science or dietetics from a U.S. regionally accredited university or college and course work approved by the Commission on Accreditation for Dietetics Education (CADE) of the American Dietetic Association (ADA). RDs have also completed a one- to two-year CADE-accredited supervised practice program (internship), which is often combined with graduate studies. Finally, RDs have passed a national registration examination—a rigorous test administered by the Commission on Dietetic Registration (CDR). RDs must also complete continuing professional education requirements to maintain their registration. Many states also require RDs to be licensed. Some RDs hold additional certifications in specialized areas of practice, such as pediatric or renal nutrition, nutrition support, and diabetes education.

A qualified nutrition expert is able and willing to provide credentials. This qualified professional will tailor individualized plans to meet patients' needs and teach them the skills to make lifestyle changes that will empower them to achieve and maintain weight loss.

To find an RD, visit the ADA Web site at www.eatright.org/find.html, or contact the ADA via mail or phone at: American Dietetic Association, 216 W. Jackson Blvd., Chicago, IL 60606-6995, (312) 899-0040.

The Consumer Nutrition Hot Line of the ADA offers the public direct access to objective, credible food and nutrition information from RDs. By dialing the toll-free number (800-366-1655), consumers can hear recorded messages about current nutrition topics, or get a referral to a registered dietitian in their area.

Summary

In applying medical nutrition therapy to the treatment of obesity, mathematical equations are often used. However, many other factors should be considered. Health care professionals need to place greater emphasis on helping patients to lose weight and at the same time teach them strategies to keep their lost weight off. Those who are ultimately successful in managing their weight are likely to have made lifestyle changes, such as choosing lower-fat cooking methods, making lower-fat substitutions when preparing foods at home, eating foods with a lower caloric density, and seeking opportunities to increase physical activity. Another predictor of long-term success is the use of a food diary to record the type and amount of foods consumed as well as emotional or psychological factors surrounding the occasion. Nutrition education and counseling can play a pivotal role in increasing a patient's success in following a prescribed calorie restricted plan, as well as for using tools such as the food guide pyramid.

References

Blackburn, G.L., Bistrian, B.R., Maini, B.S. et al. 1977. Nutritional and metabolic assessment of the hospitalized patient. *Journal of Parenteral and Enteral Nutrition* 1: 11-22.

Bowes, A.D.P., Church, C.F., and Church, H.N. 1994. *Bowes & Church's food values of portions commonly used,* 16th ed., revised by J.A.T. Pennington. Philadelphia: Lippincott.

Bray, G.A. 1976. The obese patient. *Major Problems in Internal Medicine* 9: 1-450.

Choosing a safe and successful weight-loss program. Washington, DC: U.S. Department of Health and Human Services; 1993. NIH Publication no. 94-3700.

Bray, G.A. 1998. *Contemporary diagnosis and management of obesity.* Newtown, PA: Handbooks in Health Care Company.

Consultant Dietitians in Health Care Facilities. 2001. *Pocket resource for nutrition assessment,* 5th ed. Chicago: American Dietetics Association.

Duyff, R.L. 1998. *The American Dietetic Association's complete food & nutrition guide.* Minneapolis, MN: Chronimed Publishing.

Flynn, T.J., and Walsh, M.F. 1993. Thirty-month evaluation of a popular very-low-calorie diet program. *Archives of Family Medicine* 2: 1042-1048.

Food and Nutrition Board (FNB), Institute of Medicine (IOM). 2002. Dietary reference intakes for energy, carbohydrates, fiber, fat, protein, and amino acids (macronutrients): Accessed October 23, 2002. Available at www.books.nap.edu/books.

Food Guide Pyramid: A guide to daily food choices. 1992. Leaflet No. 572. Washington, DC: U.S. Department of Agriculture, Human Nutrition Information Services.

Harris, J.A., and Benedict, F.G. 1919. *A biometric study of basal metabolism in man.* Publication No. 279. Washington, DC: Carnegie Institute of Washington.

National Task Force on the Prevention and Treatment of Obesity. 1993. Very low-calorie diets. *Journal of the American Medical Association* 270: 967-975.

The practical guide: Identification, evaluation, and treatment of overweight and obesity in adults. 2000, October. NIH Publication No. 00-4084. Washington, DC: U.S. Department of Health and Human Services; National Institutes of Health; National Heart, Lung, and Blood Institute Obesity Education Initiative; North American Association for the Study of Obesity.

Chapter 13

Physical Activity Treatment

Shawn C. Franckowiak, BS

Ross E. Andersen, PhD

Johns Hopkins School of Medicine

The latest statistics on the prevalence of obesity in the United States show that 18.9% of Americans are obese (Mokdad et al. 2000). Since researchers have discovered a strong association between long-term weight control and physical activity (Andersen et al. 1999; Kayman, Bruvold, and Stern 1990), physical activity and exercise are treatment options for overweight and obese persons seeking to reduce their body weight for improved health. Often, the overweight person (or client) seeks exercise advice from clinicians working in the field of exercise, health, and nutrition.

The objectives of exercise prescription have evolved from the conundrum of optimizing physical fitness for all adults (American College of Sports Medicine 1990) through the traditional regimen of three to five days a week of aerobic exercise at an intensity of 60 to 90% of maximum heart rate, to developing programs tailored to meet the individual needs, goals, and fitness levels of the client (Hills and Byrne 1998). To ensure that they are providing a proper exercise prescription to the overweight client, clinicians in hospitals, wellness centers, sports medicine clinics, and fitness centers must consider the unique needs of the client. In most cases, clinicians must consider disease-specific limitations (arthritis, hypertension, and cardiovascular disease and diabetes) associated with obesity (Andersen and Franckowiak 1999). While a primary goal for most overweight clients is weight loss, other goals such as improved physical fitness, health, mobility, flexibility, self-efficacy, and self-confidence may also be desired.

For the sake of simplicity, this chapter will use the terms *exercise* and *physical activity* interchangeably. Some overweight clients will receive activity prescription while others will receive prescriptions based on engaging in programmed exercise. However, these terms are different; exercise is a subset of activity and has been defined as "planned, structured, and repetitive bodily movement done to improve or maintain one or more components of physical fitness" (Caspersen, Powell, and Christensen 1985; Pate et al. 1995). Physical activity has been described as "any body movement produced by skeletal muscles that results in energy expenditure" (Caspersen et al. 1985).

This chapter will provide the clinician treating overweight individuals with an overview of the fundamentals of physical activity as a basis for exercise prescription. It will also cover the variety of issues associated with an exercise prescription for an overweight adult, such as the client interview, what has and has not worked before, the types of exercise that might be most beneficial for the individual, and how to promote adherence to a physical activity program.

Qualifications of the Clinician

To ensure that they're getting effective exercise guidance when starting an exercise or physical activity program, overweight clients should seek a clinician qualified in the areas of exercise science and personal training. The clinicians should be knowledgeable in the areas of exercise, behavioral modification, and physical activity, and be a "good match" for the client. Clinicians who are familiar with the typical needs of the overweight client may have a better understanding of some of the issues faced by the individual embarking on an exercise program. In the worst cases, clinicians that are not certified or have no experience working with overweight persons could pose undue harm to a client who simply seeks to engage in exercise.

Overweight clients should be referred to clinicians who are certified through a reputable organization that specializes in training professionals to provide safe and effective exercise programs to persons with specific diseases (Schnirring 2000). Organizations such as the American College of Sports Medicine (ACSM), the National Strength and Conditioning Association (NSCA), and the American Council on Exercise (ACE) offer personal training or strength and conditioning certifications that require professionals to complete written exams assessing their knowledge of exercise science topics such as exercise program development and prescription. Additionally, some certifications require candidates to have obtained at least a bachelor's degree in exercise science from an accredited institution. Before referring clients to a clinician that counsels individuals about exercise, physicians should ensure that the clinician is certified through a reputable organization and is qualified to work with an overweight population.

Response to Activity

Recommendations on the type and amount of physical activity that will produce health benefits focus on the idea of accumulating moderate-intensity activity throughout the day (National Institutes of Health 1995; U.S. Department of Health and Human Services 1996). These recommendations also sug-

gest that the appropriate type of activity be determined by the individual's preferences (National Institutes of Health 1995), which could potentially allow for a wide variety of physical activities. This is good news, when we think that it may be better to consider the amount of activity an individual performs rather than the specific manner in which it is performed (i.e., mode, intensity, or duration of activity bouts) (Pate et al. 1995). Overweight individuals seem to respond more favorably to the notion of engaging in physical activity and the idea that an active lifestyle may be effective in producing and maintaining weight loss.

This theory was tested in a study investigating the use of stairs or the escalator by normal weight and overweight individuals in a Baltimore mall (Andersen, Franckowiak et al. 1998). The study, which was published in the *Annals of Internal Medicine*, revealed that normal weight individuals were more likely to take the stairs than their overweight counterparts (5.4% versus 3.8%) (see figure 13.1). However, when overweight individuals were prompted by motivational signboards located at the base of stairs and adjacent escalators, they were just as likely to take the stairs as their normal weight counterparts. Stair use increased by over 65% in the overweight individuals in response to signs containing motivational slogans such as "your heart needs exercise, use the stairs" and "take the stairs for a trimmer waistline." These findings suggest that, when prompted, overweight individuals respond to the idea of engaging in physical activity. These results are inspiring when we recognize that less than a quarter of our population is currently physically active enough to derive health benefits (U.S. Department of Health and Human Services 1996), and overweight people are even more likely to be sedentary (Andersen et al. 2000).

Classic Prescription: What the Clinician Needs to Examine

A "one size fits all" approach to exercise prescription may not provide effective guidance to increase a client's activity levels. To ensure safety, a clinician should evaluate a client's medical history. Furthermore, to produce an effective activity prescription, clinicians

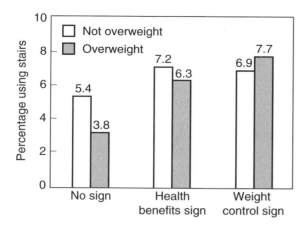

Figure 13.1 Stair use patterns of normal weight and overweight individuals.

Reprinted, by permission, from R. Andersen et al., 1998, "Can inexpensive signs encourage the use of stairs? Results from a community intervention," *Annals of Internal Medicine* 129: 363-369.

should address several important issues, discussed in the following sections.

Past Medical History

Obesity is often associated with low levels of activity (Andersen, Crespo et al. 1998; Crespo and Wright 1995). Therefore, the overweight client who is sedentary may feel overwhelmed and intimidated about engaging in vigorous, intense exercise when embarking on an exercise program. The American College of Sports Medicine (ACSM) stresses the need for screening for risk factors for various diseases before initiating an exercise program with any individual; table 13.1 lists the ACSM guidelines for clinicians to practice prior to giving an exercise prescription to any client (Franklin 2000).

These guidelines use the current health status of the client (risk factors and disease) to determine whether the client should see a physician prior to initiating any form of exercise. Table 13.1 presents recommendations on exercise testing for clients having one or more risk factors or symptoms. This table denotes when the clinician should refer the patient to a physician or progress to the exercise prescription to begin exercise or physical activity. Furthermore, patients should be screened for signs and symptoms that are suggestive of cardiovascular, pulmonary, or metabolic disease (Franklin 2000). Major symptoms include chest angina, shortness of breath with rest or

mild exertion, dizziness or syncope, orthopnea or paroxysmal nocturnal dyspnea, ankle edema, palpitations or tachycardia, intermittent claudication, known heart murmur, or unusual fatigue (shortness of breath) with usual activities (Franklin 2000).

Since 80% of type 2 diabetic clients are obese (Verity 1999), the clinician may need to follow the guidelines of the American Diabetes Association (ADA) (1998), which state that a graded exercise test may be helpful to determine the risk of underlying cardiovascular disease if a client is beginning a moderate- to high-intensity exercise program (American College of Sports Medicine 1990; Pate et al. 1995; U.S. Department of Health and Human Services 1996). The ADA recommends stress testing a diabetic client if the client

- is older than 35,
- has had type 2 diabetes for longer than 10 years,
- has had type 1 diabetes for longer than 15 years,
- has any additional risk factor for coronary artery disease,
- has microvascular disease such as retinopathy or nephropathy, or
- has peripheral vascular disease or autonomic neuropathy.

Health care providers may feel a sense of urgency to increase physical activity in the diabetic population to control diabetics' weight and medical condition. Currently, 70% of diabetics do not engage in physical activity (Ford and Herman 1995). Should there be any question regarding the health of a patient and his or her capability to exercise, clinicians should refer the person to his or her primary care physician for exercise clearance before beginning any activity.

Exercise History

Learning the patient's exercise history is important for determining the person's past involvement in activity programs and identifying the appropriate type of activity (Andersen et al. 1997). Overweight clients can differ greatly in personality and physical ability. Thus, clinicians should not use a "one size fits all" approach to exercise prescription.

Table 13.1　　　　　　*Signs and Symptoms of Risk Factors and Recommendations for At-Risk Patients*

Risk factors	Major signs/symptoms
Family history of coronary artery disease	Pain in chest, neck, arm, or jaw
Cigarette smoking	Shortness of breath at rest or relaxation
Hypertension	Dizziness or syncope
Hypercholesterolemia	Orthopnea or paroxysmal nocturnal dyspnea
Impaired fasting glucose	Ankle edema
Obesity	Palpitations or tachycardia
Sedentary lifestyle	Intermittent claudication
	Known heart murmur
	Unusual fatigue/shortness of breath with usual activities
High serum HDL cholesterol is a NEGATIVE risk factor.	

Recommendations for at-risk patients

	Moderate exercise	Vigorous exercise	Submaximal testing	Maximal testing
Low risk (Asymptomatic; no more than one risk factor from above)	–	–	–	–
Moderate risk (>45 for men; >55 for women; 2 or more risk factors from above)	–	+	–	+
High risk (Patient with one or more signs or symptoms)	+	+	+	+

+ Physician supervision of exercise testing is recommended; physician should be in close proximity in case of an emergency.

- A medical examination, exercise test, and physician supervision of exercise is not essential in prior screening of these events (however, these precautions should not be viewed as inappropriate).

Moderate exercise: Activities that are approximately 3-6 METS or the equivalent to brisk walking at 3 to 4 mph (for adults)

Vigorous exercise: Exercise above 6 METS

Adapted from the American College of Sports Medicine *ACSM's guidelines for exercise testing and prescription.*

- Did you enjoy physical activity when you were younger?
- Did you enjoy physical education class and team sports when you were younger?
- Do you have any negative feelings toward exercise, sports, or physical activity?
- Do you like the feelings associated with exercise and exertion, such as being winded or sweating?
- Do you ever have difficulty with exercises that require significant skill or coordination?
- What exercise or physical activity program has worked for you in the past, and what hasn't?
- If you had difficulty with exercise or physical acivity previously, what might you try to do differently?
- Is now a good time to start an activity program? Why is "now" a good time to begin exercising?
- Do you see any barriers to becoming and remaining active?
- Do you feel comfortable in specific exercise settings, like a fitness center or group exercise setting?
- What additional input can you provide that might help me to help you be more successful with your activity program?

Figure 13.2 Questioning the client: what to ask.

Clinicians should instead ask pertinent questions that may help them tailor an exercise and physical activity program to the individual client. Some of the questions are listed in figure 13.2.

Clinicians can begin by asking about the client's current activity levels and what the client may feel is an acceptable activity to begin with. When asking about the client's past exercise program, clinicians should be aware that the client may exhibit negative feelings or even disappointment about past exercise attempts. The information gained through this interaction between client and clinician is essential when tailoring an effective physical activity program designed to facilitate weight reduction and maintenance.

Exercise Enjoyment

Too often, clinicians make the mistake of prescribing a classical exercise routine that is vigorous and lengthy in the beginning

stages for their overweight clients. The result is often negative feelings and ultimately poor adherence to the activity program. In designing exercise programs for overweight clients, clinicians should try to incorporate safe and enjoyable forms of activity. This is especially important since a large percentage of people will not adhere to vigorous programs (Wadden et al. 1997). Before prescribing activity, the clinician should discuss alternative modes of activity with the client to determine what is most appealing to the individual. A program that the client enjoys ensures better compliance in the long term.

Activity Preferences and Accessibility

An exercise program should be realistic and focus on long-term weight loss (Andersen, Brownell, and Haskell 1992). Clients often feel a sense of empowerment when clinicians ask for their input when designing an exercise prescription. If activity and exercise goals are too lofty, feelings of bewilderment, fear, or despair may follow as the overweight client struggles to comply with the exercise prescription. The client's preferences for certain kinds of activity and exercise and the accessibility of the equipment to perform this exercise should be considered.

After inquiring about the overweight client's medical history, exercise history, and preferences, the clinician must choose the mode of activity to prescribe. Again, clients should be encouraged to provide input as to what type of exercise they prefer. Most of the time clients suggest activities that are appropriate and realistic. In some cases, however, clients will choose or suggest activities that may be inappropriate. These clients may have had previous success performing this mode of exercise when they were at or near their ideal body weight. They may therefore wish to continue this activity as a part of their regimen to produce weight loss because they either experienced pleasant feelings associated with this exercise or feel that it is the most enjoyable form of exercise. An example of this type of person would be a man in his 40s who now weighs 310 lb (140 kg) and suggests engaging in jogging outdoors to lose weight because he was formerly a college football player and remembers the joy he felt when jogging on the football field during conditioning drills as an offensive lineman. The clinician is responsible for ensuring that the exercise prescription for this gentleman is safe and effective. Jogging may not be a suitable activity in initial stages due to the high intensity of the activity, and the high-impact exercise may also result in joint injuries. Other activities to be avoided initially by the overweight person are racquetball, squash, volleyball, basketball, high-impact aerobics, and tennis. In this case, the clinician can offer a safer alternative (such as stationary cycling or walking) and gradually progress the client toward jogging after he has lost weight and improved his physical fitness.

Accessibility to exercise facilities is also an important issue to clients. Clinicians should keep in mind that not all clients have access to safe and lighted bike or walking paths, or have the option of walking outdoors in a safe neighborhood. If neighborhoods around the client's residence are unsafe, the clinician may suggest safer alternatives such as malls, school tracks, and the workplace. Similarly, clients who may not be able to afford a gym membership may have difficulty finding options for participating in aerobic exercise or strength training. Financially burdened clients may want to discuss the alternatives to joining expensive clubs and investing in machines. Low-cost solutions such as dumbbells for home strength training and used aerobic exercise equipment may make exercise more accessible to these persons.

What Worked Before, What Did Not

Often, clinicians can learn much from the client regarding the most suitable exercise or activity by simply asking about previous weight loss attempts and exercise programs. A client will often feel relieved that he or she can have some input into what new activity to try on this particular weight loss attempt. Moreover, the clinician can often discover the person's true temperament by discussing new things he or she may want to try to keep the activity program fresh and exciting. The clinician should inquire about previous modes of exercise, feelings associated with exercise, and the amount of time the client devoted to exercise in past attempts. The benefits of planning to devote a specific amount of time to exercise each day

should be discussed. Providing, thorough counseling, on how to plan for daily exercise on hectic days may be especially important since perceived lack of time is the most common excuse for not participating in an exercise program (Dishman 1982; Johnson et al. 1990; King et al. 1992).

Personality and Accountability

Personality and preferences contribute significantly to a person's response to the type of exercise prescribed. For instance, some of us are solitary exercisers, while others are group exercisers. These individual differences must be taken into account prior to supplying an exercise prescription to the overweight client. Following are four personality types and suggestions for an exercise prescription that may work best for each:

□ *Individual exerciser.* This type of individual may be ashamed to exercise or may not enjoy performing activity, often preferring home exercise in order to avoid being seen engaging in physical activity that may be difficult or undesirable to them. Group exercise to the individual exerciser may be seen as very threatening. Typically, the individual exerciser will respond well to activities performed in the own home or outdoors.

□ *Group exerciser.* This individual may not have negative feelings associated with performing exercise or physical activity in public settings. Furthermore, the group exerciser often enjoys the camaraderie of an exercise class consisting of people who have the same type of goals and frustrations. Often, group exercisers make friends in group exercise classes (such as low-impact aerobics and flexibility and strength training classes) and therefore feel a strong sense of obligation to attend class in order to avoid disappointing fellow group exercisers.

□ *Partner exerciser.* This type of person responds to the accountability of a close friend or colleague to initiate and follow through with an exercise or activity program. Partner exercise works well when the client has difficulty motivating himself to initiate and carry out the exercise. Partner exercisers enjoy exercising with people who have similar goals and attitudes toward activity. Both persons may not enjoy exercise, but they will perform the exercise if the other partner is with them every step of the way. Using partner exercise is a great way to increase the likelihood that the client will continue to be active. However, if one of the partners decides to discontinue the exercise program, the other may soon follow suit.

◻ *Exerciser needing accountability.* Some people may need a personal trainer to help them achieve fitness or weight loss goals. A qualified personal trainer can assist with providing both accountability (making sure the person shows up for an exercise session) and proper motivation and guidance through a safe and effective exercise routine. Since many first-time exercisers are novices on how to begin an exercise routine and when to increase overall intensity, frequency, and duration, a personal trainer can supply a boost of motivation and guidance to meet overall goals.

Clothing and Apparel

One of the most commonly overlooked yet essential areas of exercise counseling for overweight clients is the issue of clothing and apparel. The overweight client may perceive wearing spandex or tight-fitting exercise apparel as a barrier to publicly participating in an exercise program. The clinician must ascertain what makes the client comfortable when exercising, including clothing, equipment, and environment. When appropriate, the clinician should guide the client in the apparel selection process, suggesting that clothing be comfortable and that the client feel physically and mentally at ease wearing it. Furthermore, the clinician should inform the overweight client that outdoor clothing should be specific to the climate to reduce the risk of heat- or cold-related injuries such as heat stroke or hypothermia.

Patients do not have to change into gym clothes or spandex in order to participate in lifestyle activity that is accumulated throughout the day. Moderate-intensity physical activity can be done in almost any type of clothing; the clinician should suggest that overweight clients seize any opportunity that arises to engage in incidental physical activity.

The clinician should question the overweight client regarding the type of footwear he or she uses when performing any activity. Although the stress placed on the joints of the normal weight person performing percussive exercise may not result in joint injury, a greater amount of stress is placed on the weight-bearing joints of the overweight individual. The overweight client will often underestimate the importance of appropriate footwear in reducing the risk of injury to the ankle, knee, and hip joints. Furthermore, the diabetic overweight client is at greater risk for developing blisters or trauma to the feet. Individuals with peripheral neuropathy may experience a loss of protective sensation of the feet (American Diabetes Association 1998). Proper footwear is therefore essential.

The American Diabetes Association (1998) recommends silica gel or air insoles and polyester or blend socks since they work best to keep feet both safe and dry. It is natural for people to try to get the most out of their footwear. However, sneakers tend to work at their "joint protecting" optimum for roughly four hundred miles of walking or jogging, after which the insoles begin to lose their cushioning. Sneakers with reduced support should be replaced with new footwear with proper support and cushioning. Clinicians may want to suggest to financially burdened overweight clients that they purchase new sneakers to use specifically for their activity or exercise and use their old sneakers as casual shoes rather than throwing them away.

New Thinking About Exercise

The classic exercise prescription focuses on the frequency, intensity, and duration of exercise in order to optimize fitness in the individual (American College of Sports Medicine 1978). Organizations such as the American College of Sports Medicine, the Centers for Disease Control and Prevention (CDC) (Pate et al. 1995), and the National Institutes of Health (1996) along with the Surgeon General (U.S. Department of Health and Human Services 1996) have recommended that Americans engage in at least 30 minutes of moderate-intensity physical activity on most (preferably all) days of the week. These recommendations have arisen based on the consensus of numerous studies investigating the benefits of exercise. Although researchers and clinicians have not yet determined the optimal amount of exercise needed to maintain a healthy weight, these recommendations indicate the direction such organizations are taking to increase public awareness of the activity necessary for health benefits.

During interviews with clinicians, many overweight clients claim not to have the time to block out at least 30 to 40 minutes to exercise. Moreover, many reveal that they do not enjoy the feeling of sweating and exercising at such high intensities. Consequently, they may be predisposed to not enjoying, and not adhering to, a traditional exercise prescription. New ideas on physical activity and exercise prescription suggest prescribing shorter bouts of exercise or having the client exercise at a moderate rather than vigorous intensity.

The CDC and ACSM now suggest that activity that is of moderate intensity instead of vigorous, and accumulated rather than continuous (i.e., performed in several shorter sessions) can produce health benefits in individuals seeking to be involved in an activity program. Furthermore, these guidelines offer clinicians an added option for exercise prescription for overweight clients. Unfortunately, these new recommendations may not be reaching physicians and health care workers. Recent data suggest that only 12% of physicians are even familiar with these new recommendations (Walsh et al. 1999). The recommendations also advise that individuals currently engaging in exercise at least 30 minutes per day (or participating in higher intensity) should not seek to reduce the frequency, duration, or intensity of exercise based on these new recommendations. Currently, researchers are investigating the effectiveness of moderate-intensity activity at producing weight loss and maintenance in the obese population.

Short Bouts

Recent recommendations on the exercise necessary for developing and maintaining flexibility, cardiovascular fitness, and muscular fitness state that the recommended 20 to 60 minutes of aerobic training per day can now be done in 10-minute bouts accumulated throughout the day (American College of Sports Medicine 1998). More researchers are currently investigating the benefits of multiple short bouts of physical activity (Coleman et al. 1999; DeBusk et al. 1990; Jakicic et al. 1995, 1999) to achieve the goals of weight management and meet new physical activity recommendations (National Institutes of Health 1996; Pate et al. 1995; U.S. Department of Health and Human Services 1996). Rather than promoting the idea of one long continuous bout of exercise in order to attain health benefits, the short bouts theory recommends shorter bouts of exercise at convenient times throughout the day. Preliminary studies examining the short bouts theory have found that persons engaging in short bouts of exercise receive similar cardiovascular health benefits (Coleman et al. 1999; DeBusk et al. 1990; Jakicic et al. 1999) and weight loss (Jakicic et al. 1995, 1999) compared to those engaging in more traditional continuous exercise programs.

The short bouts concept may be an effective strategy for individuals lacking time, enabling them to stay physically active without having to perform continuous exercise in a gym setting or at home. Preliminary studies have found that prescribing multiple short bouts to individuals increases exercise participation (Jakicic et al. 1995). Furthermore, in a recent short bouts study that involved dietary modification and made engaging in activity more convenient by supplying home exercise equipment to subjects, researchers found that long-term adherence increased (Jakicic et al. 1999). Overweight clients who mention that long exercise bouts (30 to 45 minutes) are too overwhelming, difficult to fit into a busy schedule, or boring may find shorter exercise bouts more appealing.

Lifestyle Activity

Although traditional continuous vigorous exercise is the best prescription for optimizing fitness in overweight individuals, most overweight individuals may initially avoid such activity and may prefer exercise or activity producing simple and gradual improvements in health. Researchers are now investigating how lifestyle physical activity (i.e., activity that conveniently fits into a person's lifestyle and is of a moderate intensity) can be used to produce health benefits and weight loss. Since the greatest health benefits are accrued by motivating persons who are completely sedentary to simply begin any form of physical activity (Haskell 1994), this seems to be an option that could be offered to most overweight individuals. Dunn, Andersen, and Jakicic (1998) suggest that lifestyle physical activity allows individuals to tailor their physical activity programs to include a variety of activities that are of a moderate intensity and to accumulate bouts of activity in a manner that fits their circumstances.

Dunn and colleagues also found that overweight participants that were prescribed lifestyle activity for two years (intensive behavioral treatment with a maintenance period) showed improvements in blood pressure, fitness, and energy expenditure similar to their traditionally exercising (continuous vigorous bout) counterparts. Furthermore, lifestyle exercisers increased their total time engaged in moderate-intensity activity three times more than did traditional exercisers. Similarly, in a lifestyle physical activity intervention study (Andersen et al. 1999), we found that overweight individuals engaging in at least 30 minutes a day of moderate lifestyle activity and eating a low-calorie self-selected diet achieved similar reductions in weight, percentage body fat, serum lipid levels, and depressive symptoms, as well as improvements in fitness, when compared to overweight individuals participating in traditional structured, vigorous exercise (aerobic exercisers). The study also reported that lifestyle exercisers reduced their body weight by 7.9 kg (lifestyle exercisers lost 18.3 pounds, compared to 18.9 pounds lost by aerobic exercisers), and prescribed lifestyle exercise tended to keep the weight off after a one-year follow-up period.

The one problem with lifestyle activity is that patients sometimes believe that it may not have as great an effect as vigorous exercise. However, the most current findings on disease status and physical activity reveal that greater physical activity levels are associated with the reduction in risk of type 2 diabetes (Hu et al. 1999); physiological changes accompanying lifestyle activity prescribed for weight loss are very similar to those accompanying a traditional aerobic exercise program (Franckowiak et al. 1999). In a 12-week weight reduction study in which indi-

viduals consumed 1,200 to 1,500 kcal per day, patients who did lifestyle activity had reductions in body weight and resting metabolic rate similar to those engaging in traditional aerobic exercise. The lifestyle activity subjects reduced their body weight by 6.7% compared to 8.4% for the aerobic exercise group. Similarly, both lifestyle and traditional exercisers had similar decreases in their resting metabolic rate (RMR) after 12 weeks. Specifically, the lifestyle subjects had a 10.9% decrease in RMR compared to a 10.2% reduction for the traditional aerobic participants.

Some researchers suggest prescribing lifestyle activity initially when an overweight individual begins an exercise or activity program (Andersen et al. 1999). Although lifestyle physical activity may elicit better feelings when exercising for those who are overweight, clinicians should caution overweight clients that they must perform lifestyle physical activity at a purposeful pace to ensure a moderate intensity.

Lifestyle physical activity may be less daunting than traditional exercise, and unfit overweight individuals may find the intensity of exercise more easily attained (Weyer et al. 1998). Weyer and colleagues found that individuals seeking to meet the CDC and ACSM's recommendations on lifestyle physical activity were twice as likely to attain the recommended amount of activity as those seeking to engage in the more traditional vigorous recommendations (Weyer et al. 1998). Furthermore, lifestyle physical activity seems to have a long-lasting effect on physical activity behavior (Dunn, Andersen, and Jakicic 1998) (individuals continue to stay active once they begin a lifestyle physical activity program) and may be a gateway to a more vigorous exercise program in the future (Andersen 1999). After experiencing the self-efficacy of achieving a successful lifestyle activity program, an individual may be less intimidated by a more challenging vigorous exercise routine.

During intervention studies investigating dieting individuals who participated in at least 30 minutes of lifestyle physical activity (Andersen et al. 1999), overweight subjects who were advised to continue their lifestyle physical activity habits tended to keep the weight off (see figure 13.3). This further suggests that an individualized prescription recommending accumulation of moderate-intensity physical

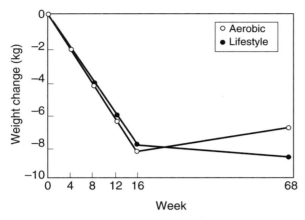

Figure 13.3 Weight changes in the diet-plus-lifestyle group and the diet-plus-aerobic group.

Reprinted, by permission, from R. Andersen, "Effects of lifestyle activity vs. structured aerobic exercise in obese women: A randomized trial," *Journal of American Medical Association* 281: 335-340. Copyright 1999, American Medical Association.

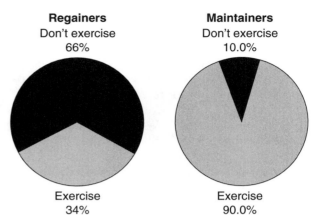

Figure 13.4 Percentage of obese women who regained or maintained lost weight.

Data from S. Kayman et al. 1990.

activity throughout the day that is convenient to the client promotes adherence to the program and may help the client maintain weight loss.

Adherence

Adherence to the exercise prescription is also an issue that a clinician must be aware of when prescribing exercise to the overweight individual. The challenge of keeping the weight off may be a far greater obstacle for the overweight individual than short-term weight loss. Clinicians should be aware of the population-specific issues that may produce noncompliance in the long term. Time constraints, fear of failure, and negative feelings toward exercise will often sabotage the overweight client's efforts to continue exercising once he or she is close to weight loss goals. Research investigating what distinguishes those that lose weight and maintain it (maintainers) and those that lose weight and regain it (regainers) suggests that maintainers report continued adherence to their exercise programs (Kayman, Bruvold, and Stern 1990) (see figure 13.4).

Strategies for Promoting Adherence

The clinician's responsibility does not end with the provision of an exercise prescription

that is effective in producing health benefits and weight loss for the overweight client. Professionals must also investigate other factors that might promote long-term adherence to the exercise or activity program. Sallis and Hovell (1990) suggest that exercise self-efficacy, a positive attitude toward exercise, an understanding of fitness, and participation in moderate-intensity exercise when starting to exercise are strong predictors of adoption of regular exercise.

Patient Readiness

To prescribe an effective exercise or activity program to the overweight client, the clinician must first determine whether now is the appropriate time for the individual to undertake an exercise program. Often, patients try to put themselves through overwhelming situations in order to lose weight. Many times, clients may try to begin dietary modification and exercise during the time of year when their work schedules are busiest or when their personal lives may not facilitate a successful weight loss attempt. Thus, proper motivation or commitment to lose weight and exercise may be lacking. The clinician would do well to ask the client, "Is this a good time to begin an exercise program?" and "Why is this a good time to begin an exercise and weight loss program?" Hopefully, the response will be yes, but if not, it may be appropriate to question whether the person is ready to begin some initial lifestyle changes consisting of increases in activity, or consult a professional specializing in behavioral treatment such as a psychologist. Some clinicians use contracts to test the readiness of the client to begin making lifestyle changes. A simple piece of paper that the client must sign stating the objectives of an activity program may be enough to motivate the client to adhere to an individualized exercise program. Additional questions that can be used to determine client readiness can be found in *The Health and Fitness Club Leader's Guide: Administering a Weight Management Program* (Andersen, Brownell, and Haskell 1992).

Social Support

Social support may be as important as patient readiness in ensuring the overweight client's long-term adherence to a physical activity program. Family support for exercise and weight loss may allow the overweight client to feel good about beginning an activity program. The overweight individual can ask a spouse or child to park farther from an entrance or to accompany him or her on the stairs instead of taking the escalator. Furthermore, reworking the family's schedule may be necessary to help the client engage in programmed exercise. The exercising client may ask that dinner be at 6:30 instead of 5:30 or that the spouse baby-sit toddlers while the client engages in exercise. Support from a spouse has been found to be positively associated with maintenance of exercise (Dishman 1982; Martin and Dubbert 1982). Social support may also involve positive reinforcement from a family member or spouse in order to continue to feel good about participating in exercise.

Clients who experience negative reinforcement from family members may need to communicate the importance of this exercise and weight loss program to their health. Frequently, family members can sabotage the efforts of the overweight client to maintain a healthy lifestyle; this form of sabotage is usually not intentional, but can involve certain behaviors that would undermine weight loss efforts such as (1) not allowing for the overweight family member to reserve a small block of time for exercise; (2) disregarding exercise as an important piece of a weight management program; and (3) specifically practicing unhealthy behaviors in front of the overweight

person, such as introducing high-fat foods to the household or exhibiting sedentary behavior. To prevent such sabotage, the overweight client should clearly state what the family can and should do to be supportive.

Family members should be urged to keep a positive attitude toward the client's weight loss efforts, keep a relaxed family atmosphere, forgive lapses, and spend time exercising with the person (Brownell 2000). Proper communication can help family members understand the importance of exercise and lifestyle change and support the overweight family member.

Exercising with a group or a partner provides the overweight individual with exercise and social support at the same time. Thus, prescribing this type of exercise may be advantageous if there is a family member or friend that has the same type of exercise objectives. As mentioned earlier, the clinician should inquire about exercise habits and suggest group or partner exercise programming if supportive family members or friends are amenable.

Contact and Accountability

Unfortunately, many clients lose focus after reaching their goal weight. Others simply lose interest in an exercise program and discontinue treatment with a clinician. By maintaining contact with the client throughout the weight loss program, the clinician establishes a climate of accountability. Clinician contact may be used for one or many of the following: performing a weigh-in, checking physical activity logs, modifying and updating the physical activity program, identifying dangerous situations of inactivity or weight gain, supplying motivation, or simply recording progress by asking about the current status of physical activity or eating patterns.

When patients experience a lapse in their weight management program, clinician contact and accountability can be valuable in helping them return to healthy lifestyles such as effective eating and exercise. In the LEARN Program for Weight Control (Brownell 1997), Brownell states that relapse prevention is an issue that needs to be addressed with individuals looking to maintain weight loss after a lifestyle intervention. Clinicians need to understand that clients will have momentary lapses in their activity programs, and should possess the confidence and ability to address them. Similarly, relapses may occur in which the client reverts to old sedentary habits. Finally, a complete collapse of the program, or total noncompliance and reversion to sedentary habits, can occur due to frustration. The clinician can assist with the maintenance phase by holding the client accountable to the exercise program through weekly, biweekly, or monthly check-ins in which he or she offers positive reinforcement to continue healthy behavior. Even frequent phone calls to the client have been found to increase engagement in physical activity (Lombard, Lombard, and Winett 1995), and may assist with the adherence to an exercise prescription.

Self-Efficacy

Strategies increasing a person's efficacy for physical activity may result in greater participation rates (Rohm-Young and King 1995). Exercise self-efficacy has previously been described as an individual's self-confidence in being able to engage in physical activity or complete an exercise program (Rohm-Young and King 1995). Self-efficacy toward a continuation of an exercise program will be an issue for certain clients. The long-term adherence to participation in physical activity may require a high level of commitment, motivation, and confidence. The clinician should address these issues and offer reinforcement progress and compliance to the overweight individual who is in the process of trying to stay physically active to manage her weight.

Finally, overweight clients may be better able to comply with a long-term activity program when they choose activities that they enjoy. Studies have revealed that exercise enjoyment is positively associated with continued exercise (McAuley et al. 1994). Activities that are perceived to be a burden of time or effort may not result in long-term compliance.

Realistic Goals

The clinician should aid with the goal-setting process by helping clients break down complex goals into short-term, simpler ones (Earley, Connolly, and Ekegren 1989). Too often, overweight clients will seek advice regarding expected and acceptable weekly weight losses when setting goals. Because they may

feel that they need to follow cultural ideals when seeking to lose weight, clients often will set unrealistic weight loss goals to attempt to look like certain models or television actors. Counseling patients on how they are progressing with more realistic goals may help to reduce negative feelings that sometimes accompany the frustration of not achieving set goals. A healthy perspective to introduce to the overweight client is that the extra weight was gained over an extended period of time, and similarly, it will take time to accomplish safe and healthy weight loss.

Self-Monitoring

Finally, self-monitoring of a physical activity program can help to optimize long-term adherence. The self-monitoring part of the approach is called individual behavioral management (U.S. Department of Health and Human Services 1996) and consists of the process of actually recording activity by using physical activity recall logs. Physical activity records can involve keeping track of the episodes of activity per week, the time spent on each episode, and the feelings associated with the activity performed (U.S. Department of Health and Human Services 1996).

Summary

Physical activity prescription is an integral part of any weight management program. Although individuals seem to be able to lose weight by simply reducing their caloric intake without engaging in exercise or activity, the addition of activity will improve health benefits during weight reduction and may be one of the most essential components to preventing weight regain. The clinician providing exercise guidance and prescription should take into account the individual differences and preferences among the various clients seeking treatment to lose weight. Individualizing the exercise prescription may involve tailoring the exercise to meet the client's needs, goals, and preferences and matching the person's lifestyle.

The goals and expectations for the individual should be reasonable and attainable; this may mean that the clinician provides the overweight client with exercise that allows for gradual progression of duration, intensity, and frequency as the individual experiences increases in fitness, strength, confidence, and self-efficacy. Clinicians should provide feedback and guidance and be able to modify the exercise prescription if feedback from the individual is negative. The focus of the prescription should center on a series of attainable short-term goals to reach an overall long-term goal. Furthermore, the activity prescription should consider that simple movement of even light to moderate intensity might be a gateway to more advanced and intense exercise that might be more enjoyable in the future.

References

American College of Sports Medicine. 1978. The recommended quantity and quality of exercise for developing and maintaining fitness in healthy adults. *Medicine and Science in Sports and Exercise* 10: vii-x.

American College of Sports Medicine. 1990. Recommended quantity and quality of exercise for developing and maintaining cardiorespiratory and muscular fitness in healthy adults. *Medicine and Science in Sports and Exercise* 22: 265-274.

American College of Sports Medicine. 1998. Position stand: The recommended quantity and quality of exercise for developing and maintaining cardiorespiratory and muscular fitness, and flexibility in healthy adults. *Medicine and Science in Sports and Exercise* 30: 975-991.

American Diabetes Association. 1998. Position statement: Diabetes mellitus and exercise. *Diabetes Care* 21: S40-S44.

Andersen, R.E. 1999. Exercise, an active lifestyle, and obesity: Making the exercise prescription work. *The Physician and Sports Medicine* 27: 41-50.

Andersen, R.E., Blair, S.N., Cheskin, L.J., and Bartlett, S.J. 1997. Encouraging patients to become more physically active: The physician's role. *Annals of Internal Medicine* 127: 395-400.

Andersen, R.E., Brownell, K.D., and Haskell, W.L. 1992. *The health & fitness club leader's guide: Administering a weight management program*. Dallas: American Health.

Andersen, R.E., Crespo, C.J., Bartlett, S.J., Cheskin, L.J., and Pratt, M. 1998. Relationship of physical activity and television watching habits among U.S. children with body weight and level of fatness: Results from the Third National Health and Nutrition Examination Survey. *Journal of the American Medical Association* 279: 938-942.

Andersen, R.E., Crespo, C.J., Franckowiak, S., Christmas, C., and Walston, J. 2000. Obesity and reports of no leisure time activity among older Americans. *Educational Gerontology* 27: 297-306.

Andersen, R.E., and Franckowiak, S. 1999. Obesity. In *Clinical exercise specialist manual: ACE's source for training special populations*, eds. R.T. Cotton and R.E. Andersen, 158-176. San Diego, CA: American Council on Exercise.

Andersen, R.E., Franckowiak, S.C., Snyder, J., Bartlett, S.J., and Fontaine, K.R. 1998. Can inexpensive signs encourage the use of stairs? Results from a community intervention. *Annals of Internal Medicine* 129: 363-369.

Andersen, R.E., Wadden, T.A., Bartlett, S.J., Zemel, B., Verde, T.J., and Franckowiak, S.C. 1999. Effects of lifestyle activity vs. structured aerobic exercise in obese women. *Journal of the American Medical Association* 281: 335-340.

Brownell, K.D. 1997. *The LEARN program for weight control*. Dallas: American Health.

Brownell, K.D. 2000. *The LEARN program for weight management 2000*. Dallas: American Health.

Caspersen, C.J., Powell, K.E., and Christenson, G.M. 1985. Physical activity, exercise, and physical fitness. *Public Health Reports* 100: 125-131.

Coleman, K.J., Raynor, H.R., Mueller, D.M., Cerny, F.J., Dorn, J.M., and Epstein, L.H. 1999. Providing sedentary adults with choices for meeting their walking goals. *Preventive Medicine* 28: 510-519.

Crespo, C.J., and Wright, J.D. 1995. Prevalence of overweight among active and inactive U.S. adults from the third National Health and Nutrition Examination Survey. *Medicine and Science in Sports and Exercise* 27: S73 (abstract).

DeBusk, R.F., Stenestrand, U., Sheehan, M., and Haskell, W.L. 1990. Training effects of long versus short bouts of exercise in healthy subjects. *American Journal of Cardiology* 65: 1010-1013.

Dishman, R.K. 1982. Compliance/adherence in health-related exercise. *Health Psychology* 1: 237-267.

Dunn, A.L., Andersen, R.E., and Jakicic, J.M. 1998. Lifestyle physical activity interventions: History, short- and long-term effects, and recommendations. *American Journal of Preventive Medicine* 15: 398-412.

Earley, P.C., Connolly, T., and Ekegren, G. 1989. Goals, strategy development and task performance: Some limits on the efficacy of goal setting. *Journal of Applied Psychology* 74: 24-33.

Ford, E.S., and Herman, W.H. 1995. Leisure-time physical activity patterns in the U.S. diabetic population. Findings from the 1990 National Health Interview Survey—Health Promotion and Disease Prevention Supplement. *Diabetes Care* 18: 27-33.

Franckowiak, S.C., Andersen, R.E., Bartlett, S.J., and Fontaine, K.R. 1999. Physiologic changes after weight reduction with vigorous exercise and moderate intensity physical activity. *Medicine and Science in Sports and Exercise* 31: S345 (abstract).

Franklin, B.A., ed. 2000. *ACSM's guidelines for exercise testing and prescription,* 6th ed. Baltimore: Lippincott Williams & Wilkins.

Haskell, W.L. 1994. Health consequences of physical activity: Understanding and challenges regarding dose-response. *Medicine and Science in Sports and Exercise* 26: 649-660.

Hills, A.P., and Byrne, N.M. 1998. Exercise prescription for weight management. *Proceedings of the Nutrition Society* 57: 93-103.

Hu, F.B., Sigal, R.J., Rich-Edwards, J.W., Colditz, G.A., Solomon, C.G., Willett, W.C., Speizer, F.E., and Manson, J.E. 1999. Walking compared with vigorous physical activity and risk of type 2 diabetes in women: a prospective study. *Journal of the American Medical Association* 282: 1433-1439.

Jakicic, J.M., Wing, R.R., Butler, B.A., and Robertson, R.J. 1995. Prescribing exercise in multiple short bouts versus one continuous bout: Effects on adherence, cardiorespiratory fitness, and weight loss in overweight women. *International Journal of Obesity and Related Metabolic Disorders* 19: 893-901.

Jakicic, J.M., Winters, C., Lang, W., and Wing, R.R. 1999. Effects of intermittent exercise and use of home exercise equipment on adherence, weight loss, and fitness in overweight women: A randomized trial. *Journal of the American Medical Association* 282: 1554-1560.

Johnson, C.A., Corrigan, S.A., Dubbert, P.M., and Gramling, S.E. 1990. Perceived barriers to exercise and weight control practices in community women. *Women and Health* 16: 177-191.

Kayman, S., Bruvold, W., and Stern, J.S. 1990. Maintenance and relapse after weight loss in women: Behavioral aspects. *American Journal of Clinical Nutrition* 52: 800-807.

King, A.C., Blair, S.N., Bild, D.E., Dishman, R.K., Dubbert, P.M., Marcus, B.H., Oldridge, N.B., Paffenbarger, R.S.J., Powell, K.E., and Yeager, K.K. 1992. Determinants of physical activity and interventions in adults. *Medicine and Science in Sports and Exercise* 24: S221-S236

Lombard, D.N., Lombard, T.N., and Winett, R.A. 1995. Walking to meet health guidelines: The effect of prompting frequency and prompt structure. *Health Psychology* 14: 164-170.

Martin, J.E., and Dubbert, P.M. 1982. Exercise applications and promotion in behavioral medicine: Current

status and future directions. *Journal of Consulting and Clinical Psychology* 50: 1004-1017.

McAuley, E., Courneya, K.S., Rudolph, D.L., and Lox, C.L. 1994. Enhancing exercise adherence in middle-aged males and females. *Preventive Medicine* 23: 498-506.

Mokdad, A.H., Serdula, M.K., Dietz, W.H., Bowman, B.A., Marks, J.S., and Koplan, J.P. 2000. The continuing epidemic of obesity in the United States. *Journal of the American Medical Association* 284: 1650-1651.

National Institutes of Health. 1995. Consensus statement 1995: Physical activity and cardiovascular health. Dec 18-20.13 (3): 1-33 (Report).

National Institutes of Health. 1996. Consensus conference on physical activity and cardiovascular health. 276: 241-246 (Conference Proceeding).

Pate, R.R., Pratt, M., Blair, S.N., Haskell, W.L., Macera, C.A., Bouchard, C., Buchner, D., Ettinger, W., Heath, G.W., King, A.C., Kriska, A., Leon, A.S., Marcus, B.H., Morris, J., Paffenbarger, R.S., Jr., Patrick, K., Pollock, M.L., Rippe, J.M., Sallis, J., and Wilmore, J.H. 1995. Physical activity and public health: A recommendation from the Centers for Disease Control and Prevention and the American College of Sports Medicine. *Journal of the American Medical Association* 273: 402-407.

Rohm-Young, D., and King, A.C. 1995. Exercise adherence: Determinants of physical activity and applications of health behavior change theories. *Medicine Exercise Nutrition and Health* 4: 335-348.

Sallis, J.F., and Hovell, M.F. 1990. Determinants of exercise behavior. In *Exercise and sport sciences reviews,* eds. J.O. Holloszy and K.B. Pandolf, 307-330. Baltimore: Williams & Wilkins.

Schnirring, L. 2000. Referring patients to personal trainers: Benefits and pitfalls. *The Physician and Sports Medicine* 28: 16-21.

U.S. Department of Health and Human Services. 1996. *Physical activity and health: A report of the Surgeon General.* Atlanta, GA: U.S. Department of Health and Human Services, Centers for Disease Control and Prevention, National Center for Chronic Disease Prevention and Health Promotion.

Verity, L.S. 1999. Diabetes mellitus. In *Clinical exercise specialist manual: ACE's source for training special populations,* eds. R.T. Cotton and R.E. Andersen, 136-157. San Diego, CA: American Council on Exercise.

Wadden, T.A., Vogt, R.A., Andersen, R.E., Bartlett, S.J., Foster, G.D., Kuehnel, R.H., Wilk, J., Weinstock, R., Buckenmeyer, P., Berkowitz, R.I., and Steen, S.N. 1997. Exercise in the treatment of obesity: Effects of four interventions on body composition, resting energy expenditure, appetite, and mood. *Journal of Consulting and Clinical Psychology* 65: 269-277.

Walsh, J.M., Swangard, D.M., Davis, T., and McPhee, S.J. 1999. Exercise counseling by primary care physicians in the era of managed care. *American Journal of Preventive Medicine* 16: 307-313.

Weyer, C., Linkeschowa, R., Heise, T., Giesen, H.T., and Spraul, M. 1998. Implications of the traditional and the new ACSM Physical Activity Recommendations on weight reduction in dietary treated obese subjects. *International Journal of Obesity and Related Metabolic Disorders* 22: 1071-1078.

Chapter 14

Physical Activity As a Therapeutic Modality

John M. Jakicic, PhD

Physical Activity and Weight Management Research
Center, School of Education, University of Pittsburgh

Preparation of this manuscript was partially supported by research grants to Dr. Jakicic from the National Institutes of Health. (HL56127, HL64991, DK58002)

Based on population surveys, it is estimated that an excess of 50 to 60% of adults in the United States are overweight (Flegal et al. 1998; Mokdad et al. 1999), and many suggest that physical activity may play a significant role in both weight loss and the prevention of weight gain. Thus, physical activity has taken on a more important role in weight management during recent years. This chapter will examine the justification for including a strong physical activity component in weight management programs and will examine (1) evidence that exercise is important for weight management, (2) factors that may explain the potential impact of physical activity for weight management, (3) activity recommendations, and (4) strategies for increasing the adoption and maintenance of physical activity behaviors.

Physical Activity and Weight Management: Is There a Link?

Many now believe that incorporating physical activity into weight management interventions, including both weight loss and the prevention of weight gain, is important. The initial evidence to support this conclusion comes from both cross-sectional and short-term (≤6 months) randomized trials. In addition, in recent years studies have shown that physical activity may be especially important for long-term weight maintenance (Pronk and Wing 1994). A summary of the evidence to support the inclusion of physical activity into programs targeting weight management follows.

Cross-Sectional Evidence

Evidence from cross-sectional and epidemiological studies supports the use of exercise in interventions targeting weight management initiatives. Kayman and colleagues (1990) reported that 76% of individuals who used exercise during a weight loss period maintained their weight loss, whereas only 36% of individuals who experienced a weight relapse initially incorporated exercise into their weight loss program. In addition, 90% of individuals who lost and maintained a minimum weight loss of 20% for a period of two years reported exercising for at least 30 minutes per day three days per week. Other investigators have also reported that participation in regular exercise is important for successful maintenance of weight loss (Colvin and Olson 1983; Gormally et al. 1980). In addition, exercise participation appears to be associated with the prevention of significant weight gain (DiPietro et al. 1998; French et al. 1994; Klesges et al. 1992; Owens et al. 1992; Taylor et al. 1994).

The National Weight Control Registry (NWCR) was established to learn more about weight loss and maintenance of weight loss from individuals who have accomplished this task, and then to track these individuals over a period of time. Initial results from the NWCR showed that individuals in the registry were maintaining a weight loss of approximately 60 to 70 lb (approximately 30 kg) for an average of five years, with 92% of these individuals indicating that exercise was a part of their weight loss program (Klem et al. 1997). Women in the NWCR were more likely than men to participate in walking and aerobic dance for exercise, with men participating in more competitive sports and weight training. In a follow-up examination of individuals in the NWCR, McGuire and colleagues (1999) reported that individuals who had started to regain their weight had lower levels of energy expenditure than did individuals who continued to maintain their weight loss.

Short-Term Interventions (≤6 Months)

When examining behavioral approaches to weight loss, one can consider the effect of changes in diet, changes in exercise, or changes in the combination of both diet and exercise. A summary of behavioral approaches to weight loss has shown that the majority of weight is lost within the initial six months of treatment (Wadden 1993; Wing 2002). Examination of these short-term (≤6 months) interventions has shown that exercise alone has a minimal impact on weight loss compared to diet alone or exercise in combination with diet. For example, in a 12-week study of women, Hagan and colleagues (1986) reported weight loss of 16.5, 13.0, and 0.4 lb (7.5, 5.9, and 0.2 kg) in the diet-plus-exercise, diet-alone, and exercise-alone interventions. Similar results were shown for men, with weight loss being 25.1, 18.5, and 0.7 lb (11.4, 8.4, and 0.3 kg) in the three groups, respectively. Moreover, Miller (1999) conducted a meta-analysis of studies over a 25-year period (1969-1994) and showed less weight loss resulting from exercise alone (–6.4 lb or –2.9 kg) when compared to diet alone (–23.6 lb or –10.7 kg) or a combination of

diet and exercise (–24.3 lb or –11.0 kg). Therefore, to maximize weight loss during short-term (<6 months) interventions using a standard behavioral approach, people would be well advised to include a dietary component in the intervention, and to add exercise to this dietary intervention to further improve weight loss.

When considering the impact of exercise on initial weight loss, it may be important to consider the level of dietary restriction. For example, in the study conducted by Hagan and colleagues (1986), dietary intake was 1,200 kcal per day, and exercise appeared to enhance the weight loss resulting from diet alone. However, the same effect may not be found when dietary intake drops significantly below this level. For example, when consuming a very low calorie diet (VLCD), the addition of exercise (either aerobic or resistance exercise) to the diet does not appear to enhance weight loss compared to diet alone during the initial 90 days of treatment (Donnelly et al. 1991). However, under VLCD conditions, aerobic exercise does appear to improve cardiorespiratory fitness, which has been shown to be important for reducing health risk in overweight adults (Wei et al. 1999). Resistance training improves strength, which may have a positive effect on functional status.

Long-Term Interventions (≥6 Months)

Despite the development of behavioral interventions that have resulted in significant weight loss within the initial six months of treatment, the maintenance of weight loss remains a challenge. A summary of behavioral interventions showed that among programs that followed participants for a minimum of 40 weeks beyond the initial short-term intervention, weight regain was approximately 33% within a one-year period, with additional weight regain in following years (Wadden 1993). Examination of data from studies conducted from 1996 to 1999, in which follow-up periods were increased to 18 months, showed weight regain rates of approximately 35 to 40% of initial weight loss (Wing 2002). However, as demonstrated by cross-sectional and epidemiological evidence presented earlier, exercise may prove to be especially important during the period when one is focusing on preventing weight regain (Colvin and Olson 1983; Gormally et al. 1980; Klem et al. 1997).

Data from clinical trials support the long-term use of exercise in behavioral weight management programs (National Institutes of Health 1998; Pronk and Wing 1994). For example, Wood and colleagues (1988) showed that exercise results in a weight loss of 8.8 lb (4.0 kg) over a one-year period compared to a 1.3-lb (0.6-kg) increase in no-treatment control subjects. In addition, Wood and colleagues (1991) showed that adding exercise to a dietary intervention can improve weight loss compared to diet alone following a one-year intervention in men (–19.2 versus –11.2 lb or –8.7 versus –5.1 kg), with an insignificant improvement in weight loss shown in women (–11.2 vs. –9.0 lb or –5.1 vs. –4.1 kg). However, exercise will only be effective if maintained over time. In a study of overweight women, Jakicic and colleagues (1999) showed that individuals who maintained exercise over the entire 18-month intervention achieved greater long-term weight loss when compared to individuals who did not maintain exercise.

Prevention of Weight Gain

As demonstrated, exercise appears to be an important factor for preventing or minimizing weight regain following initial weight loss (Pronk and Wing 1994). However, exercise may also be beneficial for preventing initial weight gain. In an examination of data from the Behavioral Risk Factor Surveillance System (BRFSS), DiPietro and colleagues (1993) reported an inverse relationship between physical activity and body mass index, a relationship that has been reported by others as well (Tyron et al. 1992). This would suggest that activity might play a role in preventing or minimizing weight gain in adults. Increasing activity that results in improvements in cardiorespiratory fitness also appears to be beneficial. Data from the Aerobics Center Longitudinal Study showed that for each minute of improvement during a fitness test, the odds of gaining ≥11.0 lb (≥5 kg) was reduced by 14% in men and 9% in women (DiPietro et al. 1998). Further evidence to support the use of physical activity for prevention of weight gain comes from the National Health and Nutrition Examination Survey (NHANES). Williamson and colleagues (1993) reported that maintaining a low level of activity or decreasing activity over a period of 10 years

was associated with an increased likelihood of significant weight gain during this period.

Some evidence indicates that increases in physical activity may be especially important for individuals who are already moderately overweight. Leermakers and colleagues (Leermakers, Jakicic et al. 1998) created a study to examine whether increasing exercise would minimize weight gain in men. Men with a BMI between 22 and 30 kg/m² were randomized to either a no-treatment control or an exercise intervention group. The exercise intervention consisted of randomization to either a clinic-based or home-based intervention, and we found no difference on outcomes between the clinic-based and home-based intervention. However, when men were divided into two groups based on BMI (22-26.9 kg/m² or 27-30 kg/m²), changes in body weight differed by BMI category. Men with a BMI of 22-26.9 kg/m² lost 2.6 lb (1.2 kg) and 1.3 lb (0.6 kg) in the intervention and control groups, respectively. Men in the intervention groups with a baseline BMI of 27-30 kg/m² had a decrease in body weight of 6.0 lb (2.7 kg), whereas those in the control group showed a 3.3-lb (1.5-kg) increase in body weight. A limitation of this study was that it was conducted over a 16-week period. However, these results appear to indicate that moderately overweight men are at risk for weight gain, and initiating an exercise program may prevent weight gain and result in modest weight loss in this group.

In summary, a review of the weight loss literature appears to suggest that the addition of exercise to a standard behavioral program has the potential for enhancing short-term weight loss. However, exercise may play an even more important role in the maintenance of weight loss, which is supported by evidence from cross-sectional, epidemiological, and clinical research studies. Moreover, some evidence supports the use of exercise for preventing weight gain. In addition, exercise can improve fitness, which has been shown to have an independent effect on health risk in overweight adults.

How Physical Activity Affects Weight Management

Exercise has been shown to influence a number of physiological parameters that can affect body weight, body composition, and energy balance. However, the scope of this section is not to examine each of these factors. Rather, this section will focus on the impact of exercise on energy expenditure during weight loss. In addition, a discussion of whether exercise is linked to other behaviors that may affect successful weight loss is included.

Energy Expenditure

Energy expenditure has typically been divided into three basic components: resting energy expenditure (REE), the thermic effect of food, and energy expenditure from physical activity (EEPA). Because EEPA is the most variable part of total daily energy expenditure, targeting increases in this component may have the greatest impact on weight management.

When examining the effect of EEPA on total daily energy expenditure (TDEE), it is important to consider the magnitude by which EEPA can influence TDEE. Consider the following example using a man weighing 198.4 lb (90 kg) and assuming that 1 metabolic equivalent (MET) is equal to 1 kcal/kg/hr. Under resting conditions, this man will expend approximately 2,160 kcal per day. If he took a 30-minute brisk walk (4.0 METs), which is the current minimal public health recommendation for physical activity (Pate et al. 1995; U.S. Department of Health and Human Services 1996), he would increase his energy expenditure by 180 kcal per day. This would result in an 8% increase in energy expenditure above resting levels. However, relying solely on this increase in energy expenditure, this man would require approximately 19 days to reduce his body weight by 1 lb (0.4 kg), which would result in a weight loss of approximately 9 lb (4 kg) during the initial 180 days of treatment (six months). However, results from randomized trials have indicated that weight loss from exercise alone is less than this amount (Hagan et al. 1986; Wood et al. 1988; Wing 1999), suggesting that energy intake does not necessarily remain stable in individuals.

In addition to its direct impact on TDEE, physical activity may also affect other components of EEPA. One factor that has been considered is that physical activity may elevate energy expenditure following periods of activity, and this has been termed EPOC (excessive postexercise oxygen consumption).

Recent research in this area has suggested that the EPOC remains significantly elevated above resting values for a relatively short period of time following exercise. In a study of individuals following an exercise bout performed at 70% of maximal oxygen consumption, EPOC returned to baseline in approximately 40 minutes in trained individuals and 50 minutes in untrained individuals (Short and Sedlock 1997). In addition, the magnitude of the EPOC was approximately 3.5 L of oxygen for both trained and untrained individuals, which would result in an increase of approximately 17.5 kcal above the exercise level. These results would suggest that people must exercise on a regular basis for their EPOC to have a significant impact on body weight regulation, and the independent impact of EPOC on weight management may be minimal.

Resting energy expenditure (REE) contributes the largest portion to TDEE. Thus, alterations in this component may have a significant impact on energy balance. Changes in REE during weight loss have been of particular concern because of the potential decrease with weight loss that has been observed. This has been particularly alarming during periods of caloric restriction. Following 90 days of a VLCD, REE decreased by approximately 138 kcal per day (579 kJ per day) (Donnelly et al. 1991), whereas a more modest decrease in energy intake has resulted in somewhat less of a decline (Kraemer et al. 1999). However, this decrease in REE may not be greater than what would be expected at this reduced body weight (Leibel et al. 1995). In addition, the effects of both aerobic and resistance exercise training on REE during weight loss have been examined. However, despite potentially minimizing the decrease in fat-free mass, neither aerobic nor resistance exercise appears to significantly affect absolute REE during periods of weight loss (Donnelly et al. 1991; Kraemer et al. 1999).

In summary, TDEE, during periods of weight loss, increased by adding exercise to the intervention. However, the majority of this increase may result from increases in energy expenditure resulting directly from the exercise. EPOC from the exercise period may also play a minimal role in increasing TDEE, and exercise does not appear to have a significant impact on REE during periods of caloric restriction that result in weight loss.

Exercise and Other Behaviors Related to Weight Loss

Exercise may be important for weight management not only because of its impact on energy expenditure but also because of its potential impact on other behaviors related to weight loss. For example, Emmons and colleagues (1998) suggested that increases in activity may be associated with high consumption of fruits and vegetables. In addition, data from the NWCR indicate that individuals successful at long-term weight loss both engage in physical activity and make significant changes in dietary intake and eating patterns, primarily related to decreases in fat intake (Klem et al. 1997). McGuire and colleagues (1999) reported similar results in a random survey of successful weight loss maintainers.

Jakicic and colleagues (2002) showed a significant positive correlation between exercise participation and improvements in eating behaviors, with both factors significantly contributing to improvements in long-term weight loss. Despite these findings, it is unclear whether changes in activity cause the adoption of these other behaviors or whether the behaviors are simply linked. Participation in physical activity may be part of a constellation of behaviors that combine to contribute to improve long-term weight loss. These findings support the need to include exercise in behavioral weight loss interventions.

Another important behavioral factor that has been linked to improvements in long-term weight loss is continued contact. In a study of overweight adults, Wadden and colleagues (1997) reported that attendance at treatment meetings accounted for 22% of the variance in weight maintenance during weeks 25 to 48 of a behavioral program. The authors examined both aerobic and resistance training exercise programs and found that neither significantly contributed to the maintenance of weight loss. Perri and colleagues (1986, 1988) also emphasized the importance of maintaining contact over long periods of time to improve long-term weight loss.

Unpublished data by Jakicic showed that individuals who report the highest levels of exercise also attend the most group sessions across an 18-month program, with these differences being noticeable during the maintenance phase (months 7 through 18) of the program. For example, individuals averaging at least 150 minutes per week of exercise during this period attended approximately 80% of the group sessions, whereas individuals exercising less than 150 minutes per week attended approximately 65% of the group sessions. Therefore, low levels of exercise may indicate less compliance with attending group sessions, or low attendance may result in poor compliance with the exercise program. Regardless of the direction of this relationship, enhancing long-term contact may be important in weight loss programs because of its link to the maintenance of exercise, and this may improve long-term weight loss outcomes.

Fitness Versus Fatness

As discussed, evidence supports the combination of both diet and exercise for weight loss. Despite some improvements in long-term treatment programs, however, few interventions have been successful at maintaining weight loss in the long term. This tendency for people to regain lost weight has led some to question whether weight loss can improve health, and this has led to the Look AHEAD Study, which is being conducted by the National Institutes of Health. Thus, in recent years a growing body of literature has suggested that improvements in fitness may reduce health risks independent of weight loss, a contention that needs further exploration.

The majority of the data that have been published in this area comes from the Cooper Clinic in Dallas, Texas (Barlow et al. 1995; Lee et al. 1998; Wei et al. 1999). In 1995 Barlow and colleagues (1995) reported that for men with a BMI of 27 to 30 kg/m^2, having moderate to high fitness reduced all-cause death rates by 40 to 60% compared to low-fit men in the same BMI category. A similar pattern of reduction in mortality rates was shown for men with a BMI of either <27 kg/m^2 or >30 kg/m^2. Lee and colleagues (1998) reported that compared to normal weight fit men, the adjusted relative risk for all-cause mortality for fit overweight men is 1.08 (95% confidence interval = 0.77-1.50). However, the adjusted relative risk for unfit normal weight men was 2.25 (95% confidence interval = 1.59-3.17), suggesting that increasing fitness in overweight adults

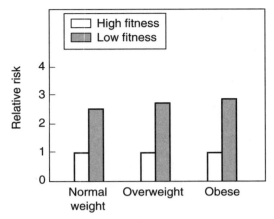

Figure 14.1 Fitness, weight, and all-cause mortality.
Data from Wei et al. 1999.

should be a focus of interventions to improve health in these individuals. Results presented by Wei and colleagues (1999) support the data of others and suggest that improvements in fitness may have a protective effect and minimize the risk of cardiovascular disease and all-causes (see figure 14.1). These findings appear to support the inclusion of exercise in interventions for overweight adults and suggest that even in the absence of weight loss or weight maintenance, exercise participation can improve health in these individuals.

Physical Activity Recommendations for Weight Management

The literature suggests that including exercise in weight loss interventions is advantageous. Clinicians must therefore evaluate the amount and types of activity to recommend in intervention programs.

Amount of Activity

When considering the amount of activity to recommend to overweight individuals, clinicians should first consider the goal of the intervention. Some have suggested that increasing fitness independent of changes in body weight can produce significant improvements in health (Barlow et al. 1995; Lee et al. 1998; Wei et al. 1999). Currently, the public health recommendation for physical activity is 30 minutes of moderate intensity on most days of the week (Pate et al. 1995; U.S. Department

of Health and Human Services 1996), which will also result in improvements in health. Thus, targeting this level of activity should be the initial focus of interventions for previously sedentary overweight adults.

Those who hope to achieve long-term weight loss must engage in levels of exercise that are greater than the minimal public health recommendations. Schoeller and colleagues (1997) used doubly labeled water to assess energy expenditure in individuals following a weight loss program. Results from this study suggest that at least 80 minutes per day of moderate-intensity activity or 35 minutes per day of vigorous-intensity activity are necessary for maintaining weight loss over the long term. Moreover, Klem and colleagues (1997) showed that individuals in the NWCR also report levels of activity that are greater than the minimal public health recommendations, with activity levels being 2,667 kcal per day and 3,488 kcal per day in women and men, respectively. Data published by Jakicic and colleagues support these findings, showing that individuals who averaged over 280 minutes per week in exercise for a period of 18 months achieved greater maintenance of weight loss compared to individuals who exercised below this level (Jakicic et al. 1999). Studies designed to specifically examine the dose-response of exercise on long-term weight loss are currently under way.

Type of Activity

In addition to being concerned about the dose of exercise for overweight individuals, clinicians must also address the type of activity that is best for the management of body weight. Aerobic forms of exercise have been the most commonly studied forms of exercise for weight loss. Common forms of aerobic exercise that have been used are walking, using stationary equipment, and aerobic dance, all of which have been shown to be beneficial for individuals engaging in weight loss efforts. One of the parameters that aerobic exercise significantly improves is cardiorespiratory fitness. In a study of both men and women, cardiorespiratory fitness significantly improved in individuals receiving diet plus exercise compared to diet alone or a no-treatment control condition across a one-year intervention (Wood et al. 1991).

Wood and colleagues (1988) also showed significant increases in fitness following a one-year exercise-only condition compared to both a diet-alone and a no-treatment control condition. In a study of 148 overweight previously sedentary women, walking was selected as the preferred form of aerobic exercise for approximately 75% of the exercise sessions across an 18-month period (Jakicic et al. 1999). When provided with a home treadmill, walking was selected for 93% of the reported sessions. These results indicate that aerobic exercise can improve cardiorespiratory fitness in overweight adults, which may significantly improve health outcomes (Barlow et al. 1995; Lee et al. 1998; Wei et al. 1999), and walking appears to be a popular form of exercise in this population (Jakicic et al. 1999).

The effectiveness of including resistance training has received increasing attention in the past decade. This may be in response to issues related to loss of lean body mass and reductions in REE during weight loss. Kraemer and colleagues (1999) showed that the addition of resistance exercise to a diet and aerobic exercise program minimized the loss of lean body mass compared to diet alone or diet combined with aerobic exercise. During periods of more severe caloric restriction, resistance exercise appears to increase the cross-sectional area of the muscle (Donnelly et al. 1993), but this does not appear to minimize the overall loss of lean body mass (Donnelly et al. 1991; Wadden et al. 1997). In addition, resistance exercise does not appear to significantly minimize the loss of REE during diet-induced weight loss, nor does it significantly improve weight loss compared to aerobic forms of exercise. One of the limitations of research examining the role of resistance training in weight loss interventions is that few long-term studies have been conducted. For example, a number of studies have been conducted in which the intervention has been less than six months in duration (Donnelly et al. 1991; Kraemer et al. 1999), with few studies examining this intervention beyond this period of time (Wadden et al. 1997).

The results of exercise studies during weight loss indicate that both aerobic and resistance forms of exercise may have very specific advantages. Therefore, the mode of exercise a person chooses during periods of weight loss may depend on the additional benefits that person desires. Ideally it is probably best to include both aerobic and resistance forms of exercise when possible in an intervention program that also includes changes in eating behavior. The duration and intensity of the activities that are selected should at minimum be consistent with the current public health recommendation of at least 30 minutes of moderate-intensity physical activity on most days of the week (Pate et al. 1995). In addition, while other forms of exercise including stretching, yoga, martial arts, and so on, are available, data to support the use of these specific activities for promotion and maintenance of weight loss are limited.

Strategies to Increase Physical Activity Adoption and Maintenance

Increasing physical activity and engaging in regular exercise appears to be beneficial to overweight adults. Exercise may improve short-term weight loss when combined with a dietary intervention, and exercise may be a key factor in preventing or minimizing weight regain following initial weight loss. In addition, exercise can improve fitness, and this has been shown to have an independent effect on health. Despite these important benefits of exercise for overweight adults, the challenge remains to get these individuals active and then to maintain this higher level of activity. Similar to other chronic diseases that have used exercise as an intervention, at least 50% of individuals initiating an exercise program will discontinue within six months, and there may be further declines beyond this period (Gwinup 1975). Thus, for exercise to be an effective intervention tool, strategies to effectively increase adoption and maintenance of this behavior need to be implemented.

Self-Directed Exercise

Many of the early exercise training studies were conducted under supervised conditions at specific facilities. However, as the field has grown increasingly concerned about the low prevalence of exercise participants and the inability of a significant number of individuals to maintain adequate levels of exercise over the long term, more information has become available regarding perceived barriers to the adoption and maintenance of exercise. One of the key factors reported is lack of time, which has led some to reexamine the need for supervised clinic-based exercise models. As a result, strategies that provide flexibility to the participant regarding when and where to exercise have been initiated, and an appropriate term for this may be "self-directed exercise." The following is a summary of the potential strategies that may lead to improvements in exercise participation. These strategies may be especially effective for individuals who are currently sedentary and can benefit from increasing their activity level.

Home-Based Versus Clinic-Based Exercise

Despite the large number of health clubs and fitness facilities available to the public, attempting to obtain all of one's activity at these facilities may not be advantageous. One of the reasons for this may be related to the lack of time that many report as a barrier to exercise. A second factor may be related to other factors such as low self-image or low self-efficacy for exercise that may affect whether an individual feels comfortable exercising in these facilities with other individuals. Thus, clinicians should consider encouraging exercise outside of these facilities if they believe that doing so will improve the participation rates of sedentary and overweight individuals.

King and colleagues (1991) examined clinic-based and home-based exercise in a study of men and women 50 to 65 years of age. This study showed that home-based exercise significantly improved cardiorespiratory fitness, and this increase was similar to what was shown in the supervised exercise condition. Of equal importance, home-based exercise seems to result in better adherence compared to clinic-based exercise. This difference was maintained during the second year of the intervention, with the difference being especially noticeable in individuals prescribed exercise at an intensity of 73 to 88% of peak treadmill heart rate (King et al. 1995).

Perri and colleagues (1997) examined the effectiveness of home-based exercise as part of a behavioral weight loss intervention in women age 40 to 60 with BMIs ranging from 27 to 45 kg/m². Results of this trial showed that home-based exercise was more effective at maintaining higher levels of exercise during months 7 through 12 of this intervention, and this may have contributed to better long-term weight loss compared to the clinic-based exercise group. Thus, the results of research trials support the use of home-based exercise interventions for improving exercise participation in adults, and this may be particularly important for previously sedentary overweight adults.

Lifestyle Physical Activity

Some have suggested encouraging individuals to incorporate more activity into other aspects of their lifestyle as an alternative to formal exercise. This would include activities such as taking the stairs rather than the elevator or getting off the bus a few blocks early and walking. Behavioral interventions have evaluated the effectiveness of such an approach.

Project Active, a randomized clinical trial, examined the effectiveness of a lifestyle approach to exercise on changes in fitness and other health-related variables (Dunn et al. 1999). Results of this trial showed that a lifestyle approach can be as effective as traditional structured exercise across a 24-month period for changes in fitness. Andersen and colleagues (1999) also showed the effectiveness of a lifestyle approach to physical activity for weight loss in a study of 40 overweight women. Results of this study showed that when combined with a dietary intervention over 12 months, lifestyle activity is as effective as structured exercise for weight loss during this period.

Despite the demonstrated effectiveness of a lifestyle intervention, questions regarding this type of intervention remain. For example, it is unclear from these trials what types of activity the participants performed that would reflect their interpretation of "lifestyle physical activity." In addition, this information would provide an understanding of how this approach differs from other home-based activity approaches that have been shown to be effective for increasing compliance, improving fitness, modifying risk factors, and decreasing body weight (King et al. 1991, 1995; Perri et al. 1997). Thus, as research in this area moves forward, quantification of activity patterns (type, frequency, duration) will be important to understanding how to recommend incorporating activity into one's lifestyle and whether certain types of lifestyle activities are more popular and more effective than others.

Intermittent Versus Continuous Exercise

The CDC and ACSM recommendations for physical activity indicate that physical activity can be accumulated throughout the day (Pate et al. 1995). At the time of these recommendations, some evidence suggested that exercise performed in as little as 10 minutes per session multiple times throughout the day could improve fitness (DeBusk et al. 1990) and may affect some cardiovascular disease risk factors (Ebisu 1985). However, these studies did not address whether this approach to exercise would improve adherence rates in previously sedentary individuals or whether this type of approach was sustainable across time.

Since the time of the CDC/ACSM recommendation, others have conducted studies looking at the effect of intermittent exercise on fitness and other risk factors, and these results have been favorable (Murphy and Hardman 1998; Snyder et al. 1997). However, our group focused on whether this approach to exercise can improve adherence when integrated into a behavioral weight loss intervention. The original work in this area focused on the short-term impact of this exercise approach. In a study of overweight women, we showed that prescribing exercise in 10-minute sessions and recommending multiple sessions per day improved exercise participation during a 20-week behavioral weight loss program (Jakicic et al. 1995). To our knowledge, this was the first study to demonstrate that this approach may be effective for increasing exercise participation in previously sedentary adults.

We have since conducted an additional 18-month trial with sedentary overweight women. When examining the initial six months of the behavioral intervention that also included a dietary component, we again showed that multiple intermittent sessions of exercise was superior to traditional continuous exercise for improving initial adoption of exercise, and was as effective for weight loss during this six-month period (Jakicic et al. 1999). However, intermittent exercise did not appear to be better than traditional continuous exercise relative to adherence or weight loss when examined over the following 12-month period. Thus, the existing research in this area suggests that intermittent exercise will improve initial exercise adoption in previously sedentary women, and that this approach is as effective as more traditional approaches to exercise when examined over longer periods of time. This provides an exercise option for individuals who may struggle to participate in traditional continuous periods of exercise.

Changing the Environment

Modifying the physical environment may play an important role in modifying activity behaviors. One method of modifying the environment would be to do this on a large scale within communities. This can potentially be accomplished by increasing access to exercise facilities (e.g., recreation centers or parks) or by ensuring that things such as sidewalks exist that promote activity. Sallis and colleagues (1990) demonstrated that proximity to exercise facilities is associated with higher levels of physical activity. In addition, using signs to prompt individuals to use the stairs in public areas such as malls and office buildings has also been shown to be effective (Andersen et al. 1998; Brownell et al. 1980). Thus, appropriate changes at the community level may have an impact on physical activity from a public health perspective.

In addition to changes at the community level, it may be as important to change the personal environment at the individual level. For example, we have demonstrated a significant correlation between activity level and the presence of exercise equipment in the home (Jakicic et al. 1997). In addition, Raynor and colleagues (1998) showed the importance of considering the proximity of activity options relative to the proximity of more sedentary options when intervening on activity behaviors. With these findings in mind, we conducted a study to examine whether providing exercise equipment (motorized treadmills) to previously sedentary overweight women is an effective intervention strategy (Jakicic et al. 1999). We chose treadmills based on an initial survey of women that indicated that they would prefer to have a treadmill in their home rather than other forms of exercise equipment. At the completion of the 18-month intervention, participants reported continuing to use the treadmill for 41.6% of their exercise sessions, which suggests that exercise equipment will continue to be used when part of a behavioral intervention. In addition, compared to individuals not receiving treadmills, more individuals completed the entire 18-month intervention, and the treadmills appear to result in high levels of exercise in the final 6 to 12 months of the intervention. Thus, modifying the home environment through the provision of home exercise equipment may be a promising intervention strategy.

Strategies to Improve Long-Term Contact

As demonstrated earlier, maintaining contact with a clinical program can be an important factor that will enhance long-term weight loss. The following is an overview of different strategies that have been used to maintain contact in behavioral interventions.

Telephone Interventions

One of the strategies that has been used in behavioral interventions to maintain contact with individuals is a telephone-based approach. This approach has been used both at the outset of an intervention and during maintenance periods to maintain patient–therapist contact. In a study of men comparing a telephone-based intervention to a clinic-based intervention, both interventions provide similar changes in physical activity and weight change during a four-month period (Leermakers, Jakicic et al. 1998). In addition, a summary of the literature has shown that others have also demonstrated the efficacy of a telephone intervention for increasing physical activity when used as the sole means of delivering the intervention or in combination with other methods of patient contact (Marcus, Owen et al. 1998).

When delivering a telephone intervention, clinicians should consider what the most appropriate message of the contact should be and in what groups this type of intervention may be most appropriate. For example, Lombard and colleagues (1995) demonstrated that the frequency of the contacts and not the structure of the contact made a significant difference in interventions targeting increases in physical activity behavior. In addition, these types of contact may be most appropriate for an individual who has difficulty participating in a face-to-face clinic-based intervention. As an example, mothers of recently born infants may be interested in minimizing postpartum weight retention, yet these individuals may find it hard to participate in a clinic-based program (Leermakers, Anglin et al. 1998). Thus, this group responds to a telephone-based intervention, which studies have shown will minimize postpartum weight retention compared to a no-treatment control condition. Clinicians should consider these factors when developing and implementing this intervention strategy.

Mail-Based Approaches

A number of studies have examined the efficacy of delivering components of behavioral interventions for physical activity via mail (Marcus, Owen et al. 1998). Materials that are individualized and matched to the individual have been shown to be more effective than standard print material. Marcus and colleagues (Marcus, Bock et al. 1998; Marcus, Emmons et al. 1998) showed that materials matched to the stage of motivation are more effective than standard print material. In addition, individualized motivationally matched materials may be most effective for individuals in the earliest stages of changing their physical activity behavior.

Approaches Using Technology

With the ever expanding technologies that are becoming available, it is important to consider whether these can be used as methods of delivering behavioral interventions for physical activity and weight loss. Currently a number of trials are underway that are examining the use of some of these techniques. Findings by Tate and colleagues (2001) have shown that the use of computers to deliver a Web-based intervention that is supplemented by electronic mail feedback may be effective in weight loss interventions (Tate et al. 2001). In addition, Harvey-Berino and colleagues (1999) have also demonstrated that the use of computer technology that integrates video support and live video chat sessions may be as effective for weight loss as therapist-led in-person sessions. However, despite these promising results, these techniques are still in their infancy and have been used only over short periods of time. Additional evaluation of these techniques may be required before definitive conclusions regarding their efficacy can be obtained.

Summary

Exercise appears to be an important component of a behavioral intervention that incorporates changes in diet and is supported by behavioral principles. This may be a result of both physiological and behavioral adaptations that occur when one initiates and maintains a more active lifestyle. In addition, exercise may be beneficial to health independent of changes in body weight. Thus, adoption and maintenance of a more active lifestyle can be beneficial to overweight adults.

Despite the benefits that exercise would have for sedentary overweight individuals, adoption and maintenance of exercise in this population is problematic. A number of behavioral strategies appear to be promising in this area. Despite some promising findings, however, the challenge remains to develop and implement strategies that effectively maintain activity over the long term, and additional research is necessary in this area. Moreover, more research is necessary to define the dose and type of activity that is most beneficial to adults seeking weight loss, weight maintenance, or both.

References

Andersen, R., Wadden, T. et al. 1999. Effects of lifestyle activity vs. structured aerobic exercise in obese women: A randomized trial. *Journal of the American Medical Association* 281: 335-340.

Andersen, R.E., Franckowiak, S. et al. 1998. Can inexpensive signs encourage the use of stairs? Results from a community intervention. *Annals of Internal Medicine* 129: 363-369.

Barlow, C.E., Kohl, H.W. et al. 1995. Physical activity, mortality, and obesity. *International Journal of Obesity* 19: S41-S44.

Brownell, K.D., Stunkard, A.J. et al. 1980. Evaluation and modifications of exercise patterns in the natural environment. *American Journal of Psychiatry* 137: 1540-1545.

Colvin, R.H., and Olson, S.B. 1983. A descriptive analysis of men and women who have lost significant weight and are highly successful at maintaining weight loss. *Addictive Behaviors* 8: 287-295.

DeBusk, R., Stenestrand, U. et al. 1990. Training effects of long versus short bouts of exercise in healthy subjects. *American Journal of Cardiology* 65: 1010-1013.

DiPietro, L., Kohl, H.W. et al. 1998. Improvements in cardiorespiratory fitness attenuate age-related weight gain in healthy men and women: the Aerobics Center Longitudinal Study. *International Journal of Obesity* 22: 55-62.

DiPietro, L., Williamson, D.F. et al. 1993. The descriptive epidemiology of selected physical activities and body weight among adults trying to lose weight: The Behavioral Risk Factor Surveillance System Survey. *International Journal of Obesity* 17 (2): 69-76.

Donnelly, J.E., Pronk, N.P. et al. 1991. Effects of a very-low-calorie diet and physical-training regimens on body composition and resting metabolic rate in obese females. *American Journal of Clinical Nutrition* 54: 56-61.

Donnelly, J.E., Sharp, T. et al. 1993. Muscle hypertrophy with large-scale weight loss and resistance training. *American Journal Clinical Nutrition* 58 (4): 561-565.

Dunn, A., Marcus, B. et al. 1999. Comparison of lifestyle and structured interventions to increase physical activity and cardiorespiratory fitness. *Journal of the American Medical Association* 281: 327-334.

Ebisu, T. 1985. Splitting the distances of endurance training: On cardiovascular endurance and blood lipids. *Japanese Journal of Physical Education* 30: 37-43.

Emmons, K., Marcus, B. et al. 1998. Physical activity: A gateway to improve dietary behaviors? *Annals of Behavioral Medicine* 20 (Suppl.): S069.

Flegal, K.M., Carroll, M.D. et al. 1998. Overweight and obesity in the United States: Prevalence and trends. *International Journal of Obesity* 22: 39-47.

French, S.A., Jeffery, R.W. et al. 1994. Predictors of weight change over two years among a population of working adults: The Healthy Worker Project. *International Journal of Obesity* 18: 145-154.

Gormally, J., Rardin, D. et al. 1980. Correlates of successful response to a behavioral weight control clinic. *Journal of Consulting and Clinical Psychology* 27: 179-191.

Gwinup, G. 1975. Effect of exercise alone on the weight of obese women. *Archives of Internal Medicine* 135: 676-680.

Hagan, R.D., Upton, S.J. et al. 1986. The effects of aerobic conditioning and/or calorie restriction in overweight men and women. *Medicine and Science in Sports and Exercise* 18 (1): 87-94.

Harvey-Berino, J., Pinauro, S.J. et al. 1999. The feasibility of using effectiveness of internet support for the maintenance of weight loss. *Obesity Research* 7 (Suppl. 1): 19S.

Jakicic, J.M., Wing, R.R. et al. 1995. Prescribing exercise in multiple short bouts versus one continuous bout: Effects on adherence, cardiorespiratory fitness, and weight loss in overweight women. *International Journal of Obesity* 19: 893-901.

Jakicic, J.M., Wing, R.R. et al. 1997. The relationship between presence of exercise equipment in the home and physical activity level. *American Journal of Health Promotion* 11 (5): 363-365.

Jakicic, J.M., Wing, R.R. et al. 2002. Relationship of physical activity to eating behaviors and weight loss in women. *Medicine and Science in Sports and Exercise* 34: 1653-1659.

Jakicic, J.M., Winters, C. et al. 1999. Effects of intermittent exercise and use of home exercise equipment on adherence, weight loss, and fitness in overweight women: A randomized trial. *Journal of the American Medical Association* 282 (16): 1554-1560.

Kayman, S., Bruvold, W. et al. 1990. Maintenance and relapse after weight loss in women: Behavioral aspects. *American Journal of Clinical Nutrition* 52: 800-807.

King, A.C., Haskell, W.L. et al. 1991. Group- versus home-based exercise training in healthy older men and women: A community-based clinical trial. *Journal of the American Medical Association* 266: 1535-1542.

King, A.C., Haskell, W.L. et al. 1995. Long-term effects of varying intensities and formats of physical activity on participation rates, fitness, and lipoproteins in men and women aged 50-65 years. *Circulation* 91: 2596-2604.

Klem, M.L., Wing, R.R. et al. 1997. A descriptive study of individuals successful at long-term maintenance of substantial weight loss. *American Journal of Clinical Nutrition* 66: 239-246.

Klesges, R.C., Klesges, L.M. et al. 1992. A longitudinal analysis of the impact of dietary intake and physical activity on weight change in adults. *American Journal of Clinical Nutrition* 55: 818-822.

Kraemer, W.J., Volek, J.S. et al. 1999. Influence of exercise training on physiological and performance changes with weight loss in men. *Medicine and Science in Sports and Exercise* 31: 1320-1329.

Lee, C.D., Blair, S.N. et al. 1998. Cardiorespiratory fitness, body composition, and all-cause and cardiovascular disease mortality in men. *American Journal of Clinical Nutrition* 69 (3): 373-380.

Leermakers, E.A., Anglin, K. et al. 1998. Reducing postpartum weight retention through a correspondence intervention. *International Journal of Obesity* 22 (11): 1103-1109.

Leermakers, E.A., Jakicic, J.M. et al. 1998. Clinic-based vs. home-based interventions for preventing weight gain in men. *Obesity Research* 6: 346-352.

Leibel, R.L., Rosenbaum, M. et al. 1995. Changes in energy expenditure resulting from altered body weight. *New England Journal of Medicine* 332: 621-628.

Lombard, D.N., Lombard, T. et al. 1995. Walking to meet health guidelines: The effect of prompting frequency and prompt structure. *Health Psychology* 14: 164-170.

Marcus, B.H., Bock, B.C. et al. 1998. Efficacy of an individualized, motivationally tailored physical activity intervention. *Annals of Behavioral Medicine* 20 (3): 174-180.

Marcus, B.H., Emmons, K.M. et al. 1998. Evaluation of motivationally-tailored versus standard self-help physical activity interventions at the workplace. *American Journal of Health Promotion* 12: 246-253.

Marcus, B.H., Owen, N. et al. 1998. Physical activity interventions using mass media, print media, and information technology. *American Journal of Preventive Medicine* 15 (4): 362-378.

McGuire, M.T., Wing, R.R. et al. 1999. What predicts weight regain in a group of successful weight losers? *Journal of Consulting and Clinical Psychology* 67 (2): 177-185.

Miller, W.C. 1999. How effective are traditional dietary and exercise interventions for weight loss? *Medicine and Science in Sports and Exercise* 31 (8): 1129-1134.

Mokdad, A.H., Serdula, M.K. et al. 1999. The spread of the obesity epidemic in the United States, 1991-1998. *Journal of the American Medical Association* 282 (16): 1519-1522.

Murphy, M.H. and Hardman, A.E. 1998. Training effects of short and long bouts of brisk walking in sedentary women. *Medicine and Science in Sports and Exercise* 30: 152-157.

National Institutes of Health. 1998. Clinical guidelines on the identification, evaluation, and treatment of overweight and obesity in adults—The evidence report. *Obesity Research* 6 (Suppl. 2).

Owens, J.F., Matthews, K.A. et al. 1992. Can physical activity mitigate the effects of aging in middle-aged women? *Circulation* 85: 1265-1270.

Pate, R.R., Pratt, M. et al. 1995. Physical activity and public health: A recommendation from the Centers for Disease Control and Prevention and the American College of Sports Medicine. *Journal of the American Medical Association* 273 (5): 402-407.

Perri, M.G., McAdoo, W.G. et al. 1986. Enhancing the efficacy of behavioral therapy for obesity: Effects of aerobic exercise and a multicomponent maintenance program. *Journal of Consulting and Clinical Psychology* 54: 670-675.

Perri, M.G., McAllister, D.A. et al. 1988. Effects of four maintenance programs on long-term management of obesity. *Journal of Consulting and Clinical Psychology* 65: 278-285.

Perri, M.G., Martin, A.D. et al. 1997. Effects of group-versus home-based exercise in the treatment of obesity. *Journal of Consulting and Clinical Psychology* 65: 278-285.

Pronk, N.P. and Wing, R.R. 1994. Physical activity and long-term maintenance of weight loss. *Obesity Research* 2 (6): 587-599.

Raynor, D.A., Coleman, K.J. et al. 1998. Effects of proximity of the choice to be physically active or sedentary. *Research Quarterly for Exercise and Sport* 69: 99-103.

Sallis, J.F., Hovell, M.F. et al. 1990. Distance between homes and exercise facilities related to frequency of exercise among San Diego residents. *Public Health Reports* 105: 179-185.

Schoeller, D.A., Shay, K. et al. 1997. How much physical activity is needed to minimize weight gain in previously obese women. *American Journal of Clinical Nutrition* 66: 551-556.

Short, K.R., and Sedlock, D.A. 1997. Excess postexercise oxygen consumption and recovery rate in trained and untrained subjects. *Journal of Applied Physiology* 83 (1): 153-159.

Snyder, K.A., Donnelly, J.E. et al. 1997. The effects of long-term, moderate intensity, intermittent exercise on aerobic capacity, body composition, blood lipids, insulin and glucose in overweight females. *International Journal of Obesity* 21: 1180-1189.

Tate, D.F., Wing, R.R. et al. 2001. Using internet technology to deliver a behavioral weight loss program. *Journal of the American Medical Association* 285 (9): 1172-1177.

Taylor, C.B., Jatulis, D.E. et al. 1994. Effects of lifestyle on body mass index change. *Epidemiology* 5: 599-603.

Tyron, W.W., Goldberg, J.L. et al. 1992. Activity decreases as percentage overweight increases. *International Journal of Obesity* 16: 591-595.

U.S. Department of Health and Human Services. 1996. *Physical activity and health: A report of the Surgeon General*. Atlanta, GA: U.S. Department of Health and Human Services, Centers for Disease Control and Prevention, National Center for Chronic Disease Prevention and Health Promotion.

Wadden, T.A. 1993. The treatment of obesity: An overview. In *Obesity: Theory and therapy*, 2nd ed., eds. A.J. Stunkard and T.A. Wadden, 197-217. New York: Raven Press.

Wadden, T.A., Vogt, R.A. et al. 1997. Exercise in the treatment of obesity: Effects of four interventions on body composition, resting energy expenditure, appetite, and mood. *Journal of Consulting and Clinical Psychology* 65: 269-277.

Wei, M.J., Kampert, J.B. et al. 1999. Relationship between low cardiorespiratory fitness and mortality in normal-weight, overweight, and obese men. *Journal of the American Medical Association* 282 (16): 1547-1553.

Williamson, D.F., Madans, J. et al. 1993. Recreational physical activity and ten-year weight change in a US national cohort. *International Journal of Obesity* 17: 279-286.

Wing, R.R. 1999. Physical activity in the treatment of adulthood overweight and obesity: Current evidence and research issues. *Medicine and Science in Sports and Exercise* 31 (11) (Suppl.): S547-S552.

Wing, R.R. 2002. Behavioral weight control. In *Handbook of obesity treatment*, eds. T.A. Wadden and A.J. Stunkard, 301-316. New York: The Guilford Press.

Wood, P.D., Stephanick, M.L. et al. 1988. Changes in plasma lipids and lipoproteins in overweight men during weight loss through dieting as compared with exercise. *New England Journal of Medicine* 319: 1173-1179.

Wood, P.D., Stephanick, M.L. et al. 1991. The effects of plasma lipoproteins of a prudent weight-reducing diet, with or without exercise, in overweight men and women. *New England Journal of Medicine* 325: 461-466.

Chapter 15

Helping Individuals Reduce Sedentary Behavior

Brian E. Saelens, PhD

Cincinnati Children's Hospital Medical Center
and the University of Cincinnati College of Medicine

The preparation of this chapter was supported in part by a grant from the National Institutes of Health DK60476.

The etiology of the epidemic rise of childhood and adult obesity (Troiano et al. 1995; Mokdad et al. 1999) has been partially attributed to the increasing sedentariness of the American lifestyle (Gortmaker, Dietz, and Cheung 1990). From the burgeoning reliance on the automobile for transportation to the increase across every age group in the amount of television watched (Comstock and Paik 1991) to the computer-based technologies that pervade our everyday lives, the energy expenditure associated with daily living has diminished over the preceding decades and continues to do so. A relevant example of this is how you came to be reading this chapter. Did you *walk* (or preferably sprint) to the bookstore or library to buy or read this book? Did you *drive* to the bookstore or library to buy or read this book? Did you *click* on a bookmarked Web site, type in your credit card number, and have the book delivered directly to your door? There are numerous illustrations of the ways that our society has recently changed in ways that chip away at energy expenditure by increasing the number of sedentary activities we have access to and engage in.

The goals of this chapter are to (1) examine the measurement and prevalence of sedentary behavior in our society, (2) detail the relationship between sedentary behavior and weight status in children and adults, (3) summarize the findings of randomized controlled and laboratory trials targeting modification of sedentary behavior, and (4) suggest strategies for reducing sedentary behavior and outline possible future directions for the empirical investigation of sedentary behavior and its impact on health and, most specifically, body weight.

Definition

For the purposes of this chapter, sedentary behaviors will be considered activities that result in energy expenditure that is close to energy expenditure "at rest," particularly when compared to vigorous physical activity. More specifically, sedentary activities will be defined as those traditionally less than or equal to 1.5 METs. A MET is a metabolic equivalent defined as the "the energy expenditure of sitting quietly, which for the average adult is approximately 1 kcal per kilogram of body weight per hour" (Ainsworth et al. 1993). Table 15.1 provides examples of sedentary activities and physical activities of various intensity levels. Clearly, this categorization is arbitrary given that energy expenditure necessarily falls along a continuum and can vary greatly even within the same category (e.g., biking can range from leisurely to racing at speeds greater than 20 mph, with MET value differences of up to 12.0 METs) (Ainsworth et al. 1993).

This definition of sedentariness as engaging in sedentary behavior at a certain rate is distinct from others' use of the term (Dietz 1996). Sedentariness in this chapter will be defined as engaging in activities deemed sedentary, rather than not engaging in physical activity at recommended levels. This is an important distinction because sedentary behavior and physical activity or physical fitness are not necessarily reciprocal or even

negatively correlated as currently measured (Katzmarzyk et al. 1998). An individual, for example, can spend the majority of the day engaged in light intensity activities (see table 15.1), thereby not exceeding the standard for either sedentary behavior or physical activity. (e.g., American College of Sports Medicine guidelines of moderate-intensity activity). Thus, reports of inactivity prevalence (Pratt, Macera, and Blanton 1999) and the disease and health cost burden of inactivity (e.g., Colditz 1999) are generally considering individuals who are not meeting some minimum level of physical activity, rather than individuals who are meeting some established rate of engaging in sedentary behaviors.

Table 15.1 — Activities of Various Intensities

Category of activity	MET level	Example activities*
Sedentary activity	≤1.5	Watching television, movies Talking on the phone Working/playing on the computer (e.g., on the Internet) Sitting or reclining, reading Playing card or board games
Light intensity activity	>1.5 to <3.0	Light cleaning (e.g., dusting) Cooking Walking-shopping (non-grocery) Playing catch (football, baseball)
Moderate intensity activity	≥3.0 to ≤4.9	Dancing, slow Bowling Heavy cleaning (e.g., washing windows) Walking downstairs
Hard intensity activity	≥5.0 to ≤6.9	Most gardening activities Golf, carrying clubs Hiking Kayaking
Very hard intensity activity	≥7.0	Running >5 mph Swimming laps Soccer Basketball, playing game Walking upstairs

* Examples were taken from Ainsworth et al. 1993.

Measurement of Sedentary Behavior

No established standards or guidelines exist for the amount of sedentary behavior below which one can maintain optimal health or healthful weight status, but research literature on the relationship between sedentary behavior and health is growing. Recommendations for television watching, a common sedentary behavior, have been established primarily for youth for violence- and academic-related reasons by professional organizations (American Academy of Pediatrics, Committee on Public Education 1999). Only recently has the amount of time engaged in sedentary behavior been addressed for the purpose of promoting physical health. Indeed, *Healthy People 2010* (U.S. Department of Health and Human Services 2000), containing guidelines and objectives for the health of the American public, details objectives for increasing the percentage of 8- to 16-year-olds watching less than two hours of television from the average of 60% to over 75%. This is the first *Healthy People* document to include recommendations about decreasing sedentary behavior.

Not only are health recommendations about the frequency of sedentary behavior in their infancy, but the measurement of sedentary behavior remains imprecise. Sedentary behavior, similar to activities of greater energy expenditure, is difficult to measure accurately and comprehensively as a result of many factors. The simultaneous engagement in multiple activities, such as vacuuming while watching television, makes it difficult to pinpoint actual energy expenditure (Do you vacuum more slowly because you were watching TV? Do you stop to take breaks in vacuuming at perceived important times during the television show you are watching?, etc.). Also, self-report surveys of sedentary behavior continue to fall behind the frequent addition of new or modified sedentary activities added to our lives (e.g., the Internet). This limits the ongoing content validity of measures of sedentary behavior. Even more objective measures of activity, including accelerometers, provide more accurate and continuous measures of activity intensity and duration, but cannot provide details about the particular type of activity engaged in.

Many investigators have attempted to get a proxy for overall sedentary behavior by measuring the amount of time spent in a common sedentary behavior, television watching. This usually involves asking individuals to recall the amount of television watched during a typical day (e.g., Sidney et al. 1996), a typical week (e.g., Gortmaker, Peterson et al. 1999), the previous day (e.g., Robinson 1999), the past week (e.g., Ching et al. 1996), or separately for weekdays and weekend days (e.g., McMurray et al. 2000). With few exceptions (e.g., Gortmaker, Peterson et al. 1999), assessments of television watching are often single-item or few-item measures and have not been tested for either reliability or validity. Some investigators have begun to question not only the validity of the subjective report of television watching, but whether television watching is indeed a proxy for the overall amount of time spent in sedentary activities (Crawford, Jeffery, and French 1999). The use of television watching as a proxy for overall sedentary behavior may be increasingly problematic given the vast expansion in the number of sedentary activities available, but television watching remains the predominant sedentary behavior particularly for children (Roberts et al. 1999). Other investigators have expanded their assessment of sedentary behavior to include sedentary activities other than television watching (e.g., video games, reading) (Epstein et al. 2000; Gordon-Larsen, McMurray, and Popkin 1999) or have more generally assessed sedentariness (e.g., "How many hours on average do you spend sitting down?") (Martinez-Gonzalez et al. 1999). Clearly, more research is needed to develop reliable and valid measures of sedentary behavior (Dietz 1996).

Prevalence of Sedentary Behavior

Whereas the measures of sedentary behavior may be incomplete using current assessment tools, information exists regarding general trends in the amount of sedentary behavior engaged in and demographic differences in the rates of sedentary behavior, particularly for television watching. First, television watching across the population increases through young childhood, peaking sometime between the ages of 10 and 14 years old (Andersen et al. 1998; Comstock and Paik 1991), and then gradually decreasing through adolescence and early adulthood (Gordon-Larsen et al. 1999). Evidence suggests that television watching is replaced by other sedentary activities during adolescence (e.g., talking on the phone, listening to music), but television often remains a daily experience. Approximately 80% of 8- to 16-year-old children reported watching more than three hours of television daily (Andersen et al. 1998). Among a national sample of 10- to 15-year-old children, the average amount of television watching in 1990 was 4.8 hours per day or approximately 34 hours per week (Gortmaker et al. 1996). In a more recent sample of older adolescents, time spent watching television and playing video games was lower, averaging between 20 and 23 hours per week for 12- to 17-year-olds. Following this decline in television watching in adolescence and young adulthood, there is a gradual increase through to older adulthood (Coakley et al. 1998; Condry 1989). Adults tend to be more stable than children in the types and amount of sedentary behavior they engage in.

In addition to age, there appear to be both gender and ethnic differences in the amount of time spent in sedentary activities. The rates of television watching and video game playing as estimated in national samples are generally lower in girls than in boys (Andersen et al. 1998; Gordon-Larsen et al. 1999), although this gender difference may not be consistent across different ethnic groups (Robinson and Killen 1995). Black children, adolescents, and adults generally report higher rates of television watching relative to white and Asian-American youth (Andersen et al. 1998; Gordon-Larsen et al. 1999; Heath et al. 1994; Myers et al. 1996; Sidney et al. 1996; Wolf et al. 1993). However, given that children's amount of television watching is consistently inversely related to parental education (Comstock and Paik 1991), these differences in rates may be confounded by unaccounted-for differences in socioeconomic status. Some evidence suggests that ethnic differences in television watching persist after controlling for other sociodemographic variables (e.g., Sidney et al. 1996). Thus, it is important to consider socioeconomic and other potentially confounding factors in the examination of the relationship between sedentary behavior and health outcomes (e.g., McMurray et al. 2000).

In summary, the rates of sedentary behavior, as estimated by the measurement of television watching, suggest that Americans, both youth (Harrell et al. 1997) and adults (Nielsen Media Research 2000), spend a considerable amount of time in these activities. Television watching and other sedentary activities are pervasive in both leisure and non-leisure time periods throughout the days of many individuals. Given this proliferation of sedentary behavior, we must understand the relationship between sedentary behavior time and health outcomes, including obesity.

Sedentary Behavior and Weight

Spending time in sedentary behavior may contribute to or help maintain a higher weight status for many reasons. First, engaging in sedentary behavior may interfere with time and opportunities to be active. Time spent in front of the television is necessary time not spent going for a bicycle ride or a walk around the block. Sedentary behavior may be particularly detrimental to accumulating moderate-intensity physical activity (Strauss et al. 2000), rather than interfering with more planned vigorous physical activity (Crespo et al. 2001). Second, sedentary behavior may set the stage for higher caloric consumption, through eating more food (e.g., snacking) or more unhealthful food. Researchers have found television watching to be positively associated with higher consumption of unhealthful foods (e.g., Coon et al. 2001; Jeffery and French 1998; Robinson and Killen 1995) and higher caloric intake (Crespo et al. 2001). Third, television watching and other sedentary behavior may reduce resting metabolic rate (Klesges, Shelton, and Klesges 1993), although support for this hypothesis remains tenuous (Buchowski and Sun 1996; Dietz et al. 1994). Alternatively, higher weight status may precede higher rates of sedentary behavior, with some prospective analysis not supporting this alternative (e.g., Gortmaker et al. 1996). The exact mechanism by which sedentary behavior may affect weight status remains unknown, but the association has been extensively explored.

Youth

Many studies with relatively large sample sizes ($N > 150$) have examined the cross-sectional and prospective relations between the amount of sedentary behavior engaged in by youth and their weight status. The citation, sample age, sedentary activities examined, sedentary behavior assessment strategies, and a brief summary of findings for these studies are provided in table 15.2 in chronological order of publication. As seen in table 15.2, findings regarding the relation between sedentary behavior time and adiposity among children are inconsistent. Dietz and Gortmaker (1985) document higher rates of obesity (>85th percentile triceps skinfold) and super obesity (>95th percentile triceps skinfold) among 6- to 11-year-old children who watch TV for more hours each day, with a significant dose-response linear relationship. Longitudinal analyses also suggest that the amount of television watching among these 6- to 11-year-olds positively predicted higher weight status when these children were 12 to 17 years old (Dietz and Gortmaker 1985). Gortmaker and colleagues (1996) provide further evidence for these cross-sectional and longitudinal findings in a separate sample of 10- to 15-year-old children, and ascribe an attributable risk estimate for obesity in childhood of over 60% for television watching, even after controlling for such factors as maternal education and household income. In contrast, others have found little or no associations between sedentary behavior time and weight status. For example, Robinson and colleagues (1993) report no significant cross-sectional or prospective relationship between television time after school and body mass index or triceps skinfold.

Given the variability across studies in the assessment of sedentary behavior and adiposity, the inconsistent controlling of other potentially confounding variables (e.g., socioeconomic status; McMurray et al. 2000), the diversity in ethnic and gender composition of samples, and the time period of measurement (e.g., some studies involved data from the 1970s), conclusions regarding the relationship between sedentary behavior and adiposity in youth are necessarily tentative. Overall, though, the majority of the studies presented in table 15.2 found some association between sedentary behavior and children's weight status. The magnitude of the relationship appears to be small to moderate, with the amount of time spent in sedentary behavior accounting for relatively low amounts of variance in adiposity, particularly after controlling for other confounding variables.

The relationship between television watching and adiposity seems least strong among younger children (<6 years old; e.g., DuRant et al. 1994) and adolescents (e.g., Berkey et al. 2000; Robinson et al. 1993; Robinson and Killen 1995; Tucker 1986), with some evidence within single studies of a decreasing magnitude with increasing age (Obarzanek et al. 1994). The largest effects were found among samples including mostly 8- to 12-year-old children (Dietz and Gortmaker 1985; Gortmaker et al. 1996).

The majority of the positive gender-specific findings were obtained among males (e.g., Guillaume et al. 1997; Katzmarzyk et al. 1998; Myers et al. 1996). These latter two findings may be partially the result of higher rates of television watching, the primary sedentary behavior measured, among this middle childhood cohort and among boys. Weight differences were also more robust when comparing groups of individuals with extreme sedentary behavior values (e.g., <2 hours per day versus >5 hours per day; Hanley et al. 2000).

Studies reported more consistent positive findings linking television watching and children's adiposity when parents, rather than the children themselves, reported the amount of television watched (Armstrong et al. 1998; Dietz and Gortmaker 1985; Gortmaker et al. 1996; Maffeis, Talamini, and Tato 1998). Whereas some concordance exists between child and parent reports of television watching (Gortmaker et al. 1996), it would be important to evaluate these reports relative to more objective measures of television watching and identify which aspects of sedentary behavior measurement (e.g., duration, frequency) are more reliably and validly reported by children than by parents (Guillaume et al. 1997).

Finally, the more recent research cited in table 15.2 more consistently documents a positive relationship between children's weight and sedentary behavior. It is unclear whether this reflects a population cohort-driven change in the impact of sedentary behavior on children's weight status, a bias against the publication of null findings, or another factor influencing results over time.

Table 15.2 *Large Studies (N >150) Examining Relations Between Sedentary Activity and Adiposity Among Youth*

Reference	Population	Sedentary activities examined	Sedentary activity assessment strategy	Summary of findings
Dietz & Gortmaker 1985	6- to 11-year-olds (N = 6,965); 12- to 17-year-olds (N = 6,671)	TV, reading books or magazines, listening to the radio	For 6- to 11-year-olds, parent report of hours per day; for 12- to 17-year-olds, self-report of hours per day	1. Higher rates of obesity and super-obesity with increasing hours of TV for younger and older children, even after controlling for family socioeconomic status and other potentially confounding variables 2. Marginally higher rates of obesity and super-obesity among older children with greater hours of TV when younger
Tucker 1986	High school males (N = 379)	TV	Self-reported daily hours (unclear if assessed categorically or continuously)	1. No differences in BMI between high (>4 TV hours), moderate (2-4 TV hours), and low (<2 TV hours) groups
Pate & Ross 1987	3rd- and 4th-graders (N = 2,372)	TV	Parent report of estimated hours per day	1. TV positively related to skinfold thickness
Gortmaker, Dietz, & Cheung 1990	6- to 17-year-olds (N = 1,900)	TV	For 6- to 11-year-olds, parent report of hours per day; for 12- to 17-year-olds, self-report of hours per day	4-year follow-up to Dietz & Gortmaker (1985) 1. Higher TV was related to higher incidence of new cases of obesity, independent of "a wide variety of social and demographic variables" 2. Obesity remission decreased at higher quartiles of TV
Shannon, Peacock, & Brown 1991	6th-graders (N = 773; 489)	TV	Self-reported typical weekly hours based on 30-minute time blocks across each day	1. TV not significantly related to concurrent BMI or triceps skinfold 2. TV significantly related to the change in BMI and triceps skinfold over a 3-year period, particularly among girls and among children from lower socioeconomic strata
Locard et al. 1992	Children entering first grade (N = 1,031)	TV	Parent report of the number of times per day child watched	1. Risk of obesity higher among children who watch TV 4 or more times per day 2. Differences between obese and non-obese children in TV watching not significant after controlling for length of sleep

Study	Subjects	Media	Measure	Findings
Robinson et al. 1993	6th- and 7th-grade girls (N = 671)	TV	Self-reported time spent after school is over	1. No cross-sectional or prospective relation between BMI, triceps skinfold, and TV 2. Similar TV time reported by obese and non-obese
Wolf et al. 1993	5th- to 12th-grade girls (N = 552)	TV	Categorical self-report on previous day (6 categories from 1 to 9.5 hr)	1. No relation between BMI and TV across all time categories of TV, since those in the "least TV" group were most obese 2. If the "least TV" group is excluded, significant positive relation between BMI and TV
DuRant et al. 1994	3- to 4-year-olds (N = 191)	TV	Direct observation of each minute over a 6- to 12-hour period up to 4 days per year	1. No relation between TV time and sum of seven skinfolds, waist/hip ratio, or BMI
Obarzanek et al. 1994; Kimm et al. 1996	9- to 10-year-old girls (N = 2,379)	TV, VCR	Self-reported specific television shows watched and number of videos watched	1. SAT related to BMI, triceps and trunk skinfolds 2. Some decrease in TV-BMI relation with increasing age among white girls 3. TV positively associated with obesity prevalence among both black and white girls, but association no longer significant for white girls after accounting for familial socioeconomic status, number of parents in home, and daily caloric intake
Robinson & Killen 1995	9th-graders (N = 1,768)	TV, VCR, VG/CG, music videos	Self-reported time on usual school day and usual weekend day	1. SAT significantly associated with BMI among white boys
Gortmaker et al. 1996	10- to 15-year-olds (N = 746)	TV	Mean of self- and parent-report of time spent on typical day	1. Higher odds of being overweight for ≥5 TV hours compared to 0-2 TV hours; higher odds of becoming overweight for ≥5 TV hours compared to 0-2 TV hours
Myers et al. 1996	5th- to 8th-graders (N = 995)	TV, VCR, VG/CG	Self-reported time spent in activities before, during, and after school on previous day	1. No relation between SAT quartile index and ponderal index 2. Among white males, larger triceps skinfold among above-median SAT
Guillaume et al. 1997	6- to 12-year-olds (N = 1,028)	TV	Self- and parent-reported days per week and duration per day (days per week used)	1. After adjusting for age and sports hours per week, significant positive TV-body weight relation for girls and boys, but TV-BMI relation only significant for boys 2. No significant TV-triceps skinfold for either boys or girls

(continued)

Table 15.2

Reference	Population	Sedentary activities examined	Sedentary activity assessment strategy	Summary of findings
Andersen et al. 1998	8- to 16-year-olds (N = 4,063)	TV	Self-reported time spent on previous day	1. >4 TV hours related to highest BMIs; <1 TV hour related to lowest BMIs 2. >4 TV hours related to highest trunk skinfolds
Armstrong et al. 1998	4th-graders (N = 588)	TV, CG, VG	Categorical self-report of typical day during summer; parent report of typical weekday during school (3 levels up to ≥3 hr)	1. For parent report, ≥3 hours of SAT related to higher BMIs than <1 or 1-2 hours for boys and girls; similar for triceps skinfold, except for girls; ≥3 hours of SAT only significantly higher skinfold than <1 hour 2. For child report, no relation between SAT and BMI
Katzmarzyk et al. 1998	9- to 18-year-olds (N = 784)	TV	Self-reported amount of time in a typical week	1. TV-BMI relation significantly positive only for 9- to 12-year-old boys, but relatively small magnitude 2. No differences in TV time between highest and lowest BMI quartile
Maffeis, Talamini, & Tato 1998	Prepubertal children (N = 298)	TV	Parent report of time spent daily	1. Obese children watched more TV than non-obese children 2. Percent above average BMI positively related to TV time 3. TV time not related to change in percent above average BMI
Filozof, Saenz, & Gonzalez 1999	8- to 11-year-olds (N = 110)	TV	TV assessment strategy was unclear	1. Positive cross-sectional association between relative weight and TV time 2. Approximately 5.2 times more likely to be overweight 30 months later if watching >31.2 TV hours vs. <11.2 TV hours 3. Relative risk of becoming overweight 4.3 times greater for children watching >31.2 TV hours (highest quartile)
Hernández et al. 1999	9- to 16-year-olds (N = 461)	TV, VCR, VG	Self-report of typical TV during each day of the week; self-report of typical VCR and VG during weekdays and weekend	1. Increasing odds ratios for obesity with increasing quartiles of TV relative to <1 TV hour per day, controlling for age, gender, physical activity, town location, and children's perception of maternal weight status 2. No increasing risk for obesity for VCR or VG time 3. 12% increase in obesity odds with each additional hour of TV

Study	Sample	Media	Measurement	Findings
Berkey et al. 2000	9- to 14-year-olds (N = 10,769)	TV, VCR, CG/VG	Self-reported typical hours separately for weekdays and weekends	1. Higher SAT before and during year between weight status measurement positively related to greater 1-year increase in BMI 2. SAT-BMI change relation higher in younger girls (9 to 11 years old)
Hanley et al. 2000	10- to 19-year-olds (N = 242)	TV, VCR, VG	Self-reported usual hours per day	1. 2.5-fold risk of overweight among children engaging in SAT >5 hours per day in comparison to those with SAT <2 hours per day
McMurray et al. 2000	10- to 16-year-olds (N = 2,389)	TV, VG	Categorical self-report of hours during typical schooldays and non-schooldays (5 categories up to >3 hr)	1. For boys, significant positive TV-BMI relation for non-school days, and significant positive VG-BMI relation for school and non-school days 2. For girls, significant positive TV-BMI relation, but no VG-BMI relation 3. For both boys and girls, no significant increase for TV or VG to risk of overweight above and beyond ethnicity, parental education, and habitual physical activity
Crespo et al. 2001	8- to 16-year-olds (N = 4,069)	TV	Average of two days self-reported hours on prior day	1. Consistent increase in obesity prevalence with increasing hours of TV
Dowda et al. 2001	8- to 16-year-olds (N = 2,791)	TV	Self-reported hours on prior day	1. For girls, 2.1 times more likely to be overweight (>85th BMI percentile) if watching ≥4 TV hours vs. >4 TV hours 2. No significant difference in rates of overweight among boys watching < or >4 TV hours per day
Dennison, Erb, & Jenkins 2002	1- to 5-year-olds (N = 2,761)	TV, VCR	Parent report of hours child usually watched on weekdays, Saturday, and Sunday	1. Prevalence of overweight (>85th BMI percentile) increased for each additional hour of TV watched
Saelens et al. 2002	6- and 12-year-olds (N = 169)	TV	Parent report of hours child typically watched on weekdays, Saturday, and Sunday	1. Positive correlation between standardized BMI values and TV hours among younger children 2. When older, children watching >2 TV hours per day had higher average standardized BMI than children watching <2 TV hours per day

BMI = body mass index; SAT = sedentary activity time; TV = television; VCR = videocassette recorder; VG = video games; CG = computer games.

Collectively, the variability in findings calls for further investigation among youth samples that solidifies the content and constructs validity of the measurement of sedentary behavior in youth and consistently examines potentially spurious associations by measuring and controlling for potential confounding variables such as familial socioeconomic status. Further, these studies would be stronger if they included more adequate measures of children's dietary intake and physical activity, which are likely other contributory factors in children's weight status. Indeed, in the studies in table 15.2 that did measure physical activity, none of them used state-of-the-art assessments of children's physical activity. The self-report measures of children's physical activity that were used lacked adequate concurrent validity with more objective measures of physical activity (e.g., accelerometers; Sallis and Saelens 2000).

Adults

Similar to the research among youth, many large studies with adult samples have examined the relation between sedentary behavior time and weight status, again primarily measuring the amount of television watching. Table 15.3 provides the citation, sample details, sedentary activities examined, sedentary behavior assessment strategy, and a summary of findings from these studies. Overall, these studies found more consistent positive cross-sectional associations between television watching and adiposity among adults than was the case for the studies involving children. As with the child samples, this association appears strongest when comparing the extremes of sedentary behavior time (e.g., Ching et al. 1996). The sedentary behavior and adiposity relation was maintained at statistically significant levels even after controlling for potentially confounding variables such as age (e.g., Tucker and Friedman 1989), education (Tucker and Bagwell 1991; Martinez-Gonzalez et al. 1999), and socioeconomic status (Sidney et al. 1996). A few studies even documented correlations between sedentary behavior time and adiposity across different levels of individuals' physical activity (Ching et al. 1996; Martinez-Gonzalez et al. 1999; Tucker and Bagwell 1991).

Although limited by the number of studies that investigated similar subsamples within the adult population (e.g., age cohorts, different ethnic groups), weight status and sedentary behavior appear to be less strongly linked cross-sectionally and prospectively among older adults (Coakley et al. 1998; Fitzgerald et al. 1997). Jeffery and French (1998) reported the strongest association between television watching and body mass index (BMI) for low-income women, but no significant association for men. These findings held cross-sectionally in a later follow-up of the same cohort, but with no evidence of prospective impact of television watching on BMI (Crawford, Jeffery, and French 1999). Sidney and colleagues (1996) documented the higher rates of obesity among individuals watching more TV across different racial groups, although studies with any ethnic and racial diversity were mostly limited to the inclusion of only black or white individuals. While some investigators found a significant relationship between TV watching and weight status only among men (Fitzgerald et al. 1997), other investigators found this association among women, but not men (Jeffery and French 1998). Still others found the relationship equally strong among men and women (Sidney et al. 1996; Tucker and Bagwell 1991; Tucker and Friedman 1989).

In summary, the cross-sectional positive relationship between participation in sedentary behavior and body mass index or obesity prevalence in adults appears to be a reliable finding. There is less evidence regarding the ability of television watching to prospectively predict weight change, with current findings suggesting a smaller prospective than cross-sectional association (Coakley et al. 1998; Crawford et al. 1999). However, keeping sedentary behavior at low levels may be important for maintaining intentional weight loss (Grodstein et al. 1996). Even though the magnitude of the relation between sedentary behavior and weight status among both children and adults to date has been small to moderate, at this point the amount of time spent in sedentary behavior is a more readily modifiable variable in the weight status equation than other obesity risk factors such as socioeconomic status and genetic predisposition. Indeed, minor reductions in sedentary behavior time may have small individual effects, but substantial effects on populations

Table 15.3   *Large Studies (N >150) Examining Relations Between Sedentary Activity and Adiposity Among Adults*

Reference	Population	Sedentary activities examined	Sedentary activity assessment strategy	Summary of findings
Tucker & Friedman 1989	≥19-year-old men (N = 6,138)	TV	Self-reported daily time spent	1. After controlling for age, fitness, smoking, weekly exercise, >4 TV hours had almost twice the risk and 3-4 TV hours had a little more than twice the risk of obesity compared with <1 TV hour. 2. After controlling for age, fitness, smoking, weekly exercise, relative risk for 3-4 TV hours for super obesity (≥31% body fat) was more than twice <1 TV hour.
Gortmaker, Dietz, & Cheung 1990	Faculty, staff, students in public health dept. (N = 778)	TV	Self-reported weekly hours	1. Higher obesity prevalence among higher quartiles of TV. 2. TV more highly associated with BMI than estimate of energy expenditure and caloric intake.
Tucker & Bagwell 1991	≥19-year-old women (N = 4,771)	TV	Self-reported daily time spent	1. After controlling for age, education, smoking status, time worked per week, and weekly exercise, >4 TV hours had more than twice the risk and 3-4 TV hours had almost twice the risk of obesity compared with <1 TV hour.
Must, Gortmaker, & Dietz 1994	16- to 28-year-olds (N = 11,591)	TV	Self-reported weekly hours	1. For Hispanic and white males, TV positively related to obesity prevalence; for Hispanic and black females, TV positively related to obesity prevalence. 2. Among white females, TV positively associated with incident shift from nonobese to obese across 5-year period. 3. Among obese males, remission of obesity lower in higher quintiles of TV watching in comparison to lowest quintile; among obese females, higher TV related to lower remission rates.

(continued)

Table 15.3

(continued)

Reference	Population	Sedentary activities examined	Sedentary activity assessment strategy	Summary of findings
Ching et al. 1996	40- to 75-year-old men (N = 22,076)	TV, VCR	Categorical self-reported hours per week (6 categories from 0 to ≥41 hr)	1. After adjusting for age and smoking status, positive dose-response, with higher risk of overweight with increasing SAT hours; ≥41 SAT had four times the risk of overweight compared to 0-1 SAT hours. 2. Within each level of physical activity, SAT hours continued to be positively related to overweight prevalence. 3. After controlling for age and smoking status, linear trend in dose-response with higher SAT related to higher incidence of becoming overweight 2 years later; ≥41 SAT hours was 56% more likely to become overweight than 0-1 SAT hours.
Sidney et al. 1996	23- to 35-year-olds (N = 4,352)	TV	Self-reported hours per day	1. After adjusting for age, education, physical activity, smoking, and alcohol use, risk of obesity was significantly higher for ≥4 TV hours relative to 0-1 TV hour across ethnicity and gender.
Fitzgerald et al. 1997	21- to 59-year-old Pima Indians (N = 2,452)	TV	Self-reported typical hours per day	1. TV significantly positively related to BMI in younger men (<40 years old), but not in younger women and not in older adults. 2. Age-adjusted BMI higher in men with >3 TV hours than in men with less than 3 TV hours, but difference not significant for women. 3. For women, age-adjusted BMI was higher among inactive/high TV group in comparison to high physically active group, regardless of latter group's television watching. 4. For men, age-adjusted BMI was higher among low physical activity/high TV group than high physical activity/low TV group. 5. After controlling for presence of diabetes and age, TV was a correlate of BMI only in men, independent of physical activity level.
Coakley et al. 1998	40- to 75-year-old men (N = 19,478)	TV, VCR	Self-reported average per week over past year	Follow-up to Ching et al. 1996 1. After controlling for baseline SAT, vigorous activity, high blood pressure, and high cholesterol, increase in SAT was significantly related to increase in weight among younger men (45-54 years old), but not among older men (>55 years old).
Jeffery & French 1998	20- to 45-year-olds (N = 1,057)	TV	Self-reported hours per average day	1. For women, TV hours related to BMI, strongest among low-income women (little change when age, education, and smoking controlled; diet and exercise variables attenuated, but did not eliminate TV-BMI relation); marginal positive prospective TV-BMI relation over 1 year for high-income women. 2. No TV-BMI cross-sectional or prospective relation for men.

Study	Sample	Media	Measurement	Results
Crawford, Jeffery, & French 1999	20- to 45-year-olds (N = 881)	TV	Self-reported hours per average day	1. After controlling for age, education, baseline smoking, positive TV–BMI relation significant for women (particularly low-income women), but not men. 2. No association between BMI change and initial or change in TV.
Martinez-Gonzalez et al. 1999	>15-year-olds (N = 14,804)	Sitting down (TV, CG, VCR, read, music, etc.)	Self-reported hours on typical weekday/ workday and weekend day/ non-workday	1. After controlling for age, education level, social class, marital status, smoking habit, recent weight loss, and country, higher SAT related to higher overweight and obesity prevalence among both women and men. 2. SAT associated with BMI independent of level of physical activity.
Salmon et al. 2000	≥18-year-olds (N = 3,392)	TV/VCR	Self-reported hours on typical weekday and weekend day	1. Higher BMI associated with higher SAT independent of level of physical activity (except among completely inactive group). 2. Higher overweight prevalence related to higher SAT independent of level of physical activity (except among completely inactive category).
Vioque, Torres, & Quiles 2000	≥15-year-olds (N = 1,772)	TV	Self-reported hours per week; then categorized into hours/day	1. Obese individuals reported more TV on average than non-obese individuals. 2. TV ≥4 hours/day were 2.36 more likely to be obese than TV ≤1 hour/day (little change after adjusting for age, marital status, education, physical activity at work and leisure, sleep, and smoking).

BMI = body mass index; SAT = sedentary activity time; TV = television; VCR = video cassette recorder; CG = computer games.

and the rising prevalence of obesity in the United States (Dietz and Gortmaker 1993). It is to this potential for decreasing the amount of sedentary behavior time that we now turn.

Targeting Reductions in Sedentary Behavior

Similar to the empirical basis regarding the link between weight status and sedentary behavior, the empirical literature on testing strategies for helping individuals reduce sedentary behavior is far from definitive. Laboratory analog studies provide more succinct and ready tools to explore activity choice and to formulate hypotheses for larger clinical trials to reduce sedentary behavior. However, the literature on reducing sedentary behavior from both laboratory and clinical trials is small. In fact, to date, only four randomized clinical trials have specifically targeted reducing sedentary activities as a method of losing weight or maintaining weight loss. Further, the majority of laboratory analog studies and all of the randomized clinical trials have been conducted with youth.

Laboratory Studies

Laboratory studies have examined individuals' choices between physical and sedentary activities following controlled manipulations of the sedentary activities (for a review, see Epstein and Saelens 2000). For instance, in a laboratory setting, Epstein and colleagues (1991) gave lean, moderately overweight, and very obese children access to various physical (stationary bike) and sedentary activities (watching videos). Children determined their access to each type of activity through their responses during a computer choice task (in this case, responding was using a joystick to "pick apples" in the computer task—a task that was designed to become tedious and boring). When sedentary and physical activities required the same amount of responding (i.e., all activities were equally easy to get as each required the same amount of computer task responding), all children worked for access to the sedentary activities. However, with increasing responses required to earn sedentary behavior time, while the response contingency was maintained at the same level

to earn physical activity time, lean and then moderately overweight children switched over to earning points for physical activity time. Very obese children did not make this switch, continuing to earn time for sedentary behavior, even with very high response costs associated with earning this access (Epstein et al. 1991). This suggests that sedentary behavior may be more relatively reinforcing than physical activity for overweight children, but this choice can be modified in more moderately overweight children.

Subsequent laboratory analog studies found that overweight children will switch to more physical activity when positively reinforced for decreasing time spent in high-rate sedentary behavior (Epstein, Saelens, and Giancola O'Brien 1995; Epstein et al. 1997). In these studies, children spent the majority of their time being sedentary when given free access to both physical and sedentary activities. When children were offered points tradable for external rewards for decreasing the time they spent on two of their four preferred sedentary activities, they reallocated time to physical activity and the other available sedentary activities. In fact, children reinforced for decreasing time in specified sedentary activities were as physically active as children directly reinforced for increasing physical activity (Epstein, Saelens, and Giancola O'Brien 1995; Epstein et al. 1997).

Examination of other ways to reduce sedentary behavior yielded similar increases in physical activity. Saelens and Epstein (1998) brought overweight children individually into the laboratory for three 90-minute sessions and provided the children with access to sedentary and physical activities. Children engaged in minimal physical activity during the first laboratory session. In subsequent sessions, for some children, researchers made playing video games and watching videos directly contingent on riding the stationary bicycle. During these latter sessions, these children had the choice of doing other sedentary activities (reading, drawing) or riding the bicycle at a minimum of 60 rotations per minute to activate the television monitor for the use of video games or videos. The other children were given continued free choice of physical and sedentary activities, similar to the first laboratory session day. Children for whom the television was directly contingent on riding the bicycle were significantly more physically active than were the children for whom the contingency was not in place (Saelens and Epstein 1998), even though other sedentary activities were freely available.

This finding was replicated among sedentary adults, where it was further clarified that the specific sedentary behavior chosen to be made contingent on being physically active affects whether the contingency will increase physical activity in an environment in which other sedentary activities are available (Saelens and Epstein 1999). In this latter study, contingent sedentary activities had to be a moderate- to high-rate sedentary behavior in order to increase physical activity, as contingent low-rate sedentary activities did not increase physical activity above baseline (with categories of rate defined separately for each individual based on how much relative time he or she spent in each sedentary behavior during the baseline session where there was equal free access to all available sedentary activities) (Saelens and Epstein 1999).

These laboratory studies provide evidence for the efficacy of positive reinforcement of decreases in sedentary behavior and for contingencies between physical and sedentary activities as ways to reduce sedentary behavior time and increase physical activity. Perhaps more important, these studies suggest that sedentary activities do not necessarily or readily substitute for each other, such that if a reduction in some particular sedentary behavior or subset of sedentary activities could occur, individuals will not necessarily replace that time with other sedentary behavior. It may not be the sedentary nature per se of a behavior that makes it reinforcing, and strategies can be employed to reduce the choice to be sedentary in these controlled settings. Although laboratory studies may encourage the development of sedentary behavior reduction techniques, clearly strategies need to be tested in more naturalistic settings with larger numbers of individuals.

Clinical Trials

Case studies and small clinical trials have evaluated strategies for reducing sedentary behavior time among children. Intervention strategies have included trading in tokens earned from doing other activities (e.g., chores,

physical activity) for time to watch television (Jason 1987), putting electronic devices on the television to regulate the amount of watching (Johnson and Jason 1996), or making television contingent on being physically active (Faith et al. 2001; Jason and Brackshaw 1999). In small studies in which overweight children earned television time by riding a stationary bicycle, children lost weight (Faith et al. 2001; Jason and Brackshaw 1999).

Larger randomized trials have not yet employed contingencies between physical and sedentary behavior, but have used other traditional behavioral and cognitive strategies to decrease children's sedentary behavior time to help them lose weight. The references, populations, sedentary activities targeted, intervention conditions, strategies for reducing sedentary behavior, and summaries of weight outcomes for these randomized trials are presented in table 15.4.

As part of a comprehensive family-based weight control program that included a significant dietary component, Epstein, Valoski, and colleagues (1995) targeted specific sedentary activities for reduction to increase children's physical activity without directly addressing increases in physical activity. Children's sedentary behavior was reduced by having them self-monitor sedentary behavior on a daily basis, set sedentary behavior time goals, and receive reinforcers for meeting sedentary behavior reduction goals. In addition, families were encouraged to reduce availability to targeted sedentary activities (e.g., putting the remote control away) and were also encouraged to reduce things that cue for targeted sedentary activities. In addition, they were encouraged to find alternative activities (not specified as sedentary or active) in which to spend time. As noted in table 15.4, children assigned to the condition targeting reductions in sedentary behavior had better long-term percent overweight change outcomes than did children assigned to the condition targeting increases in physical activity and to the condition targeting both decreases in sedentary behavior and increases in physical activity. Children had equal improvements in physical fitness across conditions, but children reinforced for reducing sedentary behavior also increased their liking of high-intensity physical activity more than did children in other conditions.

Table 15.4

Randomized Trials Targeting Reductions in Sedentary Activity and Adiposity

Reference	Population	Sedentary activities targeted	Intervention conditions	Strategies for reducing sedentary activity	Summary of weight outcomes
Epstein, Valoski et al. 1995	8- to 12-year-olds (N = 55)	TV, VCR, imaginative play, talking on phone, playing board games	Clinic-based 6-month family weight control program 1. Target SAT reduction 2. Target increasing PA 3. Target combination of SAT reduction and increasing PA	1. Reading and group content about effect of sedentary activity on weight 2. Self-monitoring of SAT 3. Decrease cues for sedentary activities 4. Weekly goal-setting and positive reinforcement for reducing SAT	Children targeted for SAT reduction had a significantly greater decrease in percent overweight than children in 1. Increasing PA to post-treatment. 2. Increasing PA or the combined condition to 1-year follow-up.
Robinson 1999	3rd- and 4th-graders (N = 192)	TV, VCR, VG	1. School-based program targeting SAT reduction 2. Assessment only	18 curriculum lessons 1. Self-monitoring 2. 10-day TV turnoff 3. Goal setting <7 SAT/wk 4. Newsletters to parents 5. Electronic TV time manager to measure and budget SAT	1. Intervention children had significantly less increase in BMI and triceps skinfold than control children. 2. Relative effects for intervention were greater among heavier children.
Epstein et al. 2000	8- to 12-year-olds (N = 90)	TV, VCR, VG/CG, talking on phone, playing board games	Clinic-based 6-month family weight control program 1. High-dose SAT reduction 2. Low-dose SAT reduction 3. High-dose increase PA 4. Low-dose increase PA	1. Reading and group content about effect of sedentary activity on weight 2. Self-monitoring of SAT 3. Decrease cues for sedentary activities 4. Weekly goal setting and positive reinforcement for reducing SAT	1. All interventions similarly reduced percent overweight to post-treatment and to 18 months after treatment cessation.

| Gortmaker, Peterson et al. 1999 | 6th- and 7th-graders ($N = 1,295$) | TV, VCR, VG/CG | 1. School-based 2-year intervention targeting SAT reduction
2. Control schools received no intervention | Classroom curriculum
1. Didactic and interactive lessons on reducing SAT
2. Goal-setting and evaluation
3. Additional cognitive and behavioral skills
4. 2-week campaign to reduce household TV time | 1. Intervention females had significantly reduced obesity prevalence, while control females had increased obesity prevalence; no difference between intervention and control males.
2. Reduction in SAT was the only mediator of intervention (greater decrease in SAT related to greater decrease in obesity prevalence).
3. Among girls obese at baseline, reductions in SAT were positively related to obesity remission. |

TV = television; VCR = videocassette recording; VG = video games; CG = computer games; SAT = sedentary activity time; PA = physical activity.

These findings suggest that children reinforced for decreasing sedentary behavior time are substituting some of the time previously spent in sedentary behavior for physical activity, and thus may be enjoying such physical activity more because they chose to do it instead of being reinforced directly for being physically active (Epstein, Valoski et al. 1995). The superiority in weight loss outcomes of the decreased sedentary behavior condition relative to the increased physical activity condition was not replicated in a more recent trial (Epstein et al. 2000), but these later findings confirm that a comprehensive family-based weight control program for overweight children that incorporates components for reducing sedentary behavior is a viable alternative to the more traditional approach of directly targeting increases in physical activity.

Using similar strategies to reduce sedentary behavior among youth not selected for being overweight, recent school-based trials with larger samples have been successful in reducing obesity prevalence among girls (Gortmaker, Peterson et al. 1999) and stemming more significant increases in body mass index among both boys and girls (Robinson 1999) relative to school children not provided intervention. It is noteworthy that these separate prevention interventions were conducted in children from different age cohorts (third- and fourth-graders versus sixth- and seventh-graders) and that among the adolescent sample the intervention effect was mediated only by the measured change in television watching (Gortmaker, Peterson et al. 1999). Another school intervention trial, although not reporting weight outcomes, provided some evidence for efficacy with television watching reductions (Gortmaker, Cheung et al. 1999). In these interventions, specific strategies to reduce sedentary behavior included sedentary behavior self-monitoring, goal setting, and other traditional cognitive-behavioral strategies. By integrating content on reducing sedentary behavior time and more specifically television watching into school curriculums, these interventions were successful novel approaches that have the potential to affect larger populations than clinic-based interventions, albeit with perhaps smaller effects per individual, but significant public health implications (Dietz and Gortmaker 1993).

Practical Applications

Considering findings from the laboratory analog studies and the promising evidence regarding the efficacy of clinic- and school-based trials for reducing weight by reducing sedentary behavior, preliminary recommendations for helping individuals reduce sedentary behavior can be derived. First, it is important to obtain an accurate evaluation of the amount of time and frequency spent in various sedentary activities. Whereas this may require daily logging of, or a detailed recall of, sedentary behavior for a period of time, more easily obtainable sedentary behavior measures do not provide good measures of time spent in various sedentary activities (e.g., rated liking or ranked preference of various sedentary activities; Saelens and Epstein 1999). Unfortunately, no empirical evidence points to an optimal length of time to assess sedentary behavior in order to generalize an overall estimate. However, a two-week diary or recall period seems adequate to estimate daily sedentary behavior time.

Specific strategies for reducing sedentary behavior should include those found to be efficacious, including stimulus control and reducing things that cue sedentary behavior (e.g., television sets in every room of one's home), specifying goals for reducing sedentary behavior, and positive reinforcement for reducing time spent in particularly high-rate sedentary behavior. An example of stimulus control would be the removal of television sets from children's bedrooms, as having a bedroom television is related to higher overall watching (Saelens et al. 2002) and child overweight (Dennison, Erb, and Jenkins 2002). Eating meals while watching television is also related to higher overall amounts of television watching in children (Saelens et al. 2002).

The elimination of all sedentary behavior is unrealistic, but it may be important to maximize enjoyment of the time spent in more limited sedentary behavior. This latter strategy could involve a careful review of the specific television shows, video games, and computer use that are most enjoyable, with a reduction in least liked aspects of these activities to reduce overall sedentary behavior time. This may decrease the likelihood of feelings of deprivation around decreasing liked activities, while increasing behavioral adherence to sedentary behavior reduction. In addition, individuals may be encouraged to increase lifestyle physical activity (e.g., walking to the store, taking the stairs), as such physical activity may be more readily integrated into a daily schedule. Whereas the more sophisticated laboratory-based contingencies between physical and sedentary behavior are not yet widely commercially available, more informal contingencies or at least simultaneous engagement in physical and traditionally sedentary behavior (e.g., watching TV while riding the stationary bicycle) can help reduce sedentary behavior, increase physical activity, and tip energy balance to be more consistent with weight loss or maintenance.

Future Directions

There are numerous potential future directions for the study of sedentary behavior and obesity. Clearly, more reliable and valid measures of sedentary behavior are needed, both for testing the effects of interventions to reduce sedentary behavior and for exploring the relationship between weight status and sedentary behavior. The refinement in measurement will also allow better examination of the link between sedentary behavior and other health outcomes (e.g., Leitzmann et al. 1999), help elucidate possible mechanisms by which sedentary behavior affects weight gain, determine whether particular sedentary activities are more obesity promoting than others, and help identify the specific correlates of sedentary behavior across the life span. Mechanisms will be further informed by intervention attempts to decrease sedentary behavior and the accurate assessment of other factors (e.g., physical activity) affecting weight gain. Controlled trials that test interventions could pinpoint the specific strategies that maximize the decrease in sedentary behavior time and increase physical activity, as not all strategies to reduce sedentary behavior may be equally efficacious (e.g., Epstein et al. 1997). We must continue to explore ways to intervene on modifiable risk factors for obesity at both the individual and population level, and to reestablish the balance between physical and sedentary behavior that promotes a more healthful lifestyle.

Summary

There is consistent evidence for an association between adults' higher discretionary sedentary behavior time and higher weight status, with some evidence for a similar association in children, particularly during middle childhood, among boys, and in more recently studied cohorts. It could be that more active transport, labor-related occupations, and more frequent and active school physical education in the past allowed for discretionary sedentary behavior time that did not contribute to positive energy balance and gradual weight gain. The shift toward reductions in energy expenditure throughout the daily lives of U.S. adults and children could now be making our current high amounts of time spent in discretionary sedentary behaviors (and a growing number of sedentary behavior options) harmful to our health. Realignment of discretionary sedentary behavior time to more physically active pursuits and infusion of physical activity back into our daily lives could contribute to long-term individual weight status and public health improvement.

References

Ainsworth, B.E., Haskell, W.L., Leon, A.S., Jacobs, D.R., Jr., Montoye, H.J., Sallis, J.F., and Paffenbarger, R.S., Jr. 1993. Compendium of physical activities: Classification of energy costs of human physical activities. *Medicine and Science in Sports and Exercise* 25: 71-80.

American Academy of Pediatrics, Committee on Public Education. 1999. Media education. *Pediatrics* 104: 341-343.

Andersen, R.E., Crespo, C.J., Bartlett, S.J., Cheskin, L.J., and Pratt, M. 1998. Relationship of physical activity and television watching with body weight and level of fatness among children: Results from the Third National Health and Nutrition Examination Study. *Journal of the American Medical Association* 279: 938-942.

Armstrong, C.A., Sallis, J.F., Alcaraz, J.E., Kolody, B., McKenzie, T.L., and Hovell, M.F. 1998. Children's television viewing, body fat, and physical fitness. *American Journal of Health Promotion* 12: 363-368.

Berkey, C.S., Rockett, H.R.H., Field, A.E., Gillman, M.W., Frazier, A.L., Camargo, C.A., and Colditz, G.A. 2000. Activity, dietary intake, and weight changes in a longitudinal study of preadolescent and adolescent boys and girls. *Pediatrics* 105, www.pediatrics.org/cgi/content/full/105/4/e56.

Buchowski, M.S., and Sun, M. 1996. Energy expenditure, television viewing and obesity. *International Journal of Obesity* 20: 236-244.

Ching, P.L.Y.H., Willett, W.C., Rimm, E.B., Colditz, G.,A., Gortmaker, S.L., and Stampfer, M.J. 1996. Activity level and risk of overweight in male health professionals. *American Journal of Public Health* 86: 25-30.

Coakley, E.H., Rimm, E.B., Colditz, G., Kawachi, I., and Willett, W. 1998. Predictors of weight change in men: Results from the Health Professionals Follow-up Study. *International Journal of Obesity* 22: 89-96.

Colditz, G.A. 1999. Economic costs of obesity and inactivity. *Medicine and Science in Sports and Exercise* 31: S663-S667.

Comstock, G.A., and Paik, H. 1991. *Television and the American child*. San Diego: Academic Press.

Condry, J. 1989. *The psychology of television*. Hillsdale, NJ: Erlbaum.

Coon, K.A., Goldberg, J., Rogers, B.L., and Tucker, K.L. 2001. Relationships between use of television during meals and children's food consumption patterns. *Pediatrics* 107, www.pediatrics.org/cgi/content/full/107/1/e7.

Crawford, D.A., Jeffrey, R.W., and French, S.A. 1999. Television viewing, physical inactivity and obesity. *International Journal of Obesity* 23: 437-440.

Crespo, C.J., Smit, E., Troiano, R.P., Bartlett, S.J., Macera, C.A., and Andersen, R.E. 2001. Television watching, energy intake, and obesity in U.S. children: Results from the Third National Health and Nutrition Examination Survey, 1988-1994. *Archives of Pediatrics and Adolescent Medicine* 155: 360-365.

Dennison, B.A., Erb, T.A., and Jenkins, P.L. 2002. Television viewing and television in bedroom associated with overweight risk among low-income preschool children. *Pediatrics* 109: 1028-1035.

Dietz, W.H. 1996. The role of lifestyle in health: The epidemiology and consequences of inactivity. *Proceedings of the Nutrition Society* 55: 829-840.

Dietz, W.H., Bandini, L.G., Morelli, J.A., Peers, K.F., and Ching, P.L. 1994. Effect of sedentary activities on resting metabolic rate. *American Journal of Clinical Nutrition* 59: 556-559.

Dietz, W.H. and Gortmaker, S.L. 1993. TV or not TV: Fat is the question. *Pediatrics* 91: 499-501.

Dietz, W.H., Jr., and Gortmaker, S.L. 1985. Do we fatten our children at the television set? Obesity and television viewing in children and adolescents. *Pediatrics* 75: 807-812.

Dowda, M., Ainsworth, B.E., Addy, C.L., Saunders, R., Reiner, W. 2001. Environmental influences, physical activity, and weight status in 8- to 16-year-olds. *Archives of Pediatric and Adolescent Medicine* 155: 711-717.

DuRant, R.H., Baranowski, T., Johnson, M., and Thompson, W.O. 1994. The relationship among television watching, physical activity, and body composition of young children. *Pediatrics* 94: 449-455.

Epstein, L.H., Paluch, R.A., Gordy, C.C., and Dorn, J. 2000. Decreasing sedentary behaviors in treating pediatric obesity. *Archives of Pediatric Adolescent Medicine* 154: 220-226.

Epstein, L.H., and Saelens, B.E. 2000. Behavioral economics of obesity: Food intake and energy expenditure. In *Reframing health behavior change with behavioral economics*, eds. W.K. Bickel and R.E. Vuchinich. Mahwah, NJ: Erlbaum.

Epstein, L.H., Saelens, B.E., and Giancola O'Brien, J. 1995. Effects of reinforcing increases in active behavior versus decreases in sedentary behavior for obese children. *International Journal of Behavioral Medicine* 2: 41-50.

Epstein, L.H., Saelens, B.E., Myers, M.D., and Vito, D. 1997. Effects of decreasing sedentary behaviors on activity choice in obese children. *Health Psychology* 16: 107-113.

Epstein, L.H., Smith, J.A., Vara, L.S., and Rodefer, J.S. 1991. Behavioral economic analysis of activity choice in obese children. *Health Psychology* 10: 311-316.

Epstein, L.H., Valoski, A.M., Vara, L.S., McCurley, J., Wisniewski, L., Kalarchian, M.A., Klein, K.R., and Shrager, L.R. 1995. Effects of decreasing sedentary behavior and increasing activity on weight change in obese children. *Health Psychology* 14: 109-115.

Faith, M.S., Berman, N., Heo, M., Pietobelli, A., Gallagher, D., Epstein, L.H., Eiden, M, and Allison, D.B. 2001. Effects of contingent television on physical activity and television viewing in obese children. *Pediatrics* 107: 1043-1048.

Filozof, C., Saenz, S., and Gonzalez, C. 1999. Television viewing and obesity in a sample of Argentinian children. *International Journal of Obesity* 23: S45.

Fitzgerald, S.J., Kriska, A.M., Pereira, M.A., and De Courten, M.P. 1997. Associations among physical activity, television watching, and obesity in adult Pima Indians. *Medicine and Science in Sports and Exercise* 29: 910-915.

Gordon-Larsen, P., McMurray, R.G., and Popkin, B.M. 1999. Adolescent physical activity and inactivity vary by ethnicity: The National Longitudinal Study of Adolescent Health. *Journal of Pediatrics* 135: 301-306.

Gortmaker, S.L., Cheung, L.W.Y., Peterson, K.E., Chomitz, G., Hammond Cradle, J., Dart, H., Kay Fox, M., Bullock, R.B., Sobol, A.M., Colditz, G., Field, A.E., and Laird, N. 1999. Impact of a school-based interdisciplinary intervention on diet and physical activity among urban primary school children: Eat well and keep moving. *Archives of Pediatrics and Adolescent Medicine* 153: 975-983.

Gortmaker, S.L., Dietz, W.H., Jr., and Cheung, L.W.Y. 1990. Inactivity, diet, and the fattening of America. *Journal of the American Dietetic Association* 90: 1247-1252, 1255.

Gortmaker, S.L., Must, A., Sobol, A.M., Peterson, K., Colditz, G.A., and Dietz, W.H. 1996. Television viewing as a cause of increasing obesity among children in the United States, 1986-1990. *Archives of Pediatrics and Adolescent Medicine* 150: 356-362.

Gortmaker, S.L., Peterson, K., Wiecha, J., Sobol, A.M., Dixit, S., Fox, M.K., and Laird, N. 1999. Reducing obesity via a school-based interdisciplinary intervention among youth. *Archives of Pediatrics and Adolescent Medicine* 153: 409-418.

Grodstein, F., Levine, R., Troy, L., Spencer, T., Colditz, G.A., and Stampfer, M.J. 1996. Three-year follow-up of participants in a commercial weight loss program: Can you keep it off? *Archives of Internal Medicine* 156: 1302-1306.

Guillaume, M., Lapidus, L., Bjorntorp, P., and Lambert, A. 1997. Physical activity, obesity, and cardiovascular risk factors in children. The Belgian Luxembourg Child Study II. *Obesity Research* 5: 549-556.

Hanley, A.J.G., Harris, S.B., Gittelsohn, J., Wolever, T.M.S., Saksvig, B., and Zinman, B. 2000. Overweight among children and adolescents in a Native Canadian community: Prevalence and associated factors. *American Journal of Clinical Nutrition* 71: 693-700.

Harrell, J.S., Gansky, S.A., Bradley, C.B., and McMurray, R.G. 1997. Leisure time activities of elementary school children. *Nursing Research* 46: 246-253.

Heath, G.W., Pratt, M., Warren, C.W., and Kann, L. 1994. Physical activity patterns in American high school students: Results from the 1990 Youth Risk Behavior Survey. *Archives of Pediatrics and Adolescent Medicine* 148: 1131-1136.

Hernández, B., Gortmaker, S.L., Colditz, G.A., Peterson, K.E., Laird, N.M., and Parra-Cabrera, S. 1999. Association of obesity with physical activity, television programs and other forms of video viewing among children in Mexico City. *International Journal of Obesity* 23: 845-854.

Jason, L.A. 1987. Reducing children's television viewing and assessing secondary changes. *Journal of Clinical Child Psychology* 16: 245-250.

Jason, L.A., and Brackshaw, E. 1999. Access to TV contingent on physical activity: Effects on reducing TV-viewing and body-weight. *Journal of Behavior Therapy and Experimental Psychiatry* 30: 145-151.

Jeffery, R.W., and French, S.A. 1998. Epidemic obesity in the United States: Are fast foods and television viewing contributing? *American Journal of Public Health* 88: 277-280.

Johnson, S.Z., and Jason, L.A. 1996. Evaluation of a device aimed at reducing children's television viewing. *Child and Family Behavior Therapy* 18: 59-61.

Katzmarzyk, P.T., Malina, R.M., Song, T.M.K., and Bouchard, C. 1998. Television viewing, physical activity, and health-related fitness of youth in the Québec Family Study. *Journal of Adolescent Health* 23: 318-325.

Kimm, S.Y.S., Obarzanek, E., Barton, B.A., Aston, C.E., Similo, S., Morrison, J.A., Sabry, Z.I., Schreiber, G.B., and McMahon, R.P. 1996. Race, socioeconomic status, and obesity in 9- to 10-year-old girls: The NHLBI Growth and Health Study. *Annals of Epidemiology* 6: 266-275.

Klesges, R.C., Shelton, M.L., and Klesges, L.M. 1993. Effects of television on metabolic rate: Potential implications for childhood obesity. *Pediatrics* 91: 281-286.

Leitzmann, M.F., Rimm, E.B., Willett, W.C., Spiegelman, D., Grodstein, F., Stampfer, M.J., Colditz, G.A., and Giovannucci, E. 1999. Recreational physical activity and the risk of cholecystectomy in women. *New England Journal of Medicine* 341: 777-784.

Locard, E., Mamelle, N., Billette, A., Miginiac, M., Munoz, F., and Rey, S. 1992. Risk factors of obesity in a five year old population: Parental versus environmental factors. *International Journal of Obesity* 16: 721-729.

Maffeis, C., Talamini, G., and Tatò, L. 1998. Influence of diet, physical activity and parents' obesity on children's adiposity: A four-year longitudinal study. *International Journal of Obesity* 22: 758-764.

Martinez-González, M.Á., Martinez, J.A., Hu, F.B., Gibney, M.J., and Kearney, J. 1999. Physical inactivity, sedentary lifestyle and obesity in the European Union. *International Journal of Obesity* 23: 1192-1201.

McMurray, R.G., Harrell, J.S., Deng, S., Bradley, C.B., Cox, L.M., and Bangdiwala, S.I. 2000. The influence of physical activity, socioeconomic status, and ethnicity on the weight status of adolescents. *Obesity Research* 8: 130-139.

Mokdad, A.H., Serdula, M.K., Dietz, W.H., Bowman, B.A., Marks, J.S., and Koplan, J.P. 1999. The spread of the obesity epidemic in the United States, 1991-1998. *Journal of the American Medical Association* 282: 1519-1522.

Must, A., Gortmaker, S.L., and Dietz, W.H. 1994. Risk factors for obesity in young adults: Hispanics, African Americans and Whites in the transition years, age 16-28 years. *Biomedicine and Pharmacotherapy* 48: 143-156.

Myers, L., Strikmiller, P.K., Webber, L.S., and Berenson, G.S. 1996. Physical and sedentary behavior in school children grades 5-8: The Bogalusa Heart Study. *Medicine and Science in Sports and Exercise* 28: 852-859.

Nielsen Media Research. 2000. *2000 report on television*. New York: Nielsen Media Research.

Obarzanek, E., Schreiber, G.B., Crawford, P.B., Goldman, S.R., Barrier, P.M., Frederick, M.M., and Lakatos, E. 1994. Energy intake and physical activity in relation to indexes of body fat: The National Heart, Lung, and Blood Institute Growth and Health Study. *American Journal of Clinical Nutrition* 60: 15-22.

Pate, R.R., and Ross, J.G. 1987. Factors associated with health-related fitness. *Journal of Physical Education, Recreation, and Dance* 58: 45-48.

Pratt, M., Macera, C.A., and Blanton, C. 1999. Levels of physical activity and inactivity in children and adults in the United States: Current evidence and research issues. *Medicine and Science in Sports and Exercise* 31: S526-S533.

Roberts, D.F., Foehr, U.G., Rideout, V.J., and Brodie, M. 1999. *Kids & media @ the new millennium*. Menlo Park, CA: A Kaiser Family Foundation Report, pp. 1-84.

Robinson, T.N. 1999. Reducing children's television viewing to prevent obesity: A randomized controlled trial. *Journal of the American Medical Association* 282: 1561-1567.

Robinson, T.N., Hammer, L.D., Killen, J.D., Kraemer, H.C., Wilson, D.M., Hayward, C., and Taylor, C.B. 1993. Does television viewing increase obesity and reduce physical activity? Cross-sectional and longitudinal analyses among adolescent girls. *Pediatrics* 91: 273-280.

Robinson, T.N., and Killen, J.D. 1995. Ethnic and gender differences in the relationships between television viewing and obesity, physical activity, and dietary fat intake. *Journal of Health Education* 26: S91-S98.

Saelens, B.E., and Epstein, L.H. 1998. Behavioral engineering of activity choice in obese children. *International Journal of Obesity* 22: 275-277.

Saelens, B.E., and Epstein, L.H. 1999. The rate of sedentary activities determines the reinforcing value of physical activity. *Health Psychology* 18: 655-659.

Saelens, B.E., Sallis, J.F., Nader, P.R., Broyles, S.L., Berry, C.C., and Taras, H.L. 2002. Home environment influences on children's television watching from early to middle childhood. *Developmental and Behavioral Pediatrics* 23: 127-132.

Sallis, J.F., and Saelens, B.E. 2000. Assessment of physical activity by self-report: Status, limitations, and future directions. *Research Quarterly for Exercise and Sport* 71: 1-14.

Salmon, J., Bauman, A., Crawford, D., Timperio, A., and Owen, N. 2000. The association between television viewing and overweight among Australian adults participating in varying levels of leisure-time physical activity. *International Journal of Obesity* 24: 600-606.

Shannon, B., Peacock, J., and Brown, M.J. 1991. Body fatness, television viewing and calorie-intake of a sample of Pennsylvania sixth grade children. *Journal of Nutrition Education* 23: 262-268.

Sidney, S., Sternfeld, B., Haskell, W.L., Jacobs, D.R., Jr., Chesney, M.A., and Hulley, S.B. 1996. Television viewing and cardiovascular risk factors in young adults: The CARDIA study. *Annals of Epidemiology* 6: 154-159.

Strauss, R.S., Loree, R., Burak, G., Rozdilsky, D., and Colin, M. 2000. Social and cognitive determinants of physical activity in children and young adolescents. *Obesity Research* 8 (Suppl.): 18S.

Troiano, R.P., Flegal, K.M., Kuczmarski, R.J., Campbell, S.M., and Johnson, C.L. 1995. Overweight prevalence and trends for children and adolescents. *Archives of Pediatrics and Adolescent Medicine* 149: 1085-1091.

Tucker, L.A. 1986. The relationship of television viewing to physical fitness and obesity. *Adolescence* 84: 797-806.

Tucker, L.A., and Bagwell, M. 1991. Television viewing and obesity in adult females. *American Journal of Public Health* 81: 908-911.

Tucker, L.A., and Friedman, G.M. 1989. Television viewing and obesity in adult males. *American Journal of Public Health* 79: 516-518.

U.S. Department of Health and Human Services. 2000. *Healthy People 2010*. Washington, DC: Author.

Vioque, J., Torres, A., and Quiles, J. 2000. Time spent watching television, sleep duration and obesity in adults living in Valencia, Spain. *International Journal of Obesity* 24: 1683-1688.

Wolf, A.M., Gortmaker, S.L., Cheung, L., Gray, H.M., Herzog, D.B., and Colditz, G.A. 1993. Activity, inactivity, and obesity: Racial, ethnic, and age differences among schoolgirls. *American Journal of Public Health* 83: 1625-1627.

Chapter 16

Physical Activity Promotion As a Public Health Strategy for Obesity Prevention

Adrian Bauman, MD, PhD

Center for Physical Activity and Health, School of
Public Health and Community Medicine, University
of New South Wales, Sydney, Australia

David Crawford, PhD

School of Health Sciences, Deakin University,
Melbourne, Australia

David Crawford is supported by a Nutrition Research Fellowship from the National Heart Foundation of Australia.

Efforts to promote physical activity and efforts to prevent obesity are important public health concerns in developed countries. To date, however, few efforts have combined them and considered how they might complement each other in making improvements in population health.

This chapter reviews the different roles physical activity might have in population approaches to weight loss and weight maintenance. In addition, we will focus on the interdependence of physical activity and obesity, and what is known about their effects on each other. A review of the population trends in activity and obesity will shed light on the possible role of inactivity in the obesity epidemic. We will review the epidemiological evidence for the health benefits attributed to regular moderate physical activity and to being of normal range body weight, as well as the interaction between the two. In addition, we

will discuss the associations between physical activity and overweight status, physical activity interventions, and the role of those interventions in weight control. Finally, we will present a rationale and framework for "environmental" and "policy" physical activity interventions. These innovative approaches may reduce the likelihood that "society is doomed to escalating obesity rates" (James 1995).

Trends in Obesity and Inactivity

Data are limited on national trends in leisure time physical activity levels. Numerous population surveys have been conducted, but changes in questions asked and instruments used have prevented trend comparisons. One such series is the Behavioral Risk Factor Surveillance System telephone surveys conducted in the United States each year. Trend data available from 1986 through 1996 demonstrate almost no change in the proportion of adults who were sedentary—the rate hovers around 30% of all adults across this period, with the rate of those meeting the U.S. Surgeon General's guidelines for physical activity also remaining remarkably constant, at around 27% of all adults (Pratt et al. 1999). The same data deficiencies exist for young Americans, but suggest possible negative trends—youth are less active and spend less time in school-based physical education classes than they did a decade ago (Pratt et al. 1999). Using different definitions of "regularly active," Mokdad and colleagues (1999) identified a similarly flat trend—with 42% being regularly active in 1991, and 43% in 1998.

Most other developed countries show similar trends in leisure time physical activity participation, with little evidence of recent change, which is contrary to the theory many held in the 1970s of a sustained fitness boom (Stephens and Casperson 1994). In Australia the different methodologies employed in surveys have made trend comparisons difficult, but little change has been noted since the mid-1980s, with recent trends suggesting decreasing physical activity (Armstrong et al. 2000; Bauman and Owen 1999).

Only two countries, Canada and Finland, have reported slight but consistent increases in measures of leisure time physical activity (LTPA) using the same questions across time. Canadians demonstrated an increase in the number who were "sufficiently active" from 21% in 1981 to 37% in 1995, approximating a percentage point increase in prevalence each year (Craig et al. 1999). Serial health behavior surveys in Finland have shown an increase among adults reporting at least 30 minutes of exercise twice a week or more, with rates increasing from 40% to over 60% between 1978 and 1999 (Helakorpi et al. 1999; Barengo et al. 2002). As for Canada, this increase was noted for both genders and across age groups. However, Finland experienced a slight decline in transportation-related physical activity (Helakorpi et al. 1999).

A conceptual model in figure 16.1 shows the energy expenditure trend pattern, with no increase in LTPA in recent years. A public health goal, as echoed in the U.S. *Healthy People 2010* objectives, is to increase this LTPA participation rate (the dashed line in figure 16.1).

While this remains an important aim, LTPA is only part of the total daily energy expenditure (Blair and Nichaman 2002). Many people in developed countries are also experiencing a substantial decline in total energy expenditure across the whole day (the dotted line in figure 16.1). This has been estimated to be as much as 800 kcal per day per person in the UK (James 1995). The public health goals to rectify this are to increase both LTPA and other components of daily energy expenditure. These are shown in the figure, as upward, dashed slopes (to the dotted and regular lines), on the right-hand side of the figure. These trends, over time, are shown as a percentage of putative 1970 values because there is no exactly comparable data available.

Total energy expenditure is related to all movement and activity throughout a 24-hour period (Blair and Nichaman 2002). Little is known about trends in aspects of physical activity other than LTPA. These additional dimensions include occupational activity, domestic activity, and other recreational and incidental physical activity as part of everyday life, as well as total time spent in sedentary activities. For many of these domains, measures have yet to be developed for use in population surveillance systems.

Evidence suggests that occupational activity has declined (Fogelholm et al. 1996; Graff-Iverson et al. 2001) and that the exposure to work-related activity was very different in the year 2001 than it was in the 1960s (Paffenbarger et al. 1970). Energy expenditure is also thought to have declined in domestic settings through the introduction of domestic labor-saving devices.

The prevalence of overweight and obesity has increased markedly over the past two de-

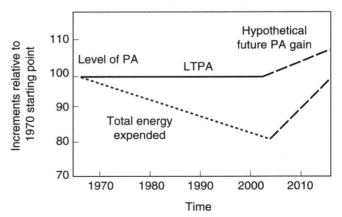

Figure 16.1 Probable trends in physical activity in developing countries across recent decades.

cades, irrespective of measurement method and the cutoff points used to define overweight or obesity. This has been described as an epidemic, occurring almost simultaneously across developed countries (WHO 1997; see chapters 1 through 3 of this volume). Depending on definitions, annual rates of change approach a 1% increase in prevalence per year in several countries. For example, different U.S. studies show similar patterns of increase (Flegal et al. 1998; Mokdad et al. 1999). In countries with already high mean BMI values, such as the United States, the prevalence increases are occurring mostly in the obese category (BMI >30).

Similar rates have occurred in the prevalence of obesity across the globe (Flegal 1999), with marked increases across countries, including Japan, Brazil, Singapore, Mauritius, and Western Samoa. Adult Australians and New Zealanders have also shown substantial increases in the prevalence of overweight (Australian Institute of Health and Welfare 1999; Simmons et al. 1996). The WHO-Monica study described rates of obesity (BMI >30) in Europe that range from around 10% in parts of France and Sweden to more than 20% of all adults in Romania, Lithuania, and Russia (Seidell 1997). An interesting trend is apparent from surveys in the Netherlands that showed the population to have stable and low obesity rates during the 1980s, hovering around 4% of adults (Seidell 1997). Since 1990, rates have gradually started to increase in the Netherlands, reaching 8 to 9% by 1995. This occurred in spite of an apparent decrease by 115 kcal per day of daily energy intake.

Canada and Finland demonstrate the complexities of assessing obesity and physical activity data. Canada has experienced increases in obesity rates (Macdonald et al. 1997) and overweight rates among adults (Craig et al. 1999; Tremblay, Katzmarzyk, and Willms 2002) in spite of monitored increases in LTPA over the decades of the 1980s and 1990s. The other country to report increasing physical activity was Finland, which also recorded increases in BMI (Kastarinen, Nissinen, and Vartiainen 2000). Even Finnish youth are becoming more overweight despite high levels of reported leisure time activity (Kautiainen et al. 2002). A population study of adults in Spain noted the same phenomenon, with slight increases in reported activity concurrent with substantial increases in obesity (Artalejo et al. 2002).

In summary, most countries have reported marked recent increases in obesity and overweight prevalence, but few have reported increases in the prevalence of leisure time physical activity. It seems that these two phenomena are not well correlated, as even where leisure time physical activity levels have increased, overweight and obesity rates have still increased by up to 1% each year.

Public Health Burden of Obesity and Inactivity

The health risks of obesity and inactivity are often considered together; combined, they are the second leading contributor to population ill health after tobacco (McGinnis and Foege 1993). The risks of inactivity and obesity overlap in some areas; for instance, both increase the risk of developing cardiovascular disease or diabetes. On the other hand, inactivity and obesity may affect disease risk in different ways. The protective effects of activity on coronary heart disease or diabetes, for example, are somewhat independent of weight and other nutrition-related factors such as cholesterol levels. For other areas, such as colon or breast cancer, both inactivity and obesity may contribute to risk, albeit through different biological mechanisms. Similarly, inactivity increases risks of falls in the elderly, which is different from the increased risk of degenerative joint disease among the obese. Finally, the mental health benefits or risks are different. Physical activity is associated with positive measures of well-being and has been an effective treatment or therapy for depression and anxiety, whereas obesity may be associated with (as a cause of) depression (Bauman and Owen 1999; U.S. Department of Health and Human Services 1996).

Over the past five years a substantial burden of epidemiological evidence has accrued for the health benefits for overweight and obese adults of being active. Blair and Brodney (1999) reviewed this evidence, mostly comparing those in the mild to moderately overweight range with those of normal weight. A consistent picture appears in these epidemiological data: Active or fit people who are overweight appear to be protected against some of the chronic disease consequences of being overweight. This appeared true for all-cause mortality, incident coronary heart disease (CHD), and diabetes. For example, all-cause mortality rates in the overweight but highest fitness group were lower than all-cause mortality rates in those who were sedentary but lean (Barlow et al. 1995; Paffenbarger et al. 1986). Even for incident diabetes, the causal risks of obesity were attenuated for those who were also active (Helmrich et al. 1991). The public health implications are that even for overweight adults, physical activity has a role in disease prevention across several chronic disease outcomes. This is not related to weight control per se, but does reinforce the need to encourage the sedentary obese to be more active, even if weight loss does not result.

The final public health issue relates to the substantial costs of obesity and inactivity, which include both the direct costs of health care and treatment and the indirect costs of lost productivity and quality of life. In the United States, estimates of the costs of obesity are as high as $70 billion, with physical-activity-related direct health care costs totaling $24 billion; together these summate to around 9% of the total U.S. health expenditure (Colditz 1999). This is greater than other country-specific estimates; the costs of obesity in France and Australia ranged around 2% of the total health expenditure (Levy et al. 1995; Segal, Carter, and Zimmet 1994). Other estimates have been reported, with limited economic modeling details, ranging from around $400 million per year in Germany, and twice this amount if co-morbidities are considered (Kurscheid and Lauterbach 1998). A British report of directs costs around $300 million has been published (James 1995). The large differences in cost estimates are based on different economic assumptions, and most do not estimate the larger indirect and societal costs. Nonetheless, the cost burden of obesity and inactivity represents a meaningful fraction of health and other budgets, which further provides a rationale for obesity prevention.

Association Between Inactivity and Obesity

Cross-sectional population-based studies have demonstrated consistent and repeated associations between inactivity and increased BMI (DiPietro 1999; Rippe and Hess 1998). Prospective studies offer some evidence that decreased physical activity may result in increased weight gain (Haapanen et al. 1997). Some studies have identified associations between sedentariness and obesity, especially for children who watch more television; this association between television watching and increased obesity has also been noted for adults (Jeffery 1998).

One important idea concerns the protective qualities of LTPA on obesity. A study of a Pima Indian community in the southwestern United States established that frequent television watchers had higher levels of obesity, across categories of physical activity (Fitzgerald et al. 1997). An Australian general population survey reached a similar conclusion: The likelihood of obesity increased across categories of television watching, particularly in the most active groups (Salmon et al. 2000). This implies that some people were overweight even though they were very active for half an hour per day. These individuals may demonstrate "compensatory sedentary behaviors" in the remaining 23.5 hours per day, with increased risks of obesity, in spite of meeting recommended "30 minute per day" goals for moderate or even vigorous levels of LTPA.

One side of the human energy balance equation is energy intake (EI), which is affected by individual metabolic differences such as basal metabolic rates and the thermic effects of food (Grilo 1995). These produce inter-individual variation, but at the population level are relatively small-scale influences. On the other side of the energy balance equation is energy expenditure (EE), which is the net amount of energy expended through all physical activities during the day. The EI and EE components are regulated physiologically, with the goal of maintaining energy balance and weight levels (Hill and Peters 1998).

Recent increases in obesity indicate that the adaptive mechanisms that work to keep our energy levels balanced have been overwhelmed. Even very small increases in daily positive energy balance, sustained over years, would lead to population shifts in obesity. The observed increases in obesity since 1980 are unlikely to have been caused by genetic shifts alone, although a small amount of genetic variability does occur in body fatness. The obesity "epidemic" suggests environmental, rather than genetic, shifts. The current culture of developed countries has been described as a "toxic" (Battle and Brownell 1996) or "obesogenic" environment (Swinburn, Egger, and Raza 1999), which has led to an epidemic of obesity.

Many experts argue that people are eating more, with positive balance accruing to the EI side of the equation. Recent analyses using ecological-level data suggest that energy intakes in the United States may have increased slightly over the past several decades (Harnack, Jeffery, and Boutelle 2000; Koplan and Dietz 1999). The paradoxical opposite observation has been made in several countries—namely, that the population is eating the same amount or less, and yet obesity rates have increased dramatically (Heini and Weinsier 1997). Some have estimated recent dietary declines of around 200 kcal per day (Grilo 1995) or 4% of total EI (Heini and Weinsier 1997). A review of food consumption patterns monitored through the USDA Food Consumption Surveys concluded that the average fat intake, as a proportion of total EI, may have also fallen, from around 41 to 37% of total kcal per day (Weinsier et al. 1998). Data from the United Kingdom show similar trends, with stable rates or a possible small decline in total food intake and total fat intake over the past four decades, despite concomitant increases in obesity (Jebb and Moore 1999; Prentice and Jebb 1995). Taken together, these data suggest that EI is not the sole or major contributor to recent obesity shifts in populations.

Given that leisure time physical activity is mostly unchanged, and moreover, that obesity has increased even where LTPA has increased, this dimension of energy expenditure is not the only component of EE responsible for obesity. The net positive energy balance must also result from small and continued decreases in activity through the remainder of the day (non-LTPA).

This decrease in non-LTPA EE has not been monitored, as there are few indicators of these components of EE. James (1995) suggested that quite small net decreases in EE, of the order of 50 kcal per day, could explain these trends. Probable contenders include declines in the energy expended in work, in domestic situations, and even in home-based recreation. Even recreation patterns now include increasing hours of watching television and videos and surfing the Internet, which contribute to a probable net decline in EE, as suggested in figure 16.1.

An analysis of LTPA (including walking) data from a national random sample of Australian adults in November 1999 is illustrative here (Armstrong, Bauman, and Davies 2000). The median time spent in all forms of LTPA was around 160 minutes in the previous week, comprised of vigorous, moderate, and walking-related activities. This represents about 2.2% of the total waking hours, assuming eight hours of sleep per night. The interquartile range for the population was from 0.06 to 4.9% of the total waking time. At most, people are carrying out LTPA or walking to get to and from places for 5% of their available time, which leaves around 105 hours per week for non-LTPA time, during which increasingly sedentary behaviors with low levels of EE occur.

The next section examines the roles of physical activity in the treatment of obesity at the individual level and reviews the effects of broader public health initiatives to increase community levels of physical activity.

Physical Activity As a Treatment for Obesity

Meta-analyses and quantitative syntheses have described the treatment efficacy of physical activity as an adjunct to dietary programs for weight loss (Glenny et al. 1997; Miller, Koceja, and Hamilton 1997). These interventions have typically been small studies using clinic patients or volunteer samples and have reported short-term effects on weight loss. Most have used aerobic, vigorous LTPA programs as the study factor and compared exercise with diet, or a combination of both, against controls. Typically, diet or diet-plus-exercise achieves the greatest weight loss, around 8 to 10 kg (17.6 to 22 lb) initially, compared to around 2 to 3 kg (4.4 to 6.6 lb) lost from exercise alone (Blix and Blix 1995; Miller, Koceja, and Hamilton 1997). One review reported a slight but insignificant benefit of diet-plus-exercise over diet alone (Wing 1999). Thus, in such clinical and selected volunteer settings, it is not appropriate to recommend LTPA programs alone.

A few clinical studies of those who have already lost weight suggest that those who remain physically active, even using LTPA measures, show reduced weight regain compared to those who are sedentary (Blair 1993; Pavlou, Krey, and Steffi 1989). This does suggest a clinical role for PA in weight maintenance.

Of even more importance is the quantity of activity required for weight loss. Most reviews suggest that at least 2,000 kcal of EE per week is required (Rippe and Hess 1998), which equates to at least one hour of moderate or half an hour of vigorous LTPA every day. Referring back to the Australian national data, only one in seven overweight people, and one in six in the normal weight range, achieve this level of more frequent LTPA (Armstrong, Bauman, and Davies 2000), and rates from other national surveys are very similar. This indicates that people have difficulty increasing the quantity of LTPA to lose weight and, as the systematic reviews suggest, also have difficulty maintaining increased levels of LTPA over the long term.

Clinical interventions often promote vigorous activity for short-term outcomes, but obese individuals are more likely to maintain moderate levels of activity (Weyer et al. 1998). In this light, we can encourage either more vigorous activity, which produces initial weight loss but is associated with low adoption and adherence rates, or more moderate home-based activity, which will have better population-level compliance but produce limited weight loss.

Community-Wide Strategies for Preventing Obesity

Public health trials have addressed the problem of obesity in community-wide studies. Nonetheless, even these programs may target volunteer samples, such as participants in worksite trials or patients who are counseled by the subsets of physicians who are enthusiastic about providing such advice. Effects are often statistically significant but usually small, and are seldom generalized or disseminated to whole populations. These include worksite interventions to promote physical activity, as well as primary care interventions (Dishman et al. 1998; Hennrikus and Jeffery 1996; Simons-Morton et al. 1998).

Great promise was suggested by whole population interventions, often focusing on multiple cardiovascular risk factors. These were implemented between the 1970s and the 1990s in the United States and elsewhere, and often had components dedicated to improving nutrition, preventing obesity, and promoting PA for the whole population (Lasater et al. 1991). The first such project was the 1970s North Karelia intervention in Finland. Although the program clearly emphasized healthy nutrition, no differences in BMI were noted at a 15-year follow-up between intervention and control provinces (Pietinen, Vartiainen, and Mannisto 1996). This was in spite of clear program effects showing a benefit for tobacco use, cholesterol levels, and the control of hypertension (Vartiainen et al. 2000).

Several of the North American projects were well designed and carefully evaluated using serial independent and cohort surveys. The first was the Stanford Three Community Study in the 1970s, which reported no increase in obesity in the intervention community, compared to increases in both comparison towns. Next was the Stanford Five City Project during the 1980s. After five years, both intervention and control communities showed increases in BMI when monitored through independent population surveys, although slightly smaller increases occurred in intervention towns (Taylor et al. 1991). There was no difference for the cohort samples (Young et al. 1993).

The Pawtucket Heart Health project in Rhode Island had some programmatic emphasis on weight control for its blue-collar target communities. Process evaluation suggested that many community members attended community "weigh-ins" and other events (Carleton et al. 1995), but there was little difference at the end of the study. Slightly more weight was gained in cross sectional comparisons of control communities compared to intervention communities, but in the panel design (cohorts of the same people followed) these differences were not significant.

The Minnesota Heart Health Program, comprising three intervention and three control communities, had the strongest emphasis on obesity prevention and management. This program used strategies such as public education, physician training, high-risk screening and patient counseling, and restaurant labeling to address obesity in a comprehensive manner (Jeffery 1993, 1995, 1998). In spite of these coordinated "best practice" efforts, there were strong upward trends in BMI for all communities, and no intervention effect. This occurred across all socioeconomic groups (Iribarren et al. 1997), with no differential change in high or moderate LTPA by intervention region. Jeffery elegantly described this lack of effect as probably the result of "the overwhelming influence (. . . and strength of the intrinsic allure) . . . of environmental pressures towards a high fat diet and a sedentary lifestyle" (Jeffery 1995).

National trends in increasing obesity were apparently greater than any intervention effects in most sites, even where nutrition or obesity control were specific community-wide initiatives, as was the case in Finland and in Minnesota (Jeffrey 1995; Kastarinen 2000). Limited effects were noted, even for maintaining population weight levels, irrespective of nutritional changes (assessed through improved cholesterol profiles) or changes to LTPA. The lack of impact of these community-wide efforts underscores the complexity of the secular increases in population obesity.

Environmental and Policy Approaches to Increasing Physical Activity

Earlier sections of this chapter provided a rationale based on energy expenditure for promoting incidental physical activity throughout the day as a necessary component of obesity prevention or weight maintenance. To understand this further, we should review dimensions of physical activity and inactivity. Leisure time physical activity is generally well understood as being comprised of organized and nonorganized activities (Sallis, Bauman, and Pratt 1998). Organized activity includes sport, regular gym classes, or other structured programs. Nonorganized LTPA may include purposive jogging, walking, cycling, or other activities. The remainder of the day is composed of non-LTPA, which is loosely described as "incidental PA." This occurs in settings specific to the individual, such as the workplace or home and domestic environments, and in traveling between these environments. Opportunities for incidental activity in work settings include activity breaks at work and restructuring work tasks

to be more active. Domestic settings include chores, gardening, yard work, and ancillary activities such as dog walking.

Beyond individual settings are broader social and physical environments. These offer opportunities for activity: using the stairs, transport-related physical activity, and supportive local environments. The converse of environments that promote physical activity are those that encourage sedentariness. These include cultural values that promote television watching or Internet use and discourage PA in the community on the grounds of lack of safety or lack of facilities or infrastructure. Koplan and Dietz (1999) argued that solutions to sedentary environments require societal reengineering to make physical activity more feasible and accessible for the whole community.

The difficult challenge is to move conceptually beyond the LTPA approach for obesity prevention solutions. For many health benefits, including cardiovascular disease and diabetes prevention, meeting the U.S. Surgeon General's recommendations for LTPA is sufficient (U.S. Department of Health and Human Services 1996). For obesity prevention, additional and incidental activity increments are necessary. Table 16.1 illustrates this, showing the potential for weight loss given different kinds and amounts of activity. It is assumed that around 7,700 kcal of EE may hypothetically result in a mean loss of 1 kg (2.2 lb) of body weight (Blix and Blix 1995). (However, this EE estimate should be reduced by around a third, as it ignores basal metabolism, the compensatory and regulatory processes when weight is lost, and overreporting of PA. This provides a conservative, and perhaps more realistic, estimate of hypothetical weight loss.)

Table 16.1 shows three hypothetical scenarios, with the first two being for recommended levels of LTPA for a normal weight individual (arbitrarily designated as 60 kg or 132 lb, scenario A) and an overweight individual (90 kg or 198 lb, scenario B). The table shows the METs (energy expenditure assigned to the activity, in multiples of the resting metabolic rate), the number of sessions, time spent per session, and energy expenditure that might result. The right-hand column shows the weight loss that might possibly accrue from these levels of activity, given other factors (energy intake and other EE) remaining unchanged.

Table 16.1   *Energy Expenditure From LTPA and Incidental PA[a]*

Physical activity	METs	Times per week	Average duration (hr) per session	Weekly estimated energy expenditure (EE) from physical activity (kcal)	Weekly EE revised [b]	Number of weeks to lose 5 kg [c]
60-kg person [c]—LTPA						
5 × 30 min U.S. Surgeon General minimum	3.5	5	0.5	525	347	111
Walk 1 hr daily	3.5	7	1	1,470	970	40
Vigorous PA 3x, 20 min each session	7.5	3	0.33	446	294	131
Vigorous PA 1 hr daily	7.5	7	1	3,150	2,079	19
90-kg person [c]—LTPA						
5 × 30 min USSG minimum	3.5	5	0.5	788	520	74
Walk 1 hr daily	3.5	7	1	2,205	1,455	26
Vigorous PA 3x, 20 min	7.5	3	0.33	668	441	87
Vigorous PA 1 hr daily	7.5	7	1	4,725	3,119	12
90-kg person—incidental PA						
Use stairs 2 flights at work	5	10	0.04	180	119	324
Walk to bus stop twice daily	3.5	10	0.25	788	520	74
Play with children	3.5	5	0.33	520	343	112
Walk to shop, walk dog	3.5	5	0.5	788	520	74
Not using the TV remote [d]	1.5	5	0.08	54	36	1,069
Walk down hall at work	2	5	0.25	225	149	258
Light gardening, yard work	3	2	0.5	270	178	217
TOTAL INCIDENTAL				2,824	1,864	21

[a] These data do not consider intraindividual variation; they are shown as hypothetical approximations of population average EE values.
[b] EE revised estimate = 0.66 EE (conservative estimate, Blix and Blix 1995)
[c] 5-kg weight loss is about 11-lb, 60-kg is about 132-lb, and 90-kg is about 198-lb.
[d] Walk 4-8 m (13-26 ft) × 15 times/night × 5 nights, active time = 5 min/night

For example, the 60 kg (132-lb) person, meeting the recommended dose of five days of 30 minutes of moderate LTPA, might expend 347 kcal per week and take 111 weeks (two years of regular activity) to lose 5 kg (11 lb). Walking for an hour per day will reduce this to 40 weeks, and vigorous activity daily will reduce this time even further. A 90-kg (198-lb) person meeting recommended PA levels for health would expend 520 kcal per week, and lose 5 kg (11 lb) in 74 weeks.

Adding all incidental physical activities can also achieve substantial EE. The example in the lower half of the table is somewhat far-fetched, but is shown for illustrative purposes (panel C). It is certainly possible to expend energy through redirecting daily activities, such as stair climbing, active transportation, or even walking down the hall at work. The TV remote is not meant to be definitive EE, but rather is symbolic of the kinds of activity changes that are possible. Overall, the incidental PA adds up to 1,864 kcal per week expended, which is more than three times the EE attributed to achieving the moderate PA recommended level. The table also shows how even slight sedentary behaviors over many years can lead to accumulating weight—using the TV channel changer only prevents 5 to 6 kcal of EE per day, but this alone could theoretically lead to a kilogram of weight increase every four years.

Incidental physical activity is an important component of total daily energy expenditure, but it is difficult to measure. Ecological associations between physical activity patterns and obesity may provide some "natural experiment" information. Some of the delay in the increase in Dutch obesity rates discussed earlier (Seidell 1997) may reflect regular naturally high population levels of transport-related activity, especially cycling, which has both good participation rates and good environmental infrastructure supports.

More structured interventions that target incidental physical activity have already begun. Projects that encourage stair climbing through "point of choice" decision prompts, such as signs, have been trialed since 1980 and are now showing consistent, albeit small, effects (Andersen et al. 1998; Blamey, Mutrie, and Aitchison 1995; Brownell, Stunkard, and Albaum 1980). Typically, signage in underground railway stations or in shopping malls result in a 3 to 10% increase in the number of people using the stairs over moving footways. Translating these modest effects across whole populations is an important strategy for increasing community EE, and is the kind of intervention likely to have a role in weight maintenance. Despite these effective trials, there have been few efforts at disseminating this kind of program throughout the community.

Other kinds of interventions are less well researched, but include "walk to school" programs, interventions promoting public transportation usage, and programs to increase access to local facilities (Humpel, Owen, and Leslie 2002). In this latter category, research in Missouri has shown that promoting local walking trails has an impact on their usage, especially by women and those from disadvantaged backgrounds (Brownson et al. 2000). Interventions in Finland have emphasized "active commuting," providing encouragement for employees to commute to their workplace by bicycle or on foot, in conjunction with public transport services (Oja, Vuori, and Paronen 1998). Underpinning this incidental physical activity is the accepted notion that short bouts of activity accumulated over time can result in weight loss (Jakicic et al. 1999).

Few interventions exist to reduce sedentarism, but one recent example is notable. A researcher in California conducted a controlled study of reduced TV watching among primary school students (Robinson 1999). He noted that children could be trained to regulate television watching, and that these children had lower increases in BMI or waist-to-hip ratio than control children over a six-month follow-up period, despite no measured vigorous physical activity differences between the groups.

The aforementioned are all examples of microenvironmental change, which are controllable and testable in interventions (Swinburn, Egger, and Raza 1999). At the macro level, it may be more difficult to conduct experiments since it would require redeveloping urban environments, changing school PE policies, organizing bike parking, or providing financial reinforcers for active transportation. These kinds of large-scale projects may be necessary to increase EE across the population and to develop regulatory and policy frameworks for making these changes possible.

In many countries, this concept of incidental PA is subsumed in the notion of "health-enhancing physical activity" or HEPA. This is clearly described in the way many Finnish national and local physical activity initiatives were developed (Vuori, Paronen, and Oja 1998). HEPA is "any form of physical activity that benefits health and functional status, without undue harm or risk." This includes sport, nonorganized LTPA, and the accumulation of incidental PA throughout the day. The HEPA initiative has been promulgated in European countries, where efforts are focused on LTPA and all other incidental forms of PA. National programs exist in Finland, England, Switzerland, and elsewhere, and include environmental change initiatives, media campaigns, and policy developments.

The concept of HEPA is analogous to an ecological approach to disease prevention (Sallis, Bauman, and Pratt 1998). This can be encapsulated in the World Health Organization principles for health promotion. Table 16.2 shows a conceptual model in which the elements of the 1986 WHO Ottawa Charter (WHO 1992) are reviewed from a HEPA perspective. Important steps include the development of coalitions and partnerships to work around the physical activity issue. Potential partners extend beyond the health sector and include government departments of transport, local government, urban planning groups, schools, sport and recreation organizations, as well as nongovernmental organizations and the private sector. These agencies can collaborate around interventions

Table 16.2   *Healthy Public Policy Framework for Promoting Incidental Physical Activity*

Health promotion concepts	Operationalized for weight loss and maintenance through environmental and policy initiatives to increase incidental physical activity
1. Develop health-related public policy	National- or state-level policies; local-level policies and ordinances; these require coalitions or partnerships from relevant sectors interested in physical activity.
2. Develop physical activity advocacy [activism] as a public health strategy	Use epidemiological evidence to influence the community, professional groups, key stakeholders, and decision makers.
3. Create supportive environments for physical activity participation in diverse urban and community settings	Environment-enhancing changes to facilitate PA; this involves government agencies and NGOs at the state or local level including health, sport, town planning, transport, schools; purpose is to build alliances for shared initiatives around improved PA environments.
4. Strengthen community action	Increase local focus on physical activity; enhance local community capacity for change; outcome is local programs or local environmental change to parks, roads, trails, or local school boards for physical education policy.
5. Educate and assist in the development of personal skills	Individual education (teaching the moderate physical activity message, encouraging physical activity behavior through skills development); professional education of health and nonhealth staff about importance of promoting LTPA and incidental physical activity for all.

Adapted for physical activity from the Ottawa Charter framework.

to enhance incidental physical activity and to make policy and regulatory directives in specific sectors to promote PA. This process extends what is usually reported in the literature, using studies which utilize PA promotion based on individual-change approaches component 5); these should be extended into interventions in the environment and policy arenas (components 1 through 4) in order to develop more effective and sustainable population change.

This process of utilizing all five components of the figure was adopted in the Australian state of New South Wales in 1996, and a five-year strategic plan was implemented (NSW State Health Department 1998). Shared approaches to cross-sectoral planning was the first step, pooling the resources and expertise of the identified stakeholders and partners (Sallis, Bauman, and Pratt 1998). The resultant task force carried out planned environmental and policy initiatives, as well as media campaigns promoting moderate activity, professional development, and school programs (Bauman et al. 2001). Similar programs have been conducted in Europe through national programs within the HEPA initiative. This approach is similar to the integrated "active living" initiatives developed in Canada (Frankish, Milligan, and Reid 1998), and through the World Health Organization between 1997 to 1998.

These intersectoral and collaborative mechanisms are probably essential for the effective population-wide dissemination of environmental changes. These often require legislation or ordinances to be developed around issues such as sidewalk width, walking trails, street lighting, traffic restriction, or the equitable provision of public transport and recreation facilities (James 1995). Policy initiatives around physical education need to be disseminated across school systems. These could all contribute to great increases in community EE, which is essential for obesity prevention.

A HEPA framework may address issues such as short trips given that almost a fifth of all trips in the United States are car journeys of less than a mile (Koplan and Dietz 1999). Many of these trips could be replaced by walking or cycling. Local interventions are needed to make the environment safe and to construct bike trails or sidewalks to facilitate short trips. Only macrolevel statewide or national dissemination of local initiatives could eventually hope to have an impact on whole population energy expenditure.

Summary

Reducing the prevalence of obesity could substantially improve population health. This would involve a reduction in population mean BMI toward the optimal 23, which has been suggested by the World Health Organization (1997). To date, most approaches to treat or prevent obesity have not been effective, and a worsening of the toxic environment for nutrition and physical activity has occurred (Battle and Brownell 1996). Efforts to address the nutritional arm of this equation are discussed elsewhere in this volume, while this chapter has concentrated on the role of physical activity. Clearly, leisure time physical activity is important for a diverse range of health outcomes (U.S. Department of Health and Human Services 1996), but the solution to the problem of obesity and overweight requires more energy expenditure than is typically provided by LTPA alone (Hill and Peters 1998). Small but consistent increases in EE are needed across domestic, occupational, and everyday environments, and at the expense of some of the current glut of sedentary time. This may produce enough population-level EE to prevent further escalation in obesity rates by shifting the whole population distribution of EE to the left.

Strategies to increase community awareness of physical activity, and to reframe the usefulness of moderate physical activity, are indispensable and an urgent first step (U.S. Department of Health and Human Services 1996). Additional community-wide education needs to target sedentary time, promote increases in incidental activity, encourage the accumulation of short bouts of walking, and facilitate alternative choices, developing more physically active modes of everyday life. These processes should involve families and children, to institutionalize nonsedentary lifestyles in the population. The physical and social environments in which people live need to be reengineered to make these changes possible and to encourage and reinforce them. Dissemination of these approaches across society is a daunting task, but intersectoral models and PA coalitions may assist with this task.

This type of work poses substantial challenges, as it defines new conceptual areas for weight control intervention, focuses primarily on physical activity, and also requires broad environmental and policy changes. Further, it extends the traditional programs targeting increases in LTPA to new strategies to address other dimensions of PA and sedentarism in everyday life. Working across all of these levels of physical activity promotion is required to increase population EE, which remains a major component of obesity prevention and control.

References

Andersen, R.E., Franckowiak, S.C., Snyder, J., Bartlett, S.J., and Fontaine, K.R. 1998. Can inexpensive signs encourage the use of stairs—Results from a community intervention. *Annals of Internal Medicine* 129 (5): 363-369.

Armstrong, T., Bauman, A., and Davies, J. 2000. Physical activity patterns of Australian adults. AIHW Catalogue CVD 10. Canberra: Australian Institute of Health and Welfare.

Artalejo, F.R., Garcia, E.L., Gutierrez-Fisac, J.L., Banegas, J.R.B., and Urdinguio, P.J.L. 2002. Changes in the prevalence of overweight and obesity and their risk factors in Spain, 1987-1997. *Preventive Medicine* 34: 72-81.

Australian Institute of Health and Welfare. 1999. Heart stroke and vascular diseases in Australia Canberra: Author.

Barengo, N.C., Nissinen, A., Tuomilehto, J., and Pekkarinen, H. 2002. Twenty-five-year trends in physical activity of 30- to 59-year-old populations in eastern Finland. *Medicine and Science in Sports and Exercise* 34: 1302-1307.

Barlow, C.E., Kohl, H.W., Gibbons, L.W., and Blair, S.N. 1995. Physical fitness, mortality and obesity. *International Journal of Obesity and Related Metabolic Disorders* 19: S41-44.

Battle, E.K., and Brownell, K.D. 1996. Confronting a rising tide of eating disorders and obesity: Treatment vs. prevention and policy. *Addictive Behaviors* 21 (6): 755-765.

Bauman, A.E., Bellew, B., Owen, N., and Vita, P. 2001. Impact of an Australian mass media campaign targeting physical activity in 1998. *American Journal of Preventive Medicine* 21: 41-47.

Bauman, A., and Owen, N. 1999. Physical activity of adult Australians: Epidemiological evidence and potential strategies for health gain. *Journal of Science in Medicine and Sport* 2: 30-41.

Blair, S.N. 1993. Evidence for success of exercise in weight loss and control. *Annals of Internal Medicine* 119: 702-706.

Blair, S.N., and Brodney, S. 1999. Effects of physical inactivity and obesity on morbidity and mortality: Current evidence and research issues. *Medicine and Science in Sports and Exercise* 31(11): S646-S662.

Blair, S.N., and Nichaman, M.Z. 2002. The public health problem of increasing prevalence rates of obesity and what should be done about it. *Mayo Clinic Proceedings* 77: 109-113.

Blamey, A., Mutrie, N., and Aitchison, T. 1995. Health promotion by encouraged use of stairs. *British Medical Journal* 311: 289-290.

Blix, G.G., and Blix, A.G. 1995. The role of exercise in weight loss. *Behavioral Medicine* 21: 31-39.

Brownell, K.D., Stunkard, A.J., and Albaum, J.M. 1980. Evaluation and modification of exercise patterns in the natural environment. *American Journal of Psychiatry* 137: 1540-1545.

Brownson, R.C., Housmann, R.A., Brown, D.R., Jackson-Thompson, J., King, A.C., Malone, B.R., and Sallis, J.F. 2000. Promoting physical activity in rural counties—Walking trails access, use and effects. *American Journal of Preventive Medicine* 18: 235-241.

Carleton, R.A., Lasater, T.M., Assaf, A.R., Feldman, H.A., and McKinlay, S. 1995. The Pawtucket Heart Health Program: Community changes in cardiovascular risk factors and projected disease risk. *American Journal of Public Health* 85 (6): 777-785.

Craig, C.L., Russell, S.J., Cameron, C., and Beaulieu, A. 1999. Foundation for joint action—Reducing physical inactivity. Ottawa: Canadian Fitness and Lifestyle Research Institute.

Colditz, G.A. 1999. Economic costs of obesity and inactivity. *Medicine and Science in Sports and Exercise:* S663-S667.

DiPietro, L. 1999. Physical activity in the prevention of obesity: Current evidence and research issues. *Medicine and Science in Sports and Exercise:* 31(11): S542-S546.

Dishman, R.K., Oldenburg, B., O'Neal, H., and Shephard, R.J. 1998. Worksite physical activity interventions. *American Journal of Preventive Medicine* 15 (4): 344-361.

Fitzgerald, S.J., Kriska, A.M., Pereira, M.A., and de Courten, M.P. 1997. Associations among physical activity, television watching, and obesity in adult Pima

Indians. *Medicine and Science in Sports and Exercise* 29 (7): 910-915.

Flegal, K.M. 1999. The obesity epidemic in children and adults: Current evidence and research issues. *Medicine and Science in Sports and Exercise:* 31(11): S509-S513.

Flegal, K.M., Carroll, M.D., Kuczmarski, R.J., and Johnson, C.L. 1998. Overweight and obesity in the United States: Prevalence and trends, 1960-1994. *International Journal of Obesity and Related Metabolic Disorders* 22 (1): 39-47

Fogelholm, M., Mannisto, S., Vartiainen, E., and Pietnen, P. 1996. Determinants of energy balance and overweight in Finland 1982 and 1992. *International Journal of Obesity and Related Metabolic Disorders* 20: 1097-1104.

Frankish, C.J., Milligan, C.D., and Reid, C. 1998. A review of relationships between active living and determinants of health. *Social Science in Medicine* 47: 287-301.

Glenny, A.M., O'Meara, S., Melville, A., Sheldon, T.A., and Wilson, C. 1997. The treatment and prevention of obesity: A systematic review of the literature. *International Journal of Obesity and Related Metabolic Disorders* 21 (9): 715-737.

Graff-Iversen, S., Skurtveit, S., Nybo, A., and Ross, G.B. 2001. Trends when it comes to occupational physical activity among Norwegians aged 40-42 years during the period 1974-94. (Abstract in English). *Tidsskr Nor Laegeforen* 121 (22): 2584-2588.

Grilo, C.M. 1995. The role of physical activity in weight loss and weight loss management. *Medicine, Exercise, Nutrition and Health* 4: 60-76.

Haapanen, N., Miiluunpalo, S., Pasanen, M., Oja, P., and Vuori, I. 1997. Association between LTPA and 10 year body mass index changes among working aged men and women. *International Journal of Obesity* 21: 288-296.

Harnack, L.J., Jeffery, R.W., and Boutelle, K.N. 2000. Temporal trends in energy intake in the United States: An ecological perspective. *American Journal of Clinical Nutrition* 71: 1478-1484.

Heini, A.F., and Weinsier, R.L. 1997. Divergent trends in obesity and fat intake patterns: The American paradox. *American Journal of Medicine* 102 (3): 259-264.

Helakorpi, S., Uutela, A., Prattala, R., and Puska, P. 1999. Suomalaisen Aikuisväestön Terveyskäyttäytyminen Ja Terveys [Health behavior survey among Finnish adults]. KTL-National Public Health Institute, Helsinki.

Helmrich, S., Ragland, D.R., Leung, R.W., and Paffenbarger, R.S. 1991. Physical activity and reduced occurrence of non insulin dependent diabetes mellitus. *New England Journal of Medicine* 325: 147-152.

Hennrikus, D.J., and Jeffery, R.W. 1996. Worksite intervention for weight control: A review of the literature. *American Journal of Health Promotion* 10: 471-498.

Hill, J.O., and Peters, J.C. 1998. Environmental contributions to the obesity epidemic. *Science* 280: 1371-1374.

Humpel, N., Owen, N., and Leslie, E. 2002. Environmental factors associated with adults' participation in physical activity. A review. *American Journal of Preventive Medicine* 22: 188-199.

Iribarren, C., Luepker, R.V., McGovern, P.G., Arnett, D.K., and Blackburn, H. 1997. Twelve-year trends in cardiovascular disease risk factors in the Minnesota Heart Survey. Are socioeconomic differences widening? *Archives of Internal Medicine* 157 (8): 873-881.

Jakicic, J.M., Winters, C., Lang, W., and Wing, R.R. 1999. Effects of intermittent exercise and use of home based exercise equipment on adherence, weight loss and fitness in overweight women—A randomized trial. *Journal of the American Medical Association* 282: 1554-1560.

James, W.P.T. 1995. A public health approach to the treatment of obesity. *International Journal of Obesity* 19: S37-S43.

Jebb, S., and Moore, M. 1999. Contribution of a sedentary lifestyle and inactivity to the ecology of overweight and obesity: Current evidence and research issues. *Medicine and Science in Sports and Exercise* 31: S534-S541.

Jeffery, R.W. 1993. Minnesota studies on community-based approaches to weight loss and control. *Annals of Internal Medicine* 119 (7): 19-21.

Jeffery, R.W. 1995. Community programs for obesity prevention: The Minnesota Heart Health Program. *Obesity Research* 3(S2): S283-288.

Jeffery, R.W. 1998. Prevention of obesity: The Minnesota experience of community-based intervention. *Appetite* 31 (3): 411-412.

Kastarinen, M.J., Nissinen, A.M., and Vartiainen, E.A. 2000. Blood pressure levels and obesity trends in hypertensive and normotensive Finnish population from 1982 to 1997. *Journal of Hypertension* 18: 255-262.

Kautiainen, S., Rimpela, A., Vikat, A., and Virtanen, S.M. 2002. Secular trends in overweight and obesity among Finnish adolescents in 1977-1999. *International Journal of Obesity and Related Metabolic Disorders* 26 (4): 544-552.

Koplan, J.P., and Dietz, W.H. 1999. Caloric imbalance and public health policy. *Journal of the American Medical Association* 282: 1579-1580.

Kurscheid, T., and Lauterbach, K. 1998. The cost implications of obesity for health care and society. *International Journal of Obesity and Related Metabolic Disorders:* 22: S3-S5.

Lasater, T.M., Sennett, L.L., Lefebvre, C.R., DeHart, K.L. et al. 1991. Community-based approach to weight loss: The Pawtucket "weigh-in." *Addictive Behaviors* 16: 175-181.

Levy, E., Levy, P., LePen, C., and Basdevant, A. 1995. Economic costs of obesity: The French situation. *International Journal of Obesity* 19: 788-792.

Macdonald, S.M., Reeder, B.A., Chen, Y., and Despres, J.P. 1997. Obesity in Canada: A descriptive analysis. Canadian Heart Health Surveys Research Group. *Canadian Medical Association Journal* 157 (Suppl. 1): S3-S9.

McGinnis, J.M., and Foege, W.H. 1993. Actual causes of death in the United States. *Journal of the American Medical Association* 270: 2207-2212.

Miller, W.C., Koceja, D.M., and Hamilton, E.J. 1997. A meta-analysis of the past 25 years of weight loss research using diet, exercise or diet plus exercise intervention. *International Journal of Obesity and Related Metabolic Disorders* 21 (10): 941-947.

Mokdad, A., Serdula, M.K., Dietz, W.H. et al. 1999. The spread of obesity in the United States 1991-1998. *Journal of the American Medical Association* 282: 1519-1522.

NSW State Health Department: Physical Activity Task Force. 1998. Simply Active Every Day: A plan to promote physical activity in NSW.

Oja, P., Vuori, I., and Paronen, O. 1998. Daily walking and cycling to work—Their utility as health enhancing physical activity (HEPA). *Patient Education and Counseling* 33: S87-S94.

Paffenbarger, R.S., Hyde, R.T., Wing, A.L., and Hsieh, C.C. 1986. Physical activity, all cause mortality and longevity of college Alumni. *New England Journal of Medicine* 314: 605-613.

Paffenbarger, R.S., Lauglin, M.E., Gima, A.S., and Black, R.A. 1970. Work activity of longshoremen and death from coronary heart disease and stroke. *New England Journal of Medicine* 282: 1109-1114.

Pavlou, K.N., Krey, S., and Steffe, W.P. 1989. Exercise as an adjunct to weight loss and maintenance in moderately obese subjects. *American Journal of Clinical Nutrition* 49: 1115-1123.

Pietinen, P., Vartiainen, E., and Mannisto, S. 1996. Trends in body mass index and obesity among adults in Finland from 1972 to 1992. *International Journal of Obesity and Related Metabolic Disorders* 20: 114-120.

Pratt, M., Macera, C.A., and Blanton, C. 1999. Level of physical activity and inactivity in children and adults in the United States: Current evidence and research issues. *Medicine and Science in Sports and Exercise* 31(11): S526-S533.

Prentice, A.M., and Jebb, S. 1995. Obesity in Britain—Gluttony or sloth? *British Medical Journal* 311: 437-439.

Rippe, J.M., and Hess, S. 1998. The role of physical activity in the prevention and management of obesity. *Journal of the American Dietetic Association* 98 (Suppl. 2): S31-S38.

Robinson, T.N. 1999. Reducing children's television viewing to prevent obesity: A randomized controlled trial. *Journal of the American Medical Association* 282: 1561-1567.

Sallis, J.F., Bauman, A., and Pratt, M. 1998. Environmental and policy interventions to promote physical activity. *American Journal of Preventive Medicine* 15 (4): 379-397.

Salmon, J., Bauman, A., Crawford, D., Timperio, A., and Owen, N. 2000.The association between television viewing and overweight among Australian adults participating in varying levels of physical activity. *International Journal of Obesity* 24: 600-606.

Segal, L., Carter, R., and Zimmet, P. 1994. The cost of obesity—The Australian perspective. *Pharmacoeconomics* 5: S45-S52.

Seidell, J.C. 1997. Time trends in obesity: An epidemiological perspective. *Hormone and Metabolic Research* 29 (4): 155-158.

Simmons, G., Jackson, R., Swinburn, B., and Yee, R.L. 1996. The increasing prevalence of obesity in New Zealand: Is it related to recent trends in smoking and physical activity? *New Zealand Medical Journal* 109 (1018): 90-92.

Simons-Morton, D., Calfas, K.J., Oldenburg, B., and Burton, N. 1998. Evaluations of interventions in health care settings on physical activity or cardiorespiratory fitness. *American Journal of Preventive Medicine* 15: 413-430.

Stephens, T., and Casperson, C. 1994. The demography of physical activity. In *Physical activity, fitness and health*, eds. C. Bouchard, R.J. Shepherd, and T. Stephens, 204-213. Champaign, IL: Human Kinetics.

Swinburn, B., Egger, G., and Raza, F. 1999. Dissecting obesogenic environments: The development and application of a framework for identifying and prioritizing environmental interventions for obesity. *Preventive Medicine* 29: 563-570.

Taylor, C.B., Fortmann, S.P., Flora, J., Kayman, S., Barrett, D.C., Jatulis, D., and Farquhar, J.W. 1991. Effect of long-term community health education on body mass index. The Stanford Five-City Project. *American Journal of Epidemiology* 134 (3): 235-249.

Tremblay, M.S., Katzmarzyk, P.T., and Willms, J.D. 2002. Temporal trends in overweight and obesity in

Canada, 1981-1996. *International Journal of Obesity and Related Metabolic Disorders* 26: 538-543.

U.S. Department of Health and Human Services. 1996. The surgeon general's report on physical activity and health. Washington, DC: U.S. Government Printing Office.

U.S. Department of Health and Human Services. 2000. *Healthy People 2010.* 2nd ed. With Understanding and Improving Health and Objectives for Improving Health. 2 vols. 11-1-2000. Washington, DC: U.S. Government Printing Office.

Vartiainen, E., Jousilahti, P., Alfthan, G., Sundvall, J., Pietnen, P., and Puska, P. 2000. Cardiovascular risk factor changes in Finland 1972-1997. *International Journal of Epidemiology* 29: 49-56.

Vuori, I., Paronen, O., and Oja, P. 1998. How to develop local physical activity programs with national support—The Finnish experience. *Patient Education and Counseling* 33: S111-S120.

Weinsier, R.L., Hunter, G.R., Heini, A.F., Goran, M.I., and Sell, S.M. 1998. The etiology of obesity: Relative contribution of metabolic factors, diet, and physical activity. *American Journal of Medicine* 105 (2): 145-150.

Weyer, C., Linkeschowa, R., Heise, T., Giesen, H.T., and Spraul, M. 1998. Implications of the traditional and the new ACSM physical activity recommendations on weight reduction in dietary treated obese subjects. *International Journal of Obesity and Related Metabolic Disorders* 22 (11): 1071-1078.

Wing, R.R. 1999, Nov. Physical activity in the treatment of adult overweight and obesity: Current evidence and research issues. *Medicine and Science in Sports and Exercise:* 31(11): S547-S552.

World Health Organization. 1992. Ottawa Charter for Health Promotion 1986, WHO Regional European Series Publications, 44: 1-7. Geneva.

World Health Organization. 1997. Obesity: Preventing and managing the global epidemic. WHO Geneva.

Young, D.R., Haskell, W.L., Jatulis, D.E., and Fortmann, S.P. 1993. Associations between changes in physical activity and risk factors for coronary heart disease in a community-based sample of men and women: The Stanford Five-City Project. *American Journal of Epidemiology* 138 (4): 205-216.

Chapter 17

Medication for Weight Management

William Hartman, PhD
Weight Management Program of San Francisco,
affiliated with California Pacific Specialty Services

Joan Saxton, MD
Weight Management Program of San Francisco,
affiliated with California Pacific Specialty Services,
and University of California at San Francisco

This chapter provides a brief overview of pharmacotherapy—the clinical use of medications—in the treatment of obesity. It is *not* a comprehensive review of the pharmacotherapy research literature, nor is it an in-depth exploration of the mechanisms of action of the various medications. Rather, our aim is to acquaint clinicians who treat obesity with the pharmacotherapy options currently available: which medications are currently used, how they are used in clinical practice, risks and benefits, realistic outcome expectations, and who is and is not a good candidate for pharmacotherapy.

Rationale for Pharmacotherapy

Obesity is now recognized as a serious, chronic medical condition with environmental, psychosocial, and *biological and genetic* components (Atkinson 1997). The prevalence of overweight is growing rapidly. As we enter the new millennium, estimates are that 63% of men and 55% of women in the United States are overweight, as defined by a body mass index of 25 kg/m² or greater (Must et al. 1999).

The association between overweight or obesity and a number of medical conditions is well documented: The incidence of type 2 diabetes; hypertension; hyperlipidemia; sleep apnea; coronary heart disease; gallbladder disease; osteoarthritis; breast, uterine, and colon cancer; and early mortality increases with increasing weight (Must et al. 1999; Wolf and Colditz 1998). Obesity and comorbid illness account for 6 to 7% of the national health care expenditure in the United States, about $46 billion in direct costs and $23 billion in indirect costs. Costs include physician visits, inpatient expenses, pharmacy and laboratory costs, and missed workdays (Brownell and Wadden 2000; Caan, Quesenberry, and Jacobson 1997; Cerulli and Malone 1998; Quesenberry, Caan, and Jacobson 1998).

There is no cure for obesity, but it is accepted that a weight loss of 5 to 10% in obese patients is associated with improvement in risk factors (Cerulli and Malone 1998; Lean 1998). A variety of treatments are available that reliably produce losses of this magnitude, including lifestyle change programs, hospital-based programs, meal-replacement regimens (low or very low calorie diets), pharmacotherapy, and surgery.

The problem is not so much how to produce the weight loss as how to sustain the weight loss: *Maintenance* is the key question facing clinicians today. Virtually all studies of weight loss show substantial regain (with the exception of some studies of surgery for the morbidly obese, e.g., Pories et al. 1995; Rabkin 1998). Although estimates of weight regain vary widely, regain following diet and behavior modification is about 33% at one year. As time passes, people regain weight, and without some form of retreatment, they will regain 75 to 100% (or more) of the weight lost in three to five years (Anderson et al. 1999; Perri 1992; Wadden et al. 1989).

We see the role of pharmacotherapy as at least twofold: Medications can produce significant weight loss when lifestyle modification alone does not, and more important, medications can produce better weight maintenance. For example, Lean (1998) estimated that diet and behavior therapy can produce significant weight loss in about 40% of patients; the success rate rises to 70% when medications are added. As we will review later, medications have been shown to sustain significant weight loss for three years or more.

A third potential benefit of pharmacotherapy is cost effectiveness. Although data are scarce, at least one clinical case study demonstrated that the use of antiobesity drugs reduced overall pharmaceutical costs among patients with diabetes, hypertension, and hyperlipidemia (Greenway et al. 1999).

A key concern of many health professionals regarding medication use is that drugs will be used instead of traditional diet-and-exercise approaches, that is, that patients will take the "lazy" way out. The National Task Force on the Prevention and Treatment of Obesity (1996) wrote, "The unjustified perception that obesity is a volitional state rather than a disease contributes to the reluctance of health professionals, patients, and regulators to accept the use of long-term pharmacotherapy for its treatment." The task force contrasts obesity treatment with the treatment of other medical conditions: "Long-term drug treatment for control of chronic health-threatening conditions, such as abnormalities in blood glucose, blood pressure, and lipids, is well established, even though many of these conditions also respond to changes in lifestyle, such as diet and exercise." However, the task force

notes that obesity "is frequently viewed as a consequence of weakness, lack of willpower, or a lifestyle 'choice'—the choice to overeat and underexercise. It should be stressed that the use of medication in obesity treatment does not change the necessity of making changes in diet and exercise; rather, it may enable patients to sustain long-term changes despite considerable environmental and biologic pressures for weight regain." It has been our experience that that is *exactly* what the medications do: They help our patients make the lifestyle changes needed to maintain a healthier weight.

In fact, it is widely accepted that pharmacological treatment should always be an adjunct to lifestyle (diet and exercise) modification efforts. Thus, almost all pharmacological research studies include a lifestyle change component, so that the comparison is drug-plus-lifestyle-change versus placebo-plus-lifestyle-change. A later section will discuss the specifics of treatment and special circumstances (e.g., solo practitioners).

A Brief History of the Use of Medications for Weight Loss

Until the widespread use of phentermine and fenfluramine began in 1993, relatively little research was conducted with antiobesity medications, and few drugs were available. Following is a very brief summary of early findings.

Early Medications

Historically, drug treatments for obesity have had a negative image, and with good reason. Drug treatment has often yielded disappointing results with serious side effects. In the 1890s, thyroid hormone was used to produce weight loss, and in the 1930s dinitrophenol was used, causing cataracts and neuropathy (Bray 1998).

From the late 1930s through the 1960s, amphetamines were widely prescribed and, of course, abused (National Task Force 1996). Amphetamines' abuse potential is likely the result of dopaminergic effects (Bray 1998). The abuse (and indiscriminant use of) the drugs probably caused the general perception that weight loss drugs are addictive, although many of the agents developed during the 1950s and 1960s were not. The result was little advance in the pharmacological treatment of obesity: The U.S. Food and Drug Administration (FDA) approved no new medications for obesity from 1973 to 1996. The FDA also limited pharmacological obesity treatment to 12 weeks (Atkinson 1997).

Four additional factors have worked against the development and use of medications in obesity treatment. First, drugs are seen as ineffective because the outcome of drug treatments is modest, especially in earlier research, which rarely exceeded 12 weeks' duration. Even when drug treatment is continued, individuals rarely continue losing weight to a low or "ideal" weight. Second, when the drugs are discontinued, weight is regained (Atkinson et al. 1997; Bray 1998). Third, any given antiobesity drug does not work for a significant number of people who take it. Finally, side effects have discouraged the use of the medications.

Drugs used to treat other chronic conditions, such as diabetes, hypertension, schizophrenia, and hyperlipidemia, can be characterized by the previous statements and yet are considered efficacious and acceptable treatments. Thus, observers have questioned whether drug treatment in obesity is held to a more rigorous standard than are drug treatments for other conditions ("Weighing the options" 1995).

The Phen/Fen Phenomenon

In 1992, Weintraub and colleagues changed the course of pharmacological treatment for obesity with the publication of a now-famous series of studies using phentermine and fenfluramine for three and half years (e.g., Weintraub 1992a, 1992b). The study was elegantly designed, including double-blind, placebo-controlled crossover features (that is, neither clinicians nor subjects knew whether subjects were taking placebo or active drugs, and subjects originally on placebo eventually received drug and vice versa), as well as an open-label portion during which participants knew that they were taking the active drugs, and a final period of no drug. Throughout, adjunctive diet, exercise, and behavioral treatment were provided. In summary, the studies showed that the drug combination showed superior weight loss to placebo; the effect was sustained for the duration of the study (although there was also regain during the latter part of the study); and full weight regain occurred when the drugs were discontinued. Weight loss was substantial, amounting to about 16% of body weight loss from baseline weight, compared to about 5% for placebo (this is higher than the weight loss that currently available drugs produce, as discussed later).

It would be difficult to overestimate the impact of Weintraub's studies on the field. Patients and professionals alike saw new hope, and "phen/fen" became part of the national vocabulary. Many established practitioners and clinics used the combination for long periods of time (e.g., Atkinson et al. 1997; Hartman, Bauchowitz, and Saxton 1997). In addition, "pill mills" sprang up, and the medications were readily and not always appropriately prescribed. The number of fenfluramine prescriptions increased from about 60,000 in 1992 to well over a million in 1995 (National Task Force 1996). The combined number of fenfluramine and phentermine prescriptions topped 18 million in 1996 (Connolly et al. 1997).

In considering the impact of the Weintraub studies, it is also worthwhile to note that while the studies were exceptionally well designed and used medications already approved for use by the FDA, the drugs were approved only for short-term (less than three months), individual use. Also, the studies began with 121 subjects; by the end of drug treatment, only 27 subjects remained on the medications. To say the least, this is a rather small data set on which to base the large-scale treatment that followed! Of course, there is little doubt that a major part of the eagerness with which consumers and professionals embraced pharmacotherapy was the generally poor long-term outcome in diet-exercise-behavior therapy ("Clinical guidelines" 1998).

During the phen/fen heyday, an isomer of fenfluramine, dexfenfluramine, was released as Redux and approved for use by the FDA, and its sales skyrocketed. In addition, over-the-counter herbal preparations, especially St. John's wort and ma huang, were touted as "herbal phen/fen" (herbal preparations and dietary supplements are discussed later in the chapter).

In August 1997, pharmacotherapy use in obesity again changed course dramatically when researchers at the Mayo Clinic reported on a number of cases of valvular heart disease, particularly abnormalities of the aortic valve, associated with fenfluramine and dexfenfluramine use (Connolly et al. 1997). By September the drugs had been voluntarily withdrawn from the market. Early estimates were that up to 30% of patients using the drugs showed heart valve changes, but later studies indicated that the percentages were somewhat lower (e.g., 7 to 14%) and dependent on the dose and length of time the drugs were taken (especially ≥60 mg, ≥3 months, or both), and that the changes stabilized or tended to reverse after discontinuing use of the drugs (Gardin et al. 2000; Hensrud et al. 1999; Li et al. 1999; Mast et al. 2001; Shively et al. 1999; Wadden et al. 1998). Although the mechanism of action of the valve changes is not known, it is possible that elevated circulating levels of serotonin, a neurotransmitter released by both fenfluramine and dexfenfluramine, caused the damage (Connolly et al. 1997; Jick 2000) (see the next section for additional information).

Guidelines for the medical follow-up for phen/fen users were established (e.g., "Interim recommendations" 1997), and legal action has been pursued. Meanwhile, American Home Products, maker of the fenfluramine drugs, has made a settlement including $4 billion to cover the costs of medical monitoring of former phen/fen users ("Weight loss drug" 1999).

Despite the discontinuation of the "phen/fen protocol," phentermine and other preexisting drugs continue to be used for obesity treatment. The FDA has also approved two more medications, sibutramine and orlistat, since 1997. The mechanism of actions of these agents is discussed in the next section.

Unrelated to the medical concerns about fenfluramine and dexfenfluramine, the only FDA-approved over-the-counter appetite suppressant medication approved to treat obesity—phenylpropanolamine—was also recently withdrawn from the market. Phenylpropanolamine, marketed as Dexatrim and Accutrim, was also a key ingredient in cough and cold remedies. It was associated with increased risk of hemorrhagic stroke in women (Kernan et al. 2000).

Action and Side Effects of Currently Used Medications

The three primary ways that medications act to cause weight loss are (1) reduction of energy intake, (2) reduction of nutrient absorption, and (3) increase in energy expenditure (National Task Force 1996).

It should be noted that the two recently approved medications, sibutramine and orlistat, have been far more rigorously tested than have their predecessors. At the time of this writing, each medication has been tested in over seven thousand obese subjects, including trials of two years in length. While they have not been in use long enough to rule out longer-term drug-related complications, standards of testing have certainly become more stringent.

Reduction of Energy Intake

Most antiobesity drugs fall into the category of reduction of energy intake. These types of drugs create their effect by increasing the availability of one or more of three neurotransmitters: dopamine, norepinephrine, and serotonin. Individuals taking the drugs experience the effect as a decrease in appetite, an increase in satiety, or both. Many patients who used phen/fen reported that cravings or preoccupation with food decreased sharply.

Table 17.1 summarizes only the medications in common current use, that is, DEA schedules IV and V medications. Table 17.1 lists the method of action, DEA schedule, generic and sample trade names, available dosage, and maximum dose of commonly used antiobesity drugs.

Amphetamine, methamphetamine, and phenmetrazine are DEA schedule II drugs that increase the availability of dopamine and norepinephrine. Their abuse potential seems to reside in the dopaminergic action, and they are not used anymore in the treatment of exogenous obesity. Similarly acting schedule III drugs include benzphetamine and phendimetrazine. These drugs are thought to have less abuse potential, but are not often prescribed by physicians.

Schedule IV drugs, with little or no abuse potential, include phentermine (e.g., Fastin, Adipex, Ionamin), mazindol (e.g., Sanorex), and diethylpropion (e.g., Tenuate). All act primarily to increase norepinephrine release. These drugs are approved for short-term use, up to about 12 weeks (*Physicians' Desk Reference* 2002).

Sibutramine (Meridia), also schedule IV, reduces the reuptake of both norepinephrine and serotonin. The FDA has approved both

Table 17.1   *Commonly Used Antiobesity Drugs*

Method of action	DEA schedule	Generic name	Sample trade names	Available dosage (mg)	Maximum dose (mg)
Increase release and/or block reuptake of norepinephrine	IV	Diethylpropion	Tenuate	25, 75	75
	IV	Phentermine HCL	Adipex Fastin Ionamin	30 37.5 15, 30	30 37.5 30
	IV	Resin Mazindol	Sanorex Mazanor	1, 2 1	3 3
Block reuptake of serotonin and norepinephrine	IV	Sibutramine	Meridia	5, 10, 15	20
Selective lipase inhibitor	V	Orlistat	Xenical	120	360

Data from Atkinson 1997; Bray 1998; and Yanovski and Yanovski 2002.

sibutramine and the other recently approved antiobesity medication orlistat (discussed in the following section) for longer-term use.

Reduction of Nutrient Absorption

The most recent drug to receive FDA approval for weight loss and maintenance is orlistat, or Xenical. Unlike the medications described in the previous section, it does not act systemically, nor does it reduce appetite. It is instead a lipase inhibitor; that is, it blocks the action of intestinal lipase, thus preventing the absorption of about one-third of the fat eaten when the medication is taken. A diet of about 30% calories from fat is recommended. Since the fat not absorbed is excreted in the stool, ingestion of a large amount of fat in a meal is likely to cause unpleasant side effects such as soft or oily stools (see the section on side effects). Some speculate that orlistat might have an aversive conditioning effect; that is, patients will choose to eat less fat to avoid gastric events (Heber 1999; Phelan and Wadden 2002).

Increase in Energy Expenditure

There are currently no drugs approved by the FDA for increasing energy expenditure, for example, by increasing thermogenesis (the body's heat-producing mechanism) or by increasing metabolism. The effects of sibutramine may be partly the result of increased energy expenditure (Astrup and Lundsgaard 1998; Scheen and Lefebvre 1999). Other agents are under development that increase energy output by increasing the activity of beta-adrenergic receptors (see the section titled Medications Under Development).

Safety and Side Effects

Clinicians should consult the *Physicians' Desk Reference* (2002) and materials provided by manufacturers regarding specific medications. This section provides a summary of safety and side effect issues.

□ Abuse. Appetite suppressants acquired their negative reputation because amphetamines are addictive. However, the schedule IV drugs that act via the norepinephrine system—phentermine, mazindol, and phenylpropanolamine—show low abuse potential. Sibutramine and orlistat have shown little or no potential for abuse (Bray 1998; National Task Force 1996).

□ Valvular heart disease and primary pulmonary hypertension. As noted earlier, fenfluramine and dexfenfluramine were withdrawn from the market because their use was associated with valvular heart disease. They are powerful serotonin "agonists"—that is, they increase the release of serotonin into the synapse. Some have speculated that their effect on heart valves was the result of an increase in serotonin circulating outside the central nervous system (Connolly et al. 1997; Jick 2000).

Sibutramine also acts on the serotonin system, but its mechanism of action is slightly different from that of the fenfluramines. Rather, it is similar to the action of the class of antidepressants known as SSRIs, or selective serotonin reuptake inhibitors, such as Prozac, Zoloft, and Paxil. Sibutramine was not observed to increase the rate of valvulopathy relative to placebo (Bach et al. 1999).

Fenfluramine and dexfenfluramine were also associated with the very rare but serious cardiopulmonary disorder, primary pulmonary hypertension (PPH). The prolonged (i.e., more than three-month) use of these drugs apparently increased the rate of PPH from one to two cases per million per year in the general population to 23 to 46 cases per million (Abenheim et al. 1996). PPH has not been observed with phentermine alone, nor with sibutramine, but because of its rare baseline occurrence, it is difficult to detect.

□ Other adverse events, side effects, and contraindications for centrally acting medications. The most common side effects for the centrally acting medications (e.g., phentermine, mazindol, sibutramine) are dry mouth, insomnia, headache, nausea, constipation, dizziness, nervousness, and depression, depending on the specific medication and individual patient differences. Increases in blood pressure and pulse rate might also occur. Vital signs should be monitored carefully. Patients with uncontrolled or poorly controlled hypertension should not use these drugs (National Task Force 1996; *Physicians' Desk Reference* 2002; Sibutramine prescribing information 1999).

Use of these medications is generally contraindicated in patients who take antidepressants, migraine medications, and some analgesics; patients who have a history of coronary artery disease, congestive heart disease, arrhythmias, or stroke; pregnant or lactating women; or children (National Task Force 1996; Sibutramine 1999). Physicians and patients should read the packing instructions of each individual medication carefully.

One reason for the concern regarding patients taking SSRI antidepressants is the possibility of serotonin syndrome, characterized by altered mental status (confusion), neuromuscular abnormalities, and autonomic dysfunction (e.g., dizziness) (Martin 1996). This syndrome is probably the result of excess stimulation of the serotonergic system. It is rare and was more of a concern when phen/fen was prescribed in conjunction with antidepressants, since both the fenfluramines and the SSRIs increase serotonin activity. Also, physicians should *not* suggest that patients discontinue antidepressants to take an antiobesity drug.

□ Adverse events, side effects, and contraindications for orlistat. Most of the side effects of orlistat are gastrointestinal, described as oily spotting, flatus with discharge, fecal urgency, fatty and oily stool, oily evacuation, and increased defecation. While such events do occur in a majority of patients who take the drug, their frequency is quite limited in individual patients (that is, while many patients experience a gastric event, most patients will experience only one or two such events). During clinical trials, gastric events were of mild to moderate intensity and were responsible for premature withdrawal from the study of a slightly higher percentage of subjects taking orlistat than of subjects taking placebo (Drent et al. 1995; Heck, Yanovski, and Calis 2000; Yanovski and Yanovski 2002).

Orlistat has also been shown to reduce the absorption of vitamins A, D, and E, and beta-carotene, and vitamin supplementation is therefore recommended (Drent et al. 1995; Yanovski and Yanovski 2002). Similarly, orlistat may interfere with the absorption of lipid-soluble medications such as cyclosporine (Colman and Fossler 2000).

□ Adverse events in drugs that increase energy expenditure. As noted earlier, the FDA has not approved the use of any drugs that increase energy expenditure. Nevertheless, over-the-counter herbal preparations of ephedrine or ma huang are popular in weight loss remedies. There are, however, reports of increased blood pressure, stroke, and other negative events, including death, associated with the use of this drug, and the FDA is strongly cautioning against its use (Atkinson 1997; Bray 1998).

▫ Drug combinations. There are no FDA-approved drug combination regimens for treating obesity. Although the phen/fen combination showed greater weight loss than any single drug applications, head-to-head comparisons were never conducted. Physicians wishing to combine drugs (for example, orlistat with sibutramine or phentermine) can do so as part of their clinical practice, but to date, few data exist regarding safety or efficacy. (However, it is important to obtain patients' consent if drug combinations are used.) Wadden and colleagues (2000) added orlistat (or placebo) to a small group of women who had already lost weight using sibutramine; the addition of the second medication did not enhance weight loss.

▫ Intermittent use of medications. Little information is available regarding the intermittent use of weight loss drugs (e.g., alternating several months on and several months off the drug). The limited research has yielded outcomes roughly equivalent to continuous medication use, with some indication of increased side effects from switching on and off drugs (Phelan and Wadden 2002; Weintraub et al. 1992; Wirth and Krause 2001; Yanovski and Yanovski 2002).

Medications Approved for Other Uses

A number of drugs approved by the FDA for indications other than obesity treatment have been and are being tested for a possible role in weight loss.

Tests were conducted with fluoxetine (Prozac), one of the antidepressants known as SSRIs, or selective serotonin reuptake inhibitors, based on the observation that weight loss occurred in some individuals taking it. In placebo-controlled studies, however, there was either no difference in weight loss between drug and placebo (Fernandez-Soto et al. 1995), or greater weight loss initially with fluoxetine, but by the end of a one-year treatment, no difference between the drug and placebo groups (Darga et al. 1991; Goldstein et al. 1994).

More recently, three additional drugs are being investigated for weight loss properties—bupropion (Wellbutrin), an antidepressant; topiramate (Topamax), an antiepileptic agent also approved for treatment of affective disorder; and metformin (Glucophage), used to treat diabetes. None of the medications are currently approved by the FDA as weight loss agents, although research results are promising (Yanovski and Yanovski 2002).

Medications Under Development

There are always antiobesity medications in various stages of development. We will consider several examples in this section.

Leptin is a peptide, or protein, that is manufactured under direction of the "ob gene." In studies that received a good deal of publicity, mice that lacked the ob gene became obese, but when they were injected with leptin, they lost weight dramatically (Halaas et al. 1995; Zhang et al. 1994). The human equivalents were identified, but subsequent studies revealed that, in general, obese humans have relatively high levels of leptin (Considine et al. 1996). Nevertheless, clinical trials have shown that subjects do lose some weight while receiving leptin injections (Bray 1998; Smith Barney 1996). Work is also under way on developing oral formulations (Hirsch 2000; Yanovski and Yanovski 2002).

Since many overweight humans have high levels of leptin, there is speculation that they may be "leptin resistant," that is, less sensitive to the effects of leptin. Ciliary neurotrophic factor (CNTF, developed as Axokine) is currently in clinical trial. CNTF stimulates other receptors in the leptin pathway and might thus circumvent leptin resistance (Hirsch 2000; Yanovski and Yanovski 2002).

Cholecystokinin (CCK) is a gut peptide that has been shown to reduce food intake in animals and humans, and efforts continue to find a means of delivery that reduces side effects. Many drug companies have been working on the problem with only limited success (Smith Barney 1996).

A recent intriguing study (Cummings et al. 2002) demonstrated that levels of ghrelin, a hormone secreted by the stomach and duodenum and associated with mealtime hunger, increases in obese persons after dieting. In contrast, persons who have undergone gastric bypass surgery (bypassing much of the area in which ghrelin is secreted) report significantly reduced hunger and have extremely low levels of ghrelin. It is believed that increased ghrelin might be a cause of dietary relapse. Thus, research efforts are likely to be focused on finding an antagonist to ghrelin.

The previously discussed approaches work to reduce to food intake. Alternatively, the adrenergic (norepinephrine) system, which controls energy expenditure and thermogenesis (burning calories for heat), is apparently mediated through various adrenergic receptors. For example, obese Pima Indians have a mutation in the β-3 adrenergic receptor. Thus, work is under way to develop β-3-agonists (Bray 1998; Hauner 1999; Smith Barney 1996; Scheen and Lefebvre 1999).

In addition, agents that inhibit gastric emptying, such as glucagon-like peptide-1 (GLP-1), may have a role in weight loss, but this is not yet well established (Scheen and Lefebvre, 1999). Trials are under way using Exendin-4, a drug similar to GLP-1 (Hirsch 2000).

Herbal Products and Dietary Supplements

This chapter is primarily concerned with medications reviewed and monitored by the FDA. However, numerous products are marketed as weight loss aids under provisions of the Dietary Supplement Health and Education Act (DSHEA) passed by Congress in 1994 (Nesheim 1999). These products are not prospectively reviewed and approved by the FDA; the DSHEA assigns product safety monitoring to the manufacturers. Hence, reliable data about these products are scarce. Examples of such products are ephedra (ma huang), chromium picolinate, dieter's tea, chitosan, and guarana.

A recent review found that studies of most of these products were poorly designed and did not convincingly demonstrate either safety or efficacy (Allison et al. 2001). There are better-designed studies of ephedrine, a compound available in over-the-counter drugs for asthma and nasal symptoms (also available in the botanical form, ma huang). These studies did demonstrate short-term weight loss (As-

trup et al. 1992; Atkinson 1997; Pasquali and Casimirri 1993). However, as indicated earlier, there have been case reports of numerous adverse events, including increased blood pressure, cardiac arrhythmia, stroke, seizure, and death; the FDA is strongly cautioning against the use of ephedra for weight loss (Atkinson 1997; Bray 1998; Haller and Benowitz 2000; Yanovski and Yanovski 2002). In summary, herbal products are not recommended for weight loss.

Medications Associated With Weight Gain

In recent years, there has been a growing recognition that weight gain—or difficulty in losing weight—may be at least in part a function of medications taken for other conditions (Cheskin et al. 1999; Heber 1999). Certain hypoglycemic drugs, psychoactive drugs, and glucocorticoids have been particularly associated with weight gain. When possible—*and without compromising treatment of the condition the drug is being used for*—adjustments might be possible to minimize weight gain. For example, in the treatment of diabetes, the sulfonylureas are associated with weight gain, whereas metformin has been shown to prevent weight gain or perhaps even cause weight loss (Fontebonne et al. 1996; Yanovski and Yanovski 2002). Similarly, some psychoactive medications are associated with relatively large amounts of weight gain (e.g., clozapine and risperidone), whereas others are not; some might even cause weight loss (e.g., bupropion and topiramate, as discussed previously). Even if medication adjustments are not feasible, the role of the concomitant medication can be taken into account in diet planning. For example, the dose of glucocorticoids is frequently reduced during periods of remission of the condition being treated. Patients may choose to plan intensive periods of active weight loss to coincide with such periods (Heber 1999).

Efficacy of Currently Used Medications

Data from clinical trials and data collected in clinical settings show a consistent, long-lasting reduction in body weight as long as medication is continued. In addition, medication can be used specifically to enhance weight loss maintenance.

Clinical Trials and Studies

Taken as a whole, the outcome of pharmacological interventions is best described as *modest*. Since studies (especially recent large sibutramine and orlistat trials) share certain characteristics, the treatment literature may be fairly summarized as follows: Patients taking medication lose on average 9 to 26 lb (4 to 12 kg), corresponding to 4 to 12% of baseline body weight, or about 4 to 18 lb (2 to 8 kg) more than is lost by subjects taking placebo. No single drug has superior efficacy, although one recent review of pharmacotherapy studies indicated a slightly larger loss for phentermine than for other currently used drugs (Glazer 2001). Maximum effect is reached within about six months; thereafter, weight loss is mostly maintained—with perhaps some regain—for as long as the drugs are taken. When the drugs are discontinued, weight regain toward baseline is rapid. Patients taking active medication are significantly (two to three times) more likely to lose and maintain more than 5 or 10% of body weight. Dropout rates vary from about 20 to 50% at one year. In clinical use, dropout rates are about 40% or more at one year, and up to 80% during the second and third year of drug use (Atkinson et al. 1997; Bray et al. 1994; "Clinical guidelines" 1998; Davidson et al. 1999; Goldstein and Potvin 1994; Jones et al. 1995; Hartman, Bauchowitz, and Saxton 1997; Scheen and Lefebvre 1999; Sjöström et al. 1998).

As noted at the beginning of this chapter, it is widely accepted that pharmacotherapy is an *adjunct* to lifestyle (diet and exercise) modification (Heber 1999; National Task Force 1996). Indeed, almost all published pharmacotherapy studies have incorporated a lifestyle modification component (e.g., Weintraub 1992a and b). Most pharmacotherapy studies have used relatively mild forms of lifestyle modification, such as monthly contact with a clinician or group leader. Studies are designed in this way at least in part to ensure that medication effects can be detected and not masked by aggressive diets (Heber 1999; Phelan and Wadden 2002). Although data are scarce, it appears that medication alone (i.e., without concomitant lifestyle modification) produces less weight loss than medication in combination with lifestyle modification. Also, it appears that total weight loss can be significantly increased up to 33 lb (15 kg) or more by using more intensive interventions and with meal replacement, either partial meal replacement while the medication is administered or full meal replacement (very low calorie diet, or VLCD) prior to medication use (Apfelbaum et al. 1999; Phelan and Wadden 2002; Stunkard, Craighead, and O'Brien 1980; Wadden et al. 2001). Medication can also be used explicitly to prevent regain of weight lost by other means, such as conventional low-calorie dieting (Hill et al. 1999).

As with weight changes, modest, significant changes in risk factors are observed among subjects taking medications. Blood lipids and glycemic control improve with sibutramine or orlistat; blood pressure improves with orlistat but not sibutramine. Some of the observed changes may be independent of the weight loss (Scheen and Lefebvre 1999).

Sjöström and colleagues (1998) found that after one year of treatment, diastolic blood pressure was significantly lower among subjects taking orlistat than among those taking placebo (80.3 mmHg versus 82.1 mmHg); after two years of treatment, LDL/HDL cholesterol ratio decreased 12.7% from baseline, relative to a decrease of 4.6% for placebo. In a different study using orlistat (Davidson et al. 1999), fasting serum insulin levels decreased significantly for medication patients, while insulin levels were unchanged for placebo recipients. Heymsfield and colleagues (2000) demonstrated that orlistat improved oral glucose tolerance and reduced the rate of progression from impaired glucose tolerance to diabetic status over a 1 1/2-year period. In a study of type 2 diabetics, Hollander and colleagues (1998) found that orlistat use was associated with improvements in HbA$_{1c}$ and lipid profile.

In a study using sibutramine (Heath et al. 1999), subjects' triglycerides decreased 11.1%, while HDL cholesterol increased 2.9%. The subset of subjects who lost ≥5% or more of body weight showed an absolute percentage change in HbA$_{1c}$ of –0.4%. For subjects losing ≥10% of body weight, fasting plasma glucose decreased 8.7% (all changes were significantly different from those of the placebo group). In a study of diabetic patients (Finer et al. 2000), sibutramine (as compared to placebo) produced similar changes in glycosylated hemoglobin and fasting plasma glucose.

Clinical Settings

In addition to clinical trials, long-term use of medication in private practice settings has been shown to produce significant, lasting weight loss. Atkinson and colleagues (1997) demonstrated with phen/fen three-year weight losses of about 12% of body weight, with concomitant reductions in blood pressure, cholesterol, and triglycerides.

Greenway and colleagues (1999) evaluated the use of phen/fen, mazindol/fenfluramine, or caffeine/ephedrine among patients with diabetes, hypertension, and/or hyperlipidemia and found that among compliant patients, weight losses of 6 to 10% were associated with reduced pharmaceutical costs. Although this was a case study and the analysis was restricted to patients following the prescribed medication and behavioral treatment regimen, it is a demonstration of potential economic—as well as clinical—benefit.

Hartman, Bauchowitz, and Saxton (1997), working with a VLCD plus behavior therapy program, made phen/fen available during the maintenance phase and demonstrated 20% body weight loss for an average of 4 1/2 years after the VLCD, including an average of three years on phen/fen, also with favorable changes in blood pressure and serum cholesterol. In this program, the medication was optional (private practice setting, not clinical trial), and patients tended to begin using the medication when they were regaining weight. In many cases the weight regain was halted or reversed. It is likely that the medication gave patients a means to cope with relapse and achieve prolonged, significant weight loss when they might not otherwise have done so. Interestingly, patients participating in the same post-VLCD maintenance program for the same amount of time but without medications also showed 20% body weight reduction. So, while traditional diet and exercise modification works well for some patients, it does not for others, and in that case the medications are a viable and useful alternative.

Patient and Clinician Expectations

In view of the modest changes in weight and risk factors, both clinicians and patients must maintain reasonable expectations for pharmacotherapy. Most individuals will not attain "ideal" body weight, that is, BMI ≤24. In contrast, it is well known that individuals embarking on a diet hope to lose more weight than they are actually likely to lose (Foster et al. 1997); it is the clinician's responsibility to address this issue. Medications are not magic bullets. They can, however, assist patients in losing medically significant amounts of weight.

Patient Selection

Not everyone is a good candidate for antiobesity drugs. A generally accepted guideline is BMI ≥30 without comorbidities, or BMI ≥27 in the presence of comorbidities, especially hypertension, dislipidemias, diabetes (or impaired glucose tolerance), sleep apnea, and osteoarthritis (Bray 1998; "Clinical guidelines" 1998). When the FDA approved sibutramine and orlistat, it recognized that the medication is useful for the *maintenance* of weight loss ("Clinical guidelines" 1998). Thus, pharmacotherapy can be considered for patients who *began* a weight loss program at or above BMI 30 (or 27), but are at a lower weight when the drug is prescribed, having lost the weight by other means.

As noted previously, not everyone responds to pharmacotherapy, and in general, clinicians should consider adjusting the dose if less than 4 lb (2 kg) is lost in the first month. If weight loss does not improve, a different medication or discontinuation of pharmacotherapy should be considered. Other than lack of initial response, there are no predictors of who will or will not respond to medication (Bray 1998; "Clinical guidelines" 1998; Kopelman 1999; National Task Force 1996; Yanovski and Yanovski 2002).

Other factors to consider in deciding whether pharmacotherapy is appropriate include failure at previous attempts to lose weight—and maintain the loss—with more traditional lifestyle modification plans; the presence of comorbidities; a family history of overweight or risk factors; and the clinician's judgment of the patient's commitment to engage in lifestyle change to "work with" the medication. As with any diet, the clinician should also take into account whether there are extenuating conditions such as depression that might make the use of anorexiant medications undesirable.

Once a patient is started on a drug, the physician should schedule a follow-up visit for two to four weeks, then monthly for three months, then every three months for the first year of treatment, after which the physician should determine ongoing follow-up. The clinical guidelines (1998) published in *Obesity Research* offer more details.

As of this writing, the use of antiobesity medications in children and adolescents is experimental and thus should be used only in specialized treatment programs or in clinical trials, with individuals whose weight is at or above the 95th percentile for age and sex and with concomitant medical concerns (Yanovski and Yanovski 2002). Although research is under way, no long-term, randomized, double-blind, placebo-controlled trials have demonstrated efficacy and safety in children and adolescents.

Incorporating Pharmacotherapy Into Diet Programs

As discussed earlier, pharmacotherapy should be used in conjunction with lifestyle change programs, and evidence shows that more intensive or aggressive interventions produce better results. A variety of options exists to meet patient needs.

Ideally, patients should participate in full multidisciplinary programs, in which they receive medical, nutritional, exercise, and behavior modification services. However, when a full program is not possible, many other less intensive options employ pharmacotherapy.

For example, in a pilot investigation to incorporate lifestyle modification programming into a primary care approach, Wadden and colleagues (1997) used phen/fen for a year and compared a regular behavior modification group with monthly 15- to 20-minute individual sessions with a physician experienced in treating obesity. Both groups were provided with the same treatment manual. At the end of the year, the groups had lost similar amounts of weight (34 lb or 15.4 kg group; 31 lb or 13.9 kg physician).

While physicians in solo practice do not realistically have even the amount of time for the monthly visits described in Wadden and colleagues (1997), they could easily provide patients with a structured manual, including materials designed explicitly for patients taking weight loss medications (Brownell and Wadden 1998). The physician's staff (nurse, physician assistant, office staff) can assist and monitor the patient. Patients can also avail themselves of auxiliary services for support, such as hospital-based weight loss programs, nutritional staff, commercial programs, self-help venues, and numerous Internet resources. Bodenheimer, Hartman, and Saxton (1994) described an office-based model of weight loss counseling that is easily adapted to incorporate antiobesity medication use.

Several certifications are available for allied health professionals who want to specialize in weight loss. Examples are the Lifestyle Counselor certification (Wolfe 1996) or the Lifestyle and Weight Management Consultant certification offered by the American Council on Exercise (1996). Individuals who earn these certificates are typically nurses, physician assistants, dietitians, exercise physiologists, and mental health counselors. These professionals can easily assist patients in weight management efforts while coordinating with a physician who provides medical monitoring for the medications.

Finally, both of the newest medications, sibutramine and orlistat, offer no-cost patient support materials, such as behavioral, exercise, and nutritional suggestions. The materials have been developed for both regular postal and Internet use.

Summary

With the limited effectiveness of currently available antiobesity drugs, pharmacotherapy is not a magic bullet, nor is it for everyone. However, in certain circumstances, medications can be an effective means of enhancing and prolonging weight loss and reducing obesity-related risk factors. For individuals who meet the overweight criteria (BMI ≥30, or BMI ≥27 with risk factors), especially those who are unable to lose significant amounts of weight or to keep the weight off once it is lost, medication can be a valuable adjunct to lifestyle modification.

It is our belief that the status of obesity medication has a number of parallels with that of antidepressant medication after the advent of the SSRIs. When SSRIs were introduced, their use spread like wildfire, and they were perhaps used in cases in which their use was not warranted. Many mental health clinicians (and patients) felt that using a drug was a lazy, easy, inappropriate way around the more difficult path of psychotherapy. Although controversy still exists about how much antidepressants can and should be used, they are widely accepted as an effective means of dealing with a disorder that has significant biological underpinnings, and they provide a useful adjunct to traditional therapy and other efforts to work with depression, anxiety, and so forth. While originally conceived as a short-term treatment, they are now routinely used over the long term: Chronic medication use is warranted when dealing with chronic medical conditions. The same things may be said of obesity drugs.

As research continues, we can expect the development of more effective medications—drugs that produce more weight loss, for longer periods of time, with fewer side effects. In the meantime, several well-tolerated medications are already available. Physicians, as well as allied health professionals working in concert with physicians, would do well by their patients to consider using the tools available to them to combat a growing and deadly disease.

References

Abenhaim, L., Moride, Y., Brenot, F., et al. 1996. Appetite-suppressant drugs and the risk of primary pulmonary hypertension. *New England Journal of Medicine* 335: 609-616.

Allison, D.B., Fontaine, D.R., Heshka, S., Mentore, J.L., and Heymsfield, S.B. 2001. Alternative treatments for weight loss: A critical review. *Critical Review of Food Science and Nutrition* 41: 1-28.

American Council on Exercise. 1996. *Lifestyle and weight management consultant manual.* San Diego: Author.

Anderson, J.W., Konz, E.C., Frederich, R.C., and Wood, C.L. 1999. Long-term weight maintenance: A meta-analysis of US studies. *Obesity Research* 7 (S1): 43S.

Apfelbaum, M., Vague, P., Ziegler, O., Hanotin, C., Thomas, F., and Leutenegger, E. 1999. Long-term maintenance of weight loss after a very-low-calorie diet: A randomized blinded trial of the efficacy and tolerability of sibutramine. *American Journal of Medicine* 106 (2): 179-184.

Astrup, A., Breum, L., Toubro, S., Hein, P., and Quaade, F. 1992. The effect and safety of an ephedrine/caffeine compound compared to ephedrine, caffeine, and placebo in obese subjects. *International Journal of Obesity Related Metabolic Disorders* 16: 269-277.

Astrup, A., and Lundsgaard, C. 1998. What do pharmacological approaches to obesity management offer? Linking pharmacological mechanisms of obesity management agents to clinical practice. *Experimental and Clinical Endocrinology of Diabetes* 106 (S2): 29-34.

Atkinson, R.L. 1997. Use of drugs in the treatment of obesity. *Annual Review of Nutrition* 17: 383-403.

Atkinson, R.L. Blank R.C., Schumacher D., Dhurandhar N.V., Ritch D.L. 1997. Long-term drug treatment of obesity in a private practice setting. *Obesity Research* 5: 578-586.

Bach, D.S., Rissanen, A.M., Mendel, C.M., Shepherd, G., Weinstein, S.P., Kelly, F., Seaton, T.B., Patel, B., Pekkarinen, T.A., and Armstrong, W.F. 1999. Absence of cardiac valve dysfunction in obese patients treated with sibutramine. *Obesity Research* 7 (4): 363-369.

Bodenheimer, T., Hartman, W.M., and Saxton, J. 1994. Helping your patients control their weight. *Internal Medicine* June: 31-40.

Bray, G.A. 1998. *Contemporary diagnosis and management of obesity.* Newtown, PA: Handbooks in Health Care.

Bray, G.A, Blackburn G.L., Ferguson J.M. et al. 1994. Sibutramine—Dose response and long-term efficacy in weight loss, a double-blind study. *International Journal of Obesity* 18 (S2): 60.

Brownell, K.D., and Wadden, T.A. 1998. *The LEARN program for weight control.* Dallas, TX: American Health Publishing.

Brownell, K.D., and Wadden, T.A. 2000. Obesity. In *Comprehensive textbook of psychiatry,* 7th ed., eds. H.T. Kaplan and B.J. Saddock, 1787-1796. Baltimore: Williams & Wilkins.

Caan, B., Quesenberry, C.P., Jr., and Jacobson, A. 1997. Increase in health care costs associated with obesity. *Obesity Research* 5: 5S.

Cerulli, J., and Malone, M. 1998. Outcomes of pharmacological and surgical treatment for obesity. *Pharmacoeconomics* 14 (3): 269-283.

Cheskin, L.J., Bartlett, S.J., Zayas, R., Twilley, C.H., Allison, D.B., and Cantoreggi, C. 1999. Prescription medications: A modifiable contributor to obesity. *Southern Medical Journal* 92 (9): 898-904.

Clinical guidelines on the identification, evaluation, and treatment of overweight and obesity in adults— The evidence report. 1998. *Obesity Research* 6 (S2).

Colman, E., and Fossler, M. 2000. Reduction in blood cyclosporine concentrations by orlistat. *New England Journal of Medicine* 342: 1141.

Connolly, H.M., Crary, J.L., McGoon, M.D., Hensrud, D.D., Edwards, B.S., Edwards, W.D., and Schaff, H.V. 1997. Valvular heart disease associated with fenfluramine-phentermine. *New England Journal of Medicine* 337: 581-588.

Considine, R.V., Sinha, M.K., Heiman, M.L., Driauciunas, A., Stephens, T.W., Nyce, M.R., Ohannesian, J.P., Marco, C.C., McKee, L.J., Bauer, T.L., et al. 1996. Serum immunoreactive-leptin concentrations in normal-weight and obese humans. *New England Journal of Medicine* 334: 292-295.

Cummings, D.E., Weigle, D.S., Frayo, R.S., Breen, P.A., Ma, M.K., Dellinger, E.P., and Purnell, J.Q. 2002. Plasma ghrelin levels after diet-induced weight loss or gastric bypass surgery. *New England Journal of Medicine* 346: 1623-1630.

Darga, L.L., Carroll-Michals, L., Botsford, S.J., and Lucas, C.P. 1991. Fluoxetine's effect on weight loss in obese subjects. *American Journal of Clinical Nutrition* 54: 321-325.

Davidson, M.H., Hauptman, J., DiGirolamo, M. et al. 1999. Weight control and risk factor reduction in obese subjects treated for two years with orlistat. A randomized controlled trial. *Journal of the American Medical Association* 281: 235-242.

Drent, M.L., Larsson, I., William-Olsson, T., Quaade, F., Czubayko, F., vonBergman, K., Strobel, W., Sjöström, L., and Van der Veen, E.A. 1995. Orlistat (RO 18-0647), a lipase inhibitor, in the treatment of human obesity: A multiple dose study. *International Journal of Obesity Related Metabolic Disorders* 19 (4): 221-226.

Fernandez-Soto, M.L., Gonzalez-Jimenez, A., Barredo-Acedo, F., Luna del Castillo, J.D., and Escobar-Jimenez, F. 1995. Comparison of fluoxetine and placebo in the treatment of obesity. *Annals of Nutrition and Metabolism* 39 (3): 159-163.

Finer, N., Bloom, S.R., Frost, G.S., Banks, L.M., and Griffiths, J. 2000. Sibutramine is effective for weight loss and diabetic control in obesity with type 2 diabetes: A randomized, double-blind, placebo-controlled study. *Diabetes, Obesity, and Metabolism* 2 (2): 195-212.

Fontebonne, A., Charles, M.A., Juhan-Vague, I., Bard, J.M., Andre, P., Isnard, F., Cohen, J.M., Grandmottet, P., Vague, P., Safar, M.E., and Eschwege, E. 1996. The effect of metformin on the metabolic abnormalities

associated with upper-body fat distribution. *Diabetes Care* 19 (9): 920-926.

Foster, G.D., Wadden, T.A., Vogt, R.A., et al. 1997. What is a reasonable weight loss? Patients' expectations and evaluations of obesity treatment outcomes. *Journal of Consulting and Clinical Psychology* 65: 79-85.

Gardin, J.M., Schumacher, K., Constantine, G., Davis, K.D., Leung, C., and Reid, C.L. 2000. Valvular abnormalities and cardiovascular status following exposure to dexfenfluramine or phentermine/fenfluramine. *Journal of the American Medical Association* 283: 1703-1709.

Glazer, G. 2001. Long-term pharmacotherapy of obesity 2000: A review of efficacy and safety. *Archives of Internal Medicine* 161: 1814-1824.

Goldstein, D.J., and Potvin, J.H. 1994. Long-term weight loss: The effect of pharmacologic agents. *American Journal of Clinical Nutrition* 60 (5): 647-657.

Goldstein, D.J., Rampey, A.H., Enas, G.G., Potvin, J.H., Fludzinski, L.A., and Levine, L.R. 1994. Fluoxetine: A randomized clinical trial in the treatment of obesity. *International Journal of Obesity Related Metabolic Disorders* 18 (3): 129-135.

Greenway, F.L., Ryan, D.H., Bray, G.A., Rood, J.C., Tucker, E.W., and Smith, S.R. 1999. Pharmaceutical cost savings of treating obesity with weight loss medications. *Obesity Research* 7: 523-531.

Halaas, J.L., Gajiwala, K.S., Maffei, M., Cohen, S.L., Chait, B.T., Rabinowitz, D., Lallone, R.L., Burley, S.K., and Friedman, J.M. 1995. Weight reducing effects of the plasma protein encoded by the obese gene. *Science* 269: 543-546.

Haller, C.A., and Benowitz, N.L. 2000. Adverse cardiovascular and central nervous system events associated with dieting supplements containing ephedra alkaloids. *New England Journal of Medicine* 343: 1833-1838.

Hartman, W.M., Bauchowitz, A., and Saxton, J. 1997. Fenfluramine/phentermine following a very low calorie diet. *Obesity Research* 5 (S1): 59S.

Hauner, H. 1999. The impact of pharmacotherapy on weight management in type 2 diabetes. *International Journal of Obesity* 23 (S7): S12-S17.

Heath, M.J. et al. 1999. Sibutramine enhances weight loss and improves glycemic control and plasma lipid profile in obese patients with Type 2 diabetes mellitus. *Diabetes* 48 (S1): A306.

Heber, D. 1999. Pharmacotherapy in the treatment of obesity. *Clinical Cornerstone* 2 (3): 33-42.

Heck, A.M., Yanovski, J.A., and Calis, K.A. 2000. Orlistat, a new lipase inhibitor for the management of obesity. *Pharmacotherapy* 20 (3): 270-279.

Hensrud, D.D., Connolly, H.M., Grogan, M., Miller, F.A., Bailey, K.R., and Jensen, M.D. 1999. Echocardiographic improvement over time after cessation of use of fenfluramine and phentermine. *Mayo Clinic Proceedings* 74: 1191-1197.

Heymsfield, S.B., Segal, K.R., Hauptman, J., Lucas, C.P., Boldrin, M.N., Rissanen, A., Wilding, J.P.H., and Sjöström, L. 2000. Effects of weight loss with orlistat on glucose tolerance and progression to type 2 diabetes in obese adults. *Archives of Internal Medicine* 160: 1321-1326.

Hill, J.O., Hauptman, J., Anderson, J.W., Fujioka, K., O'Neil, P.M., Smith, D.K., Zavoral, J.H., and Aronne, L.F. 1999. Orlistat, a lipase inhibitor for weight maintenance after conventional dieting: A 1-year study. *American Journal of Clinical Nutrition* 69 (6): 1108-1116.

Hirsch, B. 2000. Review of anti-obesity medications currently under development. *Bariatrician*:16-23.

Hollander, P.A., Elbein, S.C., Hirsch, I.B., Kelly, D., McGill, J., Taylor, T., Weiss, S.R., Crockett, S.E., Kaplan, R.A., Comstock, J., Lucas, C.P., Lodewick, P.A., Canovatchel, W., Chung, J., and Hauptman, J. 1998. Role of orlistat in the treatment of obese patients with type 2 diabetes. *Diabetes Care* 21: 1288-1294.

Interim recommendations issued for patients exposed to fenfluramine and dexfenfluramine. 1997. *Journal of the American Medical Association* 278 (21): 1728.

Jick, H. 2000. Heart valve disorders and appetite-suppressant drugs. *Journal of the American Medical Association* 283: 1738-1740.

Jones, S.P., Smith, I.G., Kelly, F. et al. 1995. Long term weight loss with sibutramine. *International Journal of Obesity* 19 (S2): 41.

Kernan, W.N., Viscoli, C.M., Brass, L.M., Broderick, J.P., Brott, T., Feldmann, E., Moregenstern, L.B., Wilterdink, J.L., and Horwitz, R.I. 2000. Phenylpropanolamine and the risk of hemorrhagic stroke. *New England Journal of Medicine* 343: 1826-1832.

Kopelman, P. 1999. Prescribing for obesity. Comment on the Royal College of Physicians' Working Party report on clinical management of overweight and obese patients with particular reference to drugs. *Journal of the Royal College of Physicians of London* 33 (1): 31-32.

Lean, M. 1998. Obesity—What are the current treatment options? *Experimental and Clinical Endocrinology of Diabetes* 106 (S2): 22-26.

Li, R., Serdula, M.K., Williamson, D.F., Bowan, B.A., Graham, D.J., and Green, L. 1999. Dose-effect of fenfluramine use on the severity of valvular heart disease among fen-phen patients with valvulopathy. *International Journal of Obesity* 23: 926-928.

Martin, T.G. 1996. Serotonin syndrome. *Annals of Emergency Medicine* 28: 520-526.

Mast, S.T., Jollis, J.G., Ryan, T., Anstrom, K.J., and Crary, J.L. 2001. The progression of fenfluramine—Associated heart disease assessed by echocardiography. *Annals of Internal Medicine* 134: 261-266.

Must, A., Spadano, J., Coakley, E.H., Field, A.E., Coldest, G., and Dietz, W.H. 1999. The disease burden associated with overweight and obesity. *Journal of the American Medical Association* 282 (16): 1523-1529.

National Task Force on the Prevention and Treatment of Obesity. 1996. Long-term pharmacotherapy in the management of obesity. *Journal of the American Medical Association* 276 (23): 1907-1915.

Nesheim, M.C. 1999. What is the research base for the use of dietary supplements? *Public Health Nutrition* 2 (1): 35-38.

Pasquali, R., and Casimirri, F. 1993. Clinical aspects of ephedrine in the treatment of obesity. *International Journal of Obesity* 17 (S1): S65-S68.

Perri, M.G. 1992. Improving maintenance of weight loss following treatment by diet and lifestyle modification. In *Treatment of the seriously obese patient*, eds. T.A. Wadden and T.B. VanItallie, 456-477. New York: Guilford Press.

Phelan, S., and Wadden, T.A. 2002. Combining behavioral and pharmacological treatments for obesity. *Obesity Research* 10 (6): 560-574.

Physicians' Desk Reference, 56th ed. 2002. Montvale, NJ: Thompson Healthcare.

Pories, W.J., Swanson, M.S., MacDonald, K.G., Long, S.B., Morris, P.G., Brown, B.M., Barakat, H.A., deRamon, R.A., Israel, G., Dolezal, J.M., et al. 1995. Who would have thought it? An operation proves to be the most effective therapy for adult-onset diabetes mellitus. *Annals of Surgery* 222: 339-350.

Quesenberry, C.P., Caan, B., and Jacobson, A. 1998. Obesity, health service use, and health care costs among members of a health maintenance organization. *Archives of Internal Medicine* 158: 466-472.

Rabkin, R. 1998. Distal gastric bypass/duodenal switch procedure, Roux-en-Y gastric bypass and biliopancreatic diversion in a community practice. *Obesity Surgery* 1: 53-59.

Scheen, A., and Lefebvre, P. 1999. Pharmacological treatment of obesity: Present status. *International Journal of Obesity Related Metabolic Disorders* 23 (S1): 47-53.

Shively, B.K., Roldan, C.A., Gill, E.A., Najarian, T., and Loar, S.B. 1999. Prevalence and determinants of valvulopathy in patients treated with dexfenfluramine. *Circulation* 100 (21): 2161-2167.

Sibutramine prescribing information. 1999. Mount Olive, NJ: Knoll Pharmaceutical Co.

Sjöström, L., Rissanen, A., Andersen, T. et al. 1998. Randomised placebo-controlled trial of orlistat for weight loss and prevention of weight regain in obese patients. *Lancet* 352: 167-172.

Smith Barney. 1996. Technology: Obesity overview, August 5, SFD08D015.

Stunkard, A.J., Craighead, L.W., and O'Brien, R. 1980. Controlled trial of behaviour therapy, pharmacotherapy, and their combination in the treatment of obesity. *Lancet* 2 (8203): 1045-1047.

Wadden, T.A., Berkowitz, R.I., Sarwer, D.B., Prus-Wisniewski, R., and Steinberg, C. 2001. Benefits of lifestyle modification in the pharmacologic treatment of obesity: A randomized trial. *Archives of Internal Medicine* 161: 218-227.

Wadden, T.A., Berkowitz, R.I., Silvestry, F., Vogt, R.A., St. John Sutton, M.G., Stunkard, A.J., Foster, G.D., and Aber, J.L. 1998. The fen-phen finale: A study of weight loss and valvular heart disease. *Obesity Research* 6 (4): 278-284.

Wadden, T.A., Berkowitz, R.I., Vogt, R.A., Steen, S.N., Stunkard, A.J., and Foster, G.D. 1997. Lifestyle modification in the pharmacological treatment of obesity: A pilot investigation of a primary care approach. *Obesity Research* 5 (3): 218-226.

Wadden, T.A., Berkowitz, R.I., Womble, L.G., Sarwer, D.B., Arnold, M.E., and Steinberg, C.M. 2000. Effects of sibutramine plus orlistat in obese women following 1 year of treatment by sibutramine alone: A placebo-controlled trial. *Obesity Research* 8: 431-437.

Wadden, T.A., Sternberg, J.A., Letizia, K.A., Stunkard, A.J., and Foster, G.D. 1989. Treatment of obesity by very low calorie diet, behavior therapy, and their combination: A five year perspective. *International Journal of Obesity* 13 (S2): 39-46.

Weighing the Options: Criteria of Evaluating Weight-Management Programs. 1995. Institute of Medicine. Washington, DC: National Academy Press.

Weight loss drug causes less severe heart damage than initially believed. 1999, November 23. *The Medical Tribune*.

Weintraub, M. 1992a Long-term weight control: The National Heart, Lung, and Blood Institute funded multi-modal intervention study. *Clinical Pharmacology and Therapeutics* 51: 581-585.

Weintraub, M. 1992b. Long-term weight control study: Conclusions. *Clinical Pharmacology and Therapeutics* 51: 642-646.

Weintraub, M., Sandaresan, P.R., Shuster, B., Ginsberg, F., Madan, M., Baldan, A., Stein, E.C., and Byrne, L. 1992. Long-term weight control study II (weeks 34 to 104). An open-label study of continuous fenfluramine plus phentermine versus targeted intermittent medication as adjuncts to behavior modification, caloric restriction, and exercise. *Clinical Pharmacology and Therapeutics* 51: 595-601.

Wirth, A., and Krause, J. 2001. Long-term weight loss with sibutramine: A randomized controlled trial. *Journal of the American Medical Association* 286: 1331-1339.

Wolf, A.M., and Colditz, G.A. 1998. Current estimates of the economic cost of obesity in the United States. *Obesity Research* 6: 97-106.

Wolfe, B.L. (ed.). 1996. *The lifestyle counselor's guide for weight control.* Dallas: American Health Publishing.

Yanovski, S.Z., and Yanovski, J.A. 2002. Obesity. *New England Journal of Medicine* 346 (8): 591-602.

Zhang, Y., Proenca, R., Maffei, M., Barone, M., Leopold, L., and Friedman, J.M. 1994. Positional cloning of the mouse obese gene and its human homologue. *Nature* 372 (6505): 425-432.

Chapter 18

Future Directions in Treating Obesity

Dana M. Catanese, BA

Melissa L. Hyder, BA

Walker S. Carlos Poston, PhD, MPH
Mid America Heart Institute and University of
Missouri at Kansas City

John P. Foreyt, PhD
Baylor College of Medicine

We have not managed to cure obesity, although attempts at sustained obesity treatment have been both prolific and creative. If successful treatments are characterized by amount of weight lost, then few remedies are successful. While health care professionals have only recently recognized obesity as a chronic disease (Kopelman 2000), it has long been a cause of cosmetic concerns and outrageously nonscientific treatments, including fat-reducing soaps, creams, and electric massagers (Stearns 1997). The observation that weight loss and maintenance are very difficult coupled with the multibillion dollar "diet" industry suggest the need for researchers to think differently about treatment options. This chapter provides several global research trends we believe will be the future of obesity treatment.

Weight loss maintenance, although highly coveted both aesthetically and medically, has been historically difficult to achieve on a consistent basis. Within five years after initial treatment, most patients regain most, if not all, of their lost weight (Haddock et al. 2002; National Task Force on the Prevention and Treatment of Obesity 1994; Wing 1998).

Surgical procedures are the most effective in treating morbid obesity (BMI ≥40), as they average weight losses of 30 to 40 kg (66 to 88 lb) (Sjöström 1995). Nonsurgical approaches, including pharmacotherapy, behavior modification, physical activity, and diet, have been disappointingly unsuccessful in producing sustained weight loss (National Institutes of Health Technology Assessment Conference Panel 1993). However, a 5 to 10% weight loss is considered medically significant, resulting in decreased health risks related to obesity and improved physical functioning. Unfortunately, this represents an aesthetically insignificant 15 to 30 lb (7 to 14 kg) to a 300-lb (136-kg) individual who is considered morbidly obese (National Institutes of Health 1998). The isolation of the obese gene and protein leptin in the ob/ob mouse provided a simplistic model for obesity etiology and treatment; however, humans appear to be more complex and resistant to the central-acting weight reduction qualities of leptin (Erickson, Hollopeter, and Palmiter 1996; Montague et al. 1997; Zhang et al. 1994). Exercise, traditional or fad diets, medications, surgery, and gene therapy have not demonstrated long-term effectiveness.

Prevalence Projections and Impact on the United States

Despite considerable attention and resources dedicated to the obesity epidemic, prevalence continues to rise and escalate health concerns (Flegal et al. 1998; WHO 1998). (The most recent overweight and obesity projections are discussed later in this chapter.) In support of this accelerating trend, examination of the third U.S. National Health and Nutrition Examination Survey (NHANES III 1998) and the most recent NHANES is enlightening. For example, approximately 54% of U.S. adults were considered overweight (BMI ≥25) and 22% (nearly 30 million people) were obese (BMI ≥30) (Flegal et al. 1998; WHO 1998). More recently, Flegal and colleagues (2002) reported that the age-adjusted prevalence of obesity was 30.5% in 1999, while the prevalence of overweight increased to 64.5%. Since NHANES II (1980), American adults have gained nearly 3.6 kg (7.9 lb) in mean body weight, and the prevalence of obesity has increased from 14.4 to 30.5%. Prior to NHANES III, the increase between each of the first three national surveys was a mere one percentage point. Thus, the growing obesity epidemic requires new thinking about treatment options.

Future Trends in Obesity Management

Obesity is increasing at alarming rates in the United States and the rest of the world. Based on past secular trends in the United States, Foreyt and Goodrick (1995) predicted that the whole U.S. population would be overweight by 2230. However, given the rapidly increasing rate of overweight (approximately 1% per year), we now predict that the entire U.S. population will be overweight by 2040 and obese by 2100. Given the extent of this problem, new ideas will be needed to address the obesity epidemic. In the rest of this chapter, we will review future directions for better managing obesity and trends we believe strongly influence the increasing prevalence.

Defining Broader Treatment Outcomes

A primary goal of obesity treatment must be to modify patients' beliefs about appropriate weight loss and improve their health status and quality of life, rather than just focusing on weight loss. For example, using patients' definitions of ideal and overweight, 82.3% of men and 95.1% of women were heavier than what they considered ideal; however, their definitions were incongruent with current recommendations (Crawford and Campbell 1999). Additionally, obese women in an obesity treatment study considered a 32% reduction in weight a success, which is substantially different from the 5 to 10% medically recommended loss typically produced by current treatments (Foster et al. 1997). Such evidence points to a need for restructuring the measurement of successful weight loss. Frustration with unreachable weight loss goals often leads clients to quit despite medical improvements.

Researchers, much like dieters, historically have viewed successful obesity treatments by the amount of pounds or kilograms lost. This primarily aesthetic goal focuses on health outcomes (e.g., reduced blood pressure and lipids) as a by-product, rather than as the primary target for treatment. As few weight reduction programs produce prolonged results, researchers are questioning the focus on weight loss as the standard indicator of success. Instead, many suggest that broader measures of medical, psychological, and behavioral success would be more meaningful (Atkinson 1993). The goals of future obesity research should focus on the improvement of health, regardless of actual pounds lost (Foreyt 1987).

Society may not be ready to reascribe the success of obesity treatment to anything but improvement in appearance, number of pounds lost, or fitting into the elusive size 6; however, the future of research is likely to focus on the reduction of "normative discontent" and weight obsession, and to use health measurements as indicators of success (Foreyt, Poston, and Goodrick 1996). Monitoring indicative health changes of blood lipids, blood pressure, diabetes, and mood instead of traditional body weight may well encourage clients to continue physical activity regardless of insignificant or unsatisfactory changes in weight.

Current and Future Drug Treatments

Obesity pharmacotherapies generally target appetite reduction and satiation enhancement, increasing energy expenditure, or nutrient partitioning (Bray and Greenway 1999; Haddock et al. 2002; Poston et al. 1998). The most recently FDA-approved drugs for long-term obesity management target fat absorption (orlistat, trade name Xenical) and appetite centers (sibutramine, trade name Meridia).

Orlistat

Orlistat is a pancreatic and gastric lipase inhibitor that prevents absorption of dietary fat in the gastrointestinal tract (Bray and Greenway 1999). The results of a 52-week randomized, double-blind clinical trial demonstrated sustained weight loss, with the treated group losing 8.6 ± 5.4 kg (18.9 ± 11.9 lb) on 120-mg tid, while the placebo group lost 5.5 ± 4.4 kg (12.1 ± 9.7 lb) (James et al. 1997). Davidson and colleagues (1999) found that orlistat-treated patients experienced significant improvements in several health parameters over a two-year period. During the first year, patients treated with 120 mg of orlistat lost more weight (mean $\pm$ SEM, 8.76 ± 0.37 kg or 19.3 ± 0.81 lb) than placebo-treated patients (5.81 ± 0.67 kg or 12.8 ± 1.5 lb) ($p < 0.001$) and regained less weight during year 2 (3.2 ± 0.45 kg or 7.0 ± 0.099 lb; 35.2% regain) than those treated with 60 mg (4.26 ± 0.57 kg or 9.4 ± 1.3 lb; 51.3% regain) or placebo (5.63 ± 0.42 kg or 12.4 ± 0.92 lb; 63.4% regain) in year 2 ($p < 0.001$). Viewed as percentages, 65.7% and 38.9% of orlistat-treated patients lost 5% and 10% of initial body weight, compared to only 43.6% and 24.8% of placebo patients, respectively. By the end of the second year, 34.1% of patients receiving orlistat maintained a 10% weight loss compared to only 17.5% of placebo patients. Treatment with orlistat also was associated with improvements in cardiovascular and diabetes risk factors including total cholesterol, low-density lipoproteins, and insulin levels (Davidson et al. 1999; Finer et al. 2000).

Similar results were reported in a two-year European trial (Sjöström et al. 1998; Rössner et al. 2000). After one year of treatment, 9.3% of orlistat-treated patients lost more than 20% of initial body weight versus only 2.1% who lost the same amount of weight in the placebo group. After two years of continuous treatment, 57.1% of orlistat patients maintained a weight loss of greater than 5%, while only 37.4% of placebo patients met this criterion. Orlistat also has been studied in obese patients with type 2 diabetes. In a one-year randomized, double-blind study of obese diabetic patients, the orlistat group lost 6.2 ± 0.45% (M $\pm$ SEM) of initial body weight versus 4.3 ± 0.49% in the placebo group (Hollander et al. 1998). In addition, these diabetic patients treated with orlistat plus diet showed significant improvements in HbA_{1c}, fasting plasma glucose, dosage reductions of sulfonylurea drugs, and lipid parameters (total cholesterol, low-density-lipoprotein [LDL] cholesterol, triglycerides [TG], apolipoprotein B, and the LDL to HDL ratio) when compared to patients treated with placebo plus diet (Hollander et al. 1998). Side effects of orlistat are minimal and primarily gastrointestinal (e.g., oily spotting, fecal urgency, fecal incontinence, flatus with discharge, fatty and oily stool, oily evacuation, and increased defecation) (Davidson et al. 1999; Rössner et al. 2000; Sjöström et al. 1998) and tend to occur more frequently in patients not adhering to the recommended low-fat (30% of calories from fat) diet (Hollander et al. 1998). Fat-soluble vitamins (A, D, and E) and carotinoids also may be affected, so the drug should be supplemented with a multivitamin (Berke and Morden 2000). Orlistat is contraindicated in patients with chronic malabsorption disorders.

Sibutramine

Sibutramine specifically inhibits the reuptake of norepinephrine and serotonin, thus having both satiating and potential preventive effects on weight-loss-related reductions in metabolism (James et al. 2000; Stock 1997; Van Gaal et al. 1998). Weight losses are dose-dependent and tend to plateau by six months (Bray et al. 1996; Hanotin et al. 1998; Lean 1997; Ryan, Kaiser, and Bray 1995; Seagle et al. 1998; Stock 1997). In a 52-week trial (conducted in the UK), patients receiving the 10-mg and 15-mg doses lost 4.8 kg (10.6 lb) and 6.1 kg (13.4 lb), respectively, while patients taking the placebo lost only 1.8 kg (4.0 lb) (Lean 1997). The proportion of patients who lost at least 5% of initial body weight over 12 months were 56 and 65% in the 10-mg-per-day and 15-mg-per-day groups, respectively, but only 29% in the placebo-treated groups.

A more recent multicenter trial (James et al. 2000) demonstrated similar efficacy. Patients were treated with sibutramine (10 mg per day) for six months during the weight loss phases of the study and then randomized to receive continued treatment or placebo for an 18-month weight maintenance phase. At the end of the study (i.e., 24 months), 43% of patients treated with sibutramine maintained 80% of their initial weight loss as compared to 16% of patients assigned to placebo after the initial weight loss phase. Expressed as percentages, by 24 months, 69% and 46% of sibutramine-maintained patients maintained 5% and 10% weight losses, while substantially fewer met these criteria in the placebo group (e.g., approximately 50% and 20%, respectively).

In addition to weight loss, treatment with sibutramine can result in favorable improvements in many obesity-related comorbidities (James et al. 2000; Van Gaal, Wauters, and De Leeuw 1998). For example, a one-year study using 10 mg per day or 15 mg per day produced significant reductions in waist-to-hip ratio compared to patients treated with placebo (Lean 1997). Sibutramine-induced weight losses also have been found to produce favorable reductions in insulin, HbA_{1c}, triglycerides, total cholesterol, LDL, and VLDL (James et al. 2000; Lean 1997). Finally, researchers have studied sibutramine in ethnic groups including African Americans and Hispanics (Cuellar et al. 2000; McMahon et al. 2000). McMahon and colleagues (2000) found that sibutramine was effective and well tolerated in both Caucasian and African American obesity patients with controlled hypertension. Substantially more sibutramine patients were 5% and 10% responders (40.1% and 13.4%) than placebo-treated patients (8.7% and 4.3%). Small increases in blood pressure were found for both ethnic groups, but both groups also experienced significant improvements in triglycerides, HDL cholesterol, and glucose compared to placebo-treated patients.

Side effects of sibutramine include mean increases of 2 mmHg in systolic and diastolic blood pressure and increases in pulse rate (Berke and Morden 2000). Blood pressure increases may be partially mitigated by sibutramine-related weight losses (Lean 1997). In controlled safety trials, 0.4% of patients treated with sibutramine and 0.4% of placebo patients were discontinued because

of hypertension (systolic blood pressure [SBP] ≥160 mmHg; diastolic blood pressure [DBP] ≥95 mmHg), while 0.4% of sibutramine-treated patients and 0.1% of placebo patients were discontinued because of tachycardia (pulse rate ≥100 bpm). In placebo-controlled trials, the most common side effects were dry mouth, anorexia, insomnia, and constipation. No cases of primary pulmonary hypertension or valvular disease have been reported with sibutramine at this time. Sibutramine should not be taken with other serotonergic drugs (Berke and Morden 2000).

Future Drug Interventions

What other possibilities exist for the future of obesity drug therapies? First, more anti-obesity agents are needed. Potential targets include drugs that agonize or antagonize neurotransmitters, neuropeptides, or hypothalamic peptides that play a role in satiation or hunger, drugs that increase energy expenditure, and drugs that interfere with nutrient absorption. While most early FDA-approved obesity drugs were centrally acting and noradrenergic or serotonergic (e.g., phentermine, diethlypropion, or fenfluramine), future drugs might target dopamine pathways, cholecystokinin, beta-endorphin, uncoupling proteins, leptin, ghrelin or other yet undiscovered pathways in weight regulation (Altman 2002; Bray and Greenway 1999; Crowley et al. 2002; Dhillo and Bloom 2001; Wang et al. 2001). In addition, antiobesity drugs also might develop from treatments for obesity-related conditions. For example, metformin, a pharmacological treatment for type 2 diabetes, has been found to induce significant weight loss and positively impact both obesity- and type 2 diabetes–related complications (e.g., myocardial infarction, mortality) in obese diabetic patients (Genuth 2000; Lee and Morley 1998). Metformin appears to reduce caloric intake in a dose-dependent manner, thus reducing weight and improving insulin sensitivity (Genuth 2000; Lee and Morley 1998).

Another possibility will be the development of more combination drug treatments. While this approach was used very effectively with respect to inducing weight loss (e.g., fenfluramine plus phentermine or ephedrine plus caffeine) (Haddock et al. 2002), significant safety concerns were raised about certain drugs in these combinations (i.e., fenfluramine and ephedrine) (Bray and Greenway 1999; Centers for Disease Control and Prevention 1997b; Haller and Benowitz 2000). Wadden and colleagues (2000) evaluated the addition of orlistat for 16 weeks among patients who had completed one year of treatment with sibutramine. Patients randomized to receive orlistat in addition to sibutramine did not evidence greater weight loss after 16 weeks of combination treatment when compared to patients receiving sibutramine plus placebo. This trial may have been limited by the fact that patients already had lost 11.6% of initial weight over one year, suggesting that there are limits to the amount of weight loss that obesity patients can achieve (Bray and Greenway 1999). Additional drug therapies will be necessary if synergistic drug combinations are to be developed.

Finally, obesity pharmacotherapy may be targeted to at-risk populations for whom lifestyle modification programs may be difficult or impossible, such as organ transplantees and patients with chronic mental illness. For example, pretransplantation obesity is a risk factor for decreased survival, decreased graft survival, and posttransplant complications for patients undergoing kidney and cardiac transplants. Meier-Kriesche and colleagues (1999) found that BMI >25 was an independent risk factor for both decreased graft survival and mortality in patients who had received renal grafts and were followed over several years. Modlin and colleagues (1997) evaluated survival status among 127 obese kidney transplantees, BMI >30, compared to matched controls. Obese patients demonstrated significantly lower five-year survival rates (i.e., 67% versus 89% for matched nonobese controls). In addition, they also experienced higher posttransplant complications and a greater incidence of new onset diabetes than nonobese transplantees. Similarly, obesity appears to negatively affect survival in cardiac transplant patients (Grady et al. 1996). Obese organ transplant patients may benefit from drug therapies prior to undergoing transplantation, and thus have improved chances of graft survival and reduced mortality risk, because physical activity programs and many dietary interventions may be too difficult for these patients.

Another patient population for whom traditional obesity interventions may not be practical are patients with chronic mental illness. For example, both conventional (e.g., thioridazine) and new generation antipsychotics (e.g., clozapine, olanzapine, risperidone) have been associated with weight gains ranging from 2 to almost 5 kg (4.4 to 11 lb) (Allison, Mentore et al. 1999; Wirshing et al. 1999). In addition, young and previously nonobese patients often demonstrate the greatest weight gains (Wetterling and Müßigbrodt 1999). Substantial weight gain among schizophrenic patients may be difficult to treat, even with rigorous diets, and may result in decreased medication adherence and increased risk for obesity-related comorbid disorders such as type 2 diabetes (Hägg et al. 1998; Wetterling and Müßigbrodt 1999; Wirshing et al. 1998).

Obesity Treatment in Primary Care

Primary care–based treatment approaches for many lifestyle-related health problems, such as tobacco use and hypertension, are standard of care (Alexander 1998; Jorenby and Fiore 1999). Many health organizations now realize the importance of addressing obesity as a health issue in primary care settings, suggesting that primary health care providers should develop obesity intervention skills and be active in identifying overweight and obese patients, providing weight loss treatments, and monitoring outcomes (Fontaine and Bartlett 2000; Gill and Carter 1999; National Health Service 1997). Because obese patients seen in primary care settings often are presenting for other less stigmatized and more socially acceptable conditions (e.g., diabetes, cardiovascular disease), intervention in this context represents an ideal "teachable moment" for providing obesity interventions.

Primary health care providers now have several resources available to them to guide their interventions including guidelines published by the World Health Organization and the National Heart, Lung, and Blood Institute of the National Institutes of Health (Anderson and Wadden 1999; Foreyt and Pendleton 2000; National Institutes of Health 1998; World Health Organization 1998). Preliminary research suggests that with adequate training, primary care physicians can increase how often they intervene with obese patients and learn relevant counseling skills (Simkin-Silverman and Wing 1997).

Wadden and colleagues (1997) demonstrated that obese patients could be treated successfully in a primary care office setting during a typical patient visit. In this study, they compared a combination of brief, individual lifestyle modification and pharmacotherapy to traditional group-based counseling. Obese patients were randomized to the primary care intervention, that is, treatment in a physician's office setting in 15- to 20-minute sessions for 52 weeks (10 office visits total) or thirty-two 75-minute group sessions led by a nutritionist. At the end of one year, patients treated with brief physician visits achieved similar weight losses as those treated in a traditional behavioral modification group program (13.9 ± 9.6 kg or 30.6 ± 21.1 lb versus 15.4 ± 7.9 kg or 33.9 ± 17.4 lb). The brief treatment also was associated with highly significant improvements in several cardiovascular risk factors, including lipids and lipoproteins.

Obesity Prevention: Addressing the Obesogenic Environment

Several authors have commented on the importance of the environment in the etiology of obesity (Crocket and Sims 1995; Hill and Peters 1998; Poston and Foreyt 1999; Richter et al. 2000; Simons-Morton et al. 1988; Swinburn, Egger, and Raza 1999). Our environment is no longer conducive to maintaining healthy weights; instead, it promotes gluttonous food consumption and discourages physical activity (Poston and Foreyt 1999).

Within the last 10 years, for example, branded lunches have been incorporated into many school cafeterias and National School Lunch Programs (NSLP), including fast-food options by some of the nation's largest franchises (e.g., Arby's, Burger King, McDonald's, Papa John's, Pizza Hut, Subway, and Taco Bell) (Gullo 1999; Gwartney 1998; Shorter 1997). While no studies have been conducted on the number of NSLP schools that provide branded fast food to students, it is likely that they tend toward high-fat, low-nutritional-value lunches—a far cry from Harry Truman's initial hopes for NSLP to provide nutritional options at subsidized prices. According to Subway's national account manager for the school lunch program, in 1997 the franchise managed 1,492 catered and 24 on-site programs in NSLP public schools (Shorter 1997).

Thus, abundant availability of fast food in educational settings that provide less physical and health education inadvertently supports an obesity-promoting environment (Pearman, Thatcher, and Valois 2000).

Healthy behaviors encouraged throughout childhood are more likely to carry over to adulthood, reducing the prevalence of obesity (Centers for Disease Control and Prevention 1997a; Iverson et al. 1985). Despite the increasing awareness of obesity as a nationwide epidemic, many children are not receiving adequate physical education classes. When faced with budget cuts, schools often cut extracurricular sports and physical education classes (Davis 2000; "School closings" 1998). For example, South Carolina legislation dictates that high school students attend only two semesters of health and physical education during high school (South Carolina Department of Education 1998), but the American Alliance for Health, Physical Education, Recreation and Dance (AAHPERD) recommends that high school students receive 225 minutes a week in health or physical education each year (1998). Thus, it is likely that the availability of energy-dense fast foods, increased portion sizes, high-fat diets, and sedentary behavior all have contributed to the rapid increase in obesity prevalence over the last several decades (Poston and Foreyt 1999).

Portion Sizes

Portion sizes have increased dramatically, doubling, tripling, and in some cases quadrupling the RDA-suggested serving size (see table 18.1) (Hill and Peters 1998). Portion sizes for meat served in restaurants is often two to three times larger than the USDA standard serving (i.e., 3 oz or 85 g) and can be as high as 22 to 38 oz (623 to 1,077 g) for one person. Some restaurants offer "it's free if you can eat it" 64-oz (1,814-g) steak specials similar to the scene in *The Great Outdoors*, where the obese John Candy gorges himself on 96 oz (almost 3 kg) of beef (gristle included) (Lenfant and Ernst 1994). While a standard serving for popped popcorn is 3 c and for soda 12 oz, a typical small movie theater popcorn consists of 5 c, a large popcorn 16 c, and soda servings can be large as 64 oz (Young and Nestle 1995).

Many restaurants and fast-food franchises offer inexpensive "supersized" portions that

Table 18.1

Nutrition Facts

Item	Suggested serving	Calories	Calories from fat	Total fat (g)	Percent Daily Value*	Saturated fat (g)	Percent Daily Value*
Fries, USDA serving size	50 g (10 fries)	158	74.7	8.3	12.7	2.5	12.5
Small fries	68 g	210	90	10	15	1.5	9
Supersized fries	176 g	540	230	26	40	4.5	23
Soda, USDA serving size	8 oz	100	0	0	0	0	0
Small soda	12 oz	150	0	0	0	0	0
Large soda	44 oz	550	0	0	0	0	0
Super Big Gulp™	64 oz	800	0	0	0	0	0
Popcorn (popped), USDA serving	1 c (11 g)	60	30	3.3	0.5	0.7	3
Small popcorn	3 c (42 g)	150	70	7	11	6	6
Large popcorn	16 c + free refills	664	310	31	47	27	28

* Percent Daily Value based on 2,000-calorie diet.

contain anywhere from two to three times the number of calories of the regular-size portion (Hill and Peters 1998). McDonald's coined the phrase "Super Size™," offering portions 2.5 times larger than the recommended RDA portions (the size of their small order of fries, which is not even listed as available).

The Outback Steakhouse offers a giant-size steak and fries dinner that contains 2,060 calories (nearly three times more calories than the regular-size portion) and Cinnabon offers a grande cinnamon bun with almost eight times the calories of the regular-size bun (800 versus 109 calories) (Fumento 1997). Chipolte Grill, a franchise specializing in burritos, offers a southwestern chicken burrito that contains 1,800 calories, weighs 1.72 lb (0.78 kg), and is 28 mm wide and 47 mm long.

Chain ice cream establishments offer low-fat and nonfat versions, but their most popular sellers are large portions that are sometimes four times larger than the RDA recommendation of one scoop. Free refills and all-you-can-eat buffets encourage financially savvy and increasingly large Americans to continue eating at the expense of their weight (see table 18.2).

While nutritional labeling has increased consumer awareness of food content, Young and Nestle contend that some labels may consistently underestimate the amount of calories contained in the product (see table 18.3) (Young and Nestle 1995). Randomly selected single-serving packaged baked goods provided an underestimation of the food weight (and caloric content) by mean differences of 14% (brownies), 16% (muffins), and 21% (cookies). Such measurement errors can account for 100 to 175 additional calories than the packaging claims, resulting in an unknown increase in caloric intake (Young and Nestle 1995). This trend in increasing portion sizes has likely played a key role in the reported increases in caloric intake over the last several decades (Life Sciences Research Office 1995; Putnam and Allshouse 1999; U.S. Department of Agriculture 1997).

Fat and Sugar Substitutes

Cheap vegetable oils and fats have made high-fat diets available to all socioeconomic classes (Drenowski and Popkin 1997). In the last 10 years, for example, the total caloric consumption per person has increased nearly 200 kcal per day (Allred 1995; Lenfant and Ernst 1994; Stephen and Wald 1990). While it is encouraging that percentage of calories consumed from fat have decreased or leveled off, grams of total fat and saturated fat may have increased over the last 5 to 10 years at the expense of nutrition (Lichtenstein et al. 1998; U.S. Department of Agriculture 1998).

In response to consumer desire for reduced-fat or nonfat foods, manufacturers often replace fat with sugar to ensure palatability; however, these modified foods often contain greater energy density than the original fat-containing foods they are meant to replace (Hill and Peters 1998). An appealing alternative for both consumers and the food industry are foods that maintain palatability and price, but have lower energy density than the original (Seidell 1999). Designer fats, such as olestra, a nondigestible, noncaloric fat substitute, are being used in snack foods because they are not metabolized and are

Table 18.2   *Economic Savings Associated With Supersizing*

Item	Price	Price/ suggested wt (oz)	Price/actual wt (oz)
Fries			
Small	$0.99	$0.41	$0.37
Supersized	$1.79	$0.29	$0.26
Soda			
Can (12 oz)	$0.69	$0.06	$0.06
Big Gulp™ (44 oz)	$0.89	$0.02	$0.02
Super Big Gulp™ (64 oz)	$0.99	$0.02	$0.02
Popcorn			
Small	$1.99	$0.11	$0.08
Large	$3.99	$0.05	$0.04

Table 18.3   *Inaccurate Serving Sizes*

Item	Suggested serving size	Actual serving size	Percentage disparity
Fries, USDA serving	10 fries		
Small fry	68 g/2.4 oz	76.5 g/2.7 oz	11.40%
Supersized	176 g/6.2 oz	192.8 g/6.8 oz	10.90%
Popcorn, USDA serving	1c/11 g		
Small popcorn	42 g/1.8 oz	70.8 g/2.5 oz	13.9%
Large popcorn	224 g/7.9 oz	238.0 g/8.4 oz	10.6%

excreted unmodified (Akoh 1995; Blackburn 1996).

The additional option of technologically reduced-fat products is not without caveat. Such foods may contain just as many calories as the full-fat product (Seidell 1999). Consumers purchasing such products to maintain weight loss or prevent weight gain must be educated against this marketing misconception. Advertisements and labeling within the food industries should be changed accordingly to reflect honest knowledge of products. The food industry should be a partner, not a competitor, in promoting healthy diets and preventing obesity. In addition to spending money and energy on technologically advanced fat alternatives, food manufacturers should be encouraged to use their marketing expertise to develop, promote, and provide more nutritionally dense food choices (World Health Organization 1990) rather than just promoting high calorie foods. For example, in 52.5 hours of television, for example, six stations presented 9,997 commercials, 56% of which advertised food. Of those food commercials, 43% were for products of high-fat oil and sugar content, 37% were for cereal and canned pasta, and only 4% were for milk products, mostly milk and yogurt (Black and Knauer 1991; Kotz and Story 1994).

Physical Activity

According to the Report of the Surgeon General (U.S. Department of Health and Human Services 1996), only 60% of the adult population in the United States is physically active, and 25% percent is completely sedentary, although there are some subgroup differences. For example, men are more physically active than women, and Caucasians are more active than are African Americans, Hispanics, and people classified as "other." The lowest percentage of physical activity is found in people with incomes less than $10,000. Education is another factor associated with physical activity; that is, people who tend to be the most active are those who have had at least 16 years of education (college graduates), while those in the lowest activity category tend to have only some high school education (U.S. Department of Health and Human Services 1996). Thus, the most physically active people seem to be Caucasian males in higher socioeconomic and education categories (U.S. Department of Health and Human Services 1996).

Physical activity alone is generally insufficient for weight loss; however, the combination of a healthy diet and an active lifestyle are the main contributing factors to maintaining any weight loss (Pavlou, Krey, and Steffee 1989; Skender et al. 1996). There are many potential mechanisms by which activity may influence weight loss and maintenance, including increased fat-free mass, elevated resting metabolic rate, increased concentrations of metabolic hormones, decreased preference for high-fat foods, energy expenditure associated with the recovery process, increased cycling of substrates, and improved psychological well-being (Ballor, Poehlman, and Toth 1998). However, comprehensive weight control programs combining diet modification with increased exercise and other lifestyle changes often are more effective in producing significant weight loss in people with mild to moderate obesity than diets alone (Grilo 1997).

One of the best examples of weight loss maintenance associated with physical activity is a classic study of overweight civil servants including policemen in Boston (Pavlou, Krey, and Steffee 1989), in which some of the participants were assigned to a diet-only treatment while others were assigned to a diet-and-exercise treatment. At the end of the treatment period, both groups had lost significantly more weight than the control group. There was a slight (but not statistically significant) difference in weight between the two experimental groups; weight loss was greater in the group engaging in exercise.

The most interesting findings were the results of the 8- and 18-month follow-ups. At 8 months, approximately 81% of the participants in the diet-and-exercise group were still exercising and had regained none of the lost weight. The other 19% of participants reported no continued exercise and had regained almost all of the weight they had lost. Participants in the diet-only group had returned quickly to baseline weight; however, 4 of the original 56 participants in the diet-only group began an exercise program at the end of the intervention. These 4 actually continued to lose a small amount of weight. At 18 months the same trend was observed; that is, the individuals in the diet-and-exercise group who had continued to exercise had maintained their weight loss, as did those in the diet-only group who had crossed over and begun exercising. Nonexercisers in the diet-only group had regained their weight, as did subjects in the diet-and-exercise group who had quit exercising.

There are two main types of physical activity, and each may offer its own health benefits. Resistance training (e.g., weightlifting) has gained appeal because it increases muscular strength, preserves fat-free mass, and increases daily expenditure (Ballor, Poehlman, and Toth 1998). The American College of Sports Medicine recommends performing strength-developing activities at least twice a week (U.S. Department of Health and Human Services 1996). Aerobic activity, according to the U.S. Surgeon General's Report on Physical Activity (U.S. Department of Health and Human Services 1996), is defined as "training that improves the efficiency of aerobic energy-producing systems and that can improve cardiorespiratory endurance" (p. 21). The American College of Sports Medicine now recommends that all people should accu-

mulate at least 30 minutes of endurance-type physical activity, of at least moderate intensity (equivalent to walking 3 to 4 mph), on most, but preferably all, days of the week (U.S. Department of Health and Human Services 1996). It is important to note the addition of the word *accumulate*. Unfortunately, only approximately 22% of American adults meet these recommendations for physical activity. More recently, the Institute of Medicine (IOM 2002) recommended that all Americans accumulate at least one hour of physical activity each day.

Regular physical activity confers substantial health benefits in terms of reducing the risk of mortality and morbidity. For example, Barlow and colleagues (1995) found that moderately and highly fit men, regardless of BMI, experienced significantly lower age-adjusted risk for all-cause mortality compared to sedentary or low-fit men. In particular, men with BMIs between 27 and 30 and with BMIs greater than 30 who were moderately to highly fit experienced from 30 to 60% of the risk for all-cause mortality of low-fit men in any BMI category.

Similarly, Wei and colleagues (1999) found that low cardiorespiratory fitness (using age-specific cutoff points from maximal treadmill testing) was independently associated with both all-cause and cardiovascular-related mortality among normal weight, overweight, and obese adults. For example, using active, normal weight individuals as the reference group (RR = 1.00), the relative risk of cardiovascular disease-related mortality (RR; 95% confidence interval) was 3.1 (2.2-4.5), 4.5 (3.4-6.0), and 5.0 (3.6-7.0) greater among low-fit normal weight, overweight, and obese participants, respectively. The moderately-to-highly-fit groups experienced lower mortality risk, (1.5 [1.1-2.0] for overweight, 1.6 [1.0-2.8] for obese), suggesting that cardiorespiratory fitness mitigates much of the mortality risk associated with obesity. The same BMI-related gradient was found for all-cause mortality except that the magnitude of the risk ratios was somewhat smaller (i.e., ranging from 2.2 to 3.1) (Wei et al. 1999). These data support the notion of "healthy obesity" or metabolic fitness, that is, individuals who are clinically obese, but physically active with minimal obesity-related health risk (Donnelly et al. 2000; Tremblay et al. 1999).

Numerous studies (Blair et al. 1995; Stofan et al. 1998; Wannamethee, Shaper, and Walker 1998) also have demonstrated that physical activity can reduce morbidity. Physical activity may reduce the risk of developing illnesses such as cardiovascular disease (CVD), coronary heart disease (CHD), hypertension, high cholesterol, colon cancer, type 2 diabetes, obesity, and mental health problems (Barlow et al. 1995; Giovannucci et al. 1995; Helmrich et al. 1991; Sandvik et al. 1993; Stofan et al. 1998; U.S. Department of Health and Human Services 1996; Wannamethee, Shaper, and Walker 1998). It is important to note that studies have found that even one bout of physical activity can result in an improved blood lipid profile that may last for days (Durstine and Haskell 1994).

Another benefit physical activity may offer is the positive distribution of body fat (U.S. Department of Health and Human Services 1996). Physical activity also has been shown to have a beneficial effect on relieving symptoms of depression and anxiety, improving mood and psychological well-being, increasing satisfaction with life, and decreasing anger (Bahrke and Morgan 1978; Camacho et al. 1991; Farmer et al. 1988; Gauvin and Spence 1996; Peturzzello et al. 1991; Rejeski, Brawley, and Shumaker 1996; Ross and Hayes 1988; Stephens 1988; U.S. Department of Health and Human Services 1996; Weyerer 1992).

Increasing lifestyle activity may offer similar health benefits as regular aerobic activity, even when accumulated in brief bouts (U.S. Department of Health and Human Services 1996). Lifestyle activity includes many common activities that people can easily do every day such as climbing stairs, parking farther from the door at work or the store, increasing housework or yard work, and brisk walking. Because such activities are more accessible and cheaper, and foster greater independence in the exercise regimen, they can provide important opportunities for increasing physical activity for obese patients. Dunn and colleagues (1999) noted that lifestyle physical intervention is as effective as structured exercise programs in increasing physical activity, increasing cardiorespiratory fitness, lowering blood pressure, and improving body composition. In addition, Andersen and colleagues (1999) found that obese women who were treated with a 16-week lifestyle intervention

program experienced similar weight losses when compared to women who received a more traditional aerobic exercise program (i.e., 7.9 ± 4.2 kg or 17.4 ± 9.2 lb versus 8.3 ± 3.8 kg or 18.3 ± 8.4 lb, respectively). In addition, at a one-year follow-up, women in the lifestyle program experienced less weight regain than those in the aerobic program, suggesting that benefits were more sustainable (Andersen et al. 1999). Thus, lifestyle interventions may offer easier adherence, as they do not require radical life changes, but small adjustments to daily activities. Encouraging activities that patients enjoy reinforces the idea that exercise should promote health instead of weight loss.

Reducing sedentary behavior also has produced promising results (Epstein and Roemmich 2001). For example, Epstein and colleagues (2002) recently evaluated the results of an intervention aimed at reducing sedentary behavior, rather than focusing on increasing activity, in a within-subjects crossover study. Families were provided inducements for reducing their sedentary behavior (e.g., television watching, playing video games, etc.) by at least 25 or 50% and attended three meetings that provided instruction on reinforcement and stimulus control strategies for reducing sedentary behavior. During the phase of the study focused on reducing sedentary behavior, participants reduced targeted sedentary behaviors by 53% from baseline.

Similarly, Robinson's (1999) randomized controlled trial focused solely on reducing television watching in intervention schools in one school district and found statistically significant relative decreases in BMI, triceps skinfold thickness, waist circumference, and waist-to-hip ratio. Specifically, he found that treated children experienced a -0.45 kg/m^2 reduction in BMI relative to children in the control group (Robinson 1999). This is the first study to test the causal relationship of television viewing and obesity directly and represents the strongest evidence to date that reducing television watching may help decrease obesity and childhood obesity in particular.

In conclusion, lifestyle activity programs and interventions focused on reducing sedentary behavior may offer obese patients the most promise in the future. This is because they are easier behavior changes to sustain, and in the case of reducing sedentary behavior, require little preparation, special equipment, or other considerations that are common for more traditional physical activity programs. Future research should focus on expanding these interventions to high-risk populations such as ethnic minority groups and individuals for whom traditional physical activity programs are not a practical option. In addition, because the sedentary behavior–reducing interventions focused on children, future research should address their application to adults.

Gene and Lifestyle or Environmental Interactions

Biological factors play a role in the etiology of obesity; however, none of the numerous genetic loci that have been identified and associated with obesity act in a simple Mendelian fashion (Bouchard 1994; Bouchard and Pérusse 1998; Comuzzie and Allison 1998). Genes increase our susceptibility to obesity, but none appear to be necessary or sufficient for obesity to manifest itself (Bouchard 1995). Genes may influence obesity by interacting with different environmental or lifestyle factors and result in individual and population differences in energy intake or expenditure, taste preferences (particularly for fats or vegetables), and muscle fiber and metabolic characteristics, thus helping to explain the differences in obesity prevalence found in genetically similar populations living in different environments (Comuzzie and Allison 1998; Goran and Weinsier 2000).

Fox and colleagues (1998) examined resting metabolic rate in rural Mexican Pima Indians who had not been exposed to affluent Western diets, in contrast to Pima Indians in Arizona, and compared them to non-Pima Mexicans in the same environment. They found no differences in plasma leptin or resting metabolic rate between the two groups, suggesting that Pima Indians are not more likely to exhibit genetic characteristics that increase their risk for obesity, at least with respect to leptin and resting metabolic rate. Esparza and colleagues (2000) compared energy expenditure in rural Mexican (mean weight = 66 ± 13 kg or 145 ± 29 lb) and U.S. Pima Indians (mean weight = 93 ± 22 kg or 205 ± 48 lb) and found that Mexican Pimas were significantly more physically active and exhibited higher total energy expenditure and energy expenditure adjusted for

body weight. These data suggest that differences in activity level are important factors in the etiology of obesity in U.S. Pima Indians.

Luke and colleagues (2000) evaluated resting energy expenditure in African Americans and Nigerians. While they did not study any specific genes, they found that the relationship between resting metabolic rate and fat-free mass was identical in both groups even though they found striking differences in BMI and percent body fat. African Americans (mean BMI = 31.4 and 27.7; percent obese = 51.3% and 35.4% for women and men, respectively) were substantially heavier than Nigerians (mean BMI = 23.3 and 21.6; percent obese = 5.3% and 4.0% in women and men, respectively) and had greater body fat percentage.

Similarly, Poston and colleagues (2001) studied first-generation African immigrants and African Americans and found significant differences in BMI (27.3 versus 30.2) and hypertension prevalence (33.1% versus 42.8%) even though the populations were genetically similar with respect to several loci thought to play a role in obesity and hypertension (e.g., G-protein 825, AGT-235, ACE I/D). In addition, BMI and hypertension prevalence in the African immigrants was intermediate to that reported for African Americans and Africans living in African nations (Cooper et al. 1997; Kaufman et al. 1996), suggesting that environmental and lifestyle differences between Africa and the United States substantially contribute to the greater obesity risk among African Americans. Thus, the interaction between "thrifty" genes that conferred survival advantages at one point in human evolution and an environment that now is overabundant in food and sedentary activities is the primary factors increasing risk for obesity and related diseases (Eaton et al. 1988).

Because the environment appears to play such a strong role in the rapidly increasing obesity trends in both developed and developing nations (Poston and Foreyt 1999), research that systematically investigates the determinants and distribution of environmental risk factors is needed. For example, area of residence may influence health behaviors and body weight through several potential mechanisms. Neighborhood factors and socioeconomic status likely influence food shopping practices and food choices (i.e., health behaviors that mediate the relationship between the physical environment and obesity prevalence) (French et al. 2001). Lower income neighborhoods have fewer fruits and vegetables and more foods high in fat available than higher income neighborhoods (Sooman et al. 1993). Lower income neighborhoods also have greater density of fast-food outlets and fewer grocery stores (Morland et al. 2002). Thus, future research and policy initiatives will need to focus on how these types of environmental factors can be practically modified in order to reduce the incidence of obesity. For example, it has been suggested that the sales of soft drinks, candy bars, and other foods with low nutritional value should be banned in schools (Nestle 2002). Recently, the city of Los Angeles banned the sale of sodas in public schools after 2004. Future research will be needed to document the impact of policy suggestions and implementations of such bans.

Economic Costs of Obesity

Obesity is estimated to account for approximately 280,000 deaths per year (nearly 14%) in the United States (Allison, Fontaine et al. 1999; McGinnis and Foege 1993). Similarly, there are consistent reports of a significant linear relationship between BMI and all-cause mortality risk (Linstead and Singh 1998; National Institutes of Health 1998). Although some studies indicate a curvilinear association between BMI and mortality, it is likely the result of increased health risks among underweight individuals (BMI <18.5) because of smoking or significant weight loss related to a chronic medical condition (Linstead and Singh 1998). The adverse medical and psychosocial consequences of obesity result in significant health care costs. Thompson and colleagues (1999) estimated an additional increase of $10,000 in medical care costs for five diseases affected by obesity. Sturm (2002) reported that the effects of obesity on reductions in the health-related quality of life, and increased health care and medication costs, were larger than those seen with smoking or alcoholism. Between 0.89% and 4.32% of total U.S. health care costs or $99.2 billion U.S. dollars (in 1995) can be attributed to obesity (Allison, Fontaine et al. 1999; Wolf and Colditz 1998). Given the current trends of rapidly increasing obesity prevalence in adults and children, health care costs associated with obesity also will likely increase progressively and become a larger portion of health care costs.

Summary

The development of new obesity treatments will be challenging and rewarding as we gain more knowledge about the molecular and environmental basis of obesity and how this information can be applied to new interventions (Pi-Sunyer 2000). We believe that a larger arsenal of pharmacotherapies addressing a variety of molecular targets will improve the management of obesity. In addition, better treatment delivery will occur by placing obesity within a primary care context and training primary care physicians in obesity management. Current primary care physicians should review the National Institutes of Health (1998) treatment guidelines and become familiar with treatment outcomes associated with behavioral, dietary, physical activity, medical, and surgical interventions. However, these improvements are not likely to stem the obesity epidemic because their focus is on already affected individuals.

Much more importance must be given to the environmental basis of obesity and examining interactions between biological risk factors and our lifestyles. Greater emphasis should be placed on systematically evaluating the frequency and geography of specific environmental obesity risk factors for different populations. In addition, understanding how specific genotypes interact with lifestyle and environmental factors also should grow in importance. Once these factors are better understood, policy level interventions can be implemented and studied.

Parents and community leaders will need to be made more aware of their role in obesity prevention. Schools could be pressed to provide adequate nutrition and opportunities for physical activity, as well as to educate students about the need for both in leading a healthy life. School-based intervention programs can have positive behavioral changes in the dietary habits and physical activity levels of children that will reinforce health behaviors into adulthood (Gortmaker et al. 1999). Educators must fight to keep daily physical activity programs in schools and to partner with the community and parents to involve children in after-school recreational programs.

Additionally, parents must be made aware of the influence model behavior can play on encouraging children to consume healthy snacks, avoid sugar-based cereals, and replace television and video games with outdoor activities. Adults will have to make changes in their own physical and eating patterns and avoid relying on labor-saving devices such as escalators, remote controls, automobiles, power-driven lawn mowers, and other devices. Only by first making changes in our personal environments and then addressing broader societal practices will we be able to begin to counter the effects of the obesogenic environment.

References

Akoh, C.C. 1995. Lipid based fat substitutes. *Crit. Rev. Food Sci. Nutr.* 35: 405-430.

Alexander, L.M. 1998. Guidelines for hypertension treatment: Applications for primary care practice—A review of the JNC VI Report. *Lippincott's Primary Care Practice* 2: 485-497.

Allison, D.B., Fontaine, K.R., Manson, J.E., Stevens, J., and VanItallie, T.B. 1999. Annual deaths attributable to obesity in the United States. *JAMA* 282 (16): 1530-1538.

Allison, D.B., Mentore, J.L., Moonseng, H., Chandler, L.P., Cappelleri, J.C., Infante, M.C., and Weiden, P.J. 1999. Antipsychotic-induced weight gain: A comprehensive research synthesis. *Am. J. Psychiatry* 156: 1686-1696.

Allred, J.B. 1995. Too much of a good thing? An overemphasis on eating low-fat foods may be contributing to the alarming increase in overweight among U.S. adults. *J. Am. Diet. Assoc.* 95: 417-418.

Altman, J. 2002. Weight in the balance. *Neuroendocrinol* 76: 131-136.

American Alliance for Health, Physical Education, Recreation and Dance (AAHPERD). 1998. *Shape of the nation.* Reston, VA: American Alliance for Health, Physical Education, Recreation and Dance: 1-5.

Andersen, R.E., Wadden, T.A., Bartlett, S.J., Zemel, B., Verde, T.J., and Franckowiak, S.C. 1999. Effect of lifestyle activity vs. structured aerobic exercise in obese women: A randomized trial. *JAMA* 281: 335-340.

Anderson, D.A., and Wadden, T.A. 1999. Treating the obese patient: Suggestions for primary care practice. *Arch. Fam. Med.* 8: 156-167.

Atkinson, R.L. 1993. Propose standards for judging the success of the treatment of obesity. *Ann. Intern. Med.* 119: 677-680.

Bahrke, M.S., and Morgan, W.P. 1978. Anxiety reduction following exercise and meditation. *Cog. Ther. Res.* 2: 323-333.

Ballor, D.L., Poehlman, E.P., and Toth, M.J. 1998. Exercise as a treatment for obesity. In *Handbook of obesity*, eds. G.A. Bray, C. Bouchard, and W.P.T. James. New York: Marcel Dekker.

Barlow, C.E., Kohl, H.W., Gibbons, L.W., and Blair, S.N. 1995. Physical fitness, mortality, and obesity. *Int. J. Obes. Relat. Metab. Disord.* 19: S41-S44.

Berke, E.M., and Morden, N.E. 2000. Medical management of obesity. *Am. Fam. Physician* 62: 419-426.

Black, D.M., and Knauer, S.L. 1991. The legal implications of dietary fats: Risks of cardiovascular disease and the duty of food manufacturers. *J. Nutr.* 121: 578-582.

Blackburn, H. 1996. Olestra and the FDA. *N. Engl. J. Med.* 334: 984-986.

Blair, S.N., Kohl, H.W. III, Barlow, C.E., Paffenbarger, R.S. Jr., Gibbons, L.W., and Macera, C.A. 1995. Changes in physical fitness and all-cause mortality: A prospective study of healthy and unhealthy men. *JAMA* 273: 1093-1098.

Bouchard, C. 1994. Genetics of obesity: Overview and research direction. In *The genetics of obesity*, ed. C.B. Bouchard, 223-233. Boca Raton, FL: CRC Press.

Bouchard, C. 1995. Genetics of obesity: An update on molecular markers. *Int. J. Obes. Relat. Metab. Disord.* 19 (Suppl. 3): S10-S13.

Bouchard, C., and Pérusse, L. 1998. The genetics of human obesity. In *Handbook of obesity*, eds. G.A. Bray, C. Bouchard, W.P.T. James, 157-190. New York: Marcel Dekker.

Bray, G.A., and Greenway, F.L. 1999. Current and potential drugs for treatment of obesity. *Endocr. Rev.* Dec. 20(6): 805-875.

Bray, G.A., Ryan, D.H., Gordon, D. et al. 1996. A double-blind, randomized placebo-controlled trial of sibutramine. *Obes. Res.* 4: 263-270.

Camacho, T.C., Roberts, R.E., Lazarus, N.B. et al. 1991. Physical activity and depression: Evidence from the Alameda County study. *Am. J. Epidemiol.* 134: 220-231.

Centers for Disease Control and Prevention (CDCP). 1997a. Guidelines for school and community programs to promote lifelong physical activity among young people. *MMWR* 46 (No.RR-6).

Centers for Disease Control and Prevention (CDCP). 1997b. Cardiac valvulopathy associated with exposure to fenfluramine or dexfenfluramine: U.S. Department of Health and Human Services Interim Public Health Recommendations, November, 1997. *MMWR* 46: 1061-1066.

Comuzzie, A.G., and Allison, D.B. 1998. The search for human obesity genes. *Science* 280: 1374-1377.

Cooper, R., Rotimi, C., Ataman, S. et al. 1997. The prevalence of hypertension in seven populations of West African origin. *Am. J. Public Health* 87: 160-168.

Crawford, D. and Campbell, K. 1999. Lay definitions of ideal weight and overweight. *Int. J. Obes.* 23: 738-745.

Crockett, S.J., and Sims, L.S. 1995. Environmental influences on children's eating. *J. Prev. Nutr. Educ.* 27: 235-249.

Crowley, V.E., Yeo, G.S., and O'Rahilly, S. 2002. Obesity therapy: Altering the energy intake-and-expenditure balance sheet. *Nature Rev. Drug Discov.* 4: 276-286.

Cuellar, G.E.M., Ruiz, A.M., Monsalve, M.C.R., and Berber, A. 2000. Six-month treatment of obesity with sibutramine 15 mg: A double-blind, placebo-controlled monocenter clinical trial in a Hispanic population. *Obes. Res.* 8: 71-82.

Davidson, M.H., Hauptman, J., DiGirolamo, M., Foreyt, J.P., Halsted, C.H., Heber, D., Heimburger, D.C., Lucas, C.P., Robbins, D.C., Chung, J., and Heymsfield, S.B. 1999. Weight control and risk factor reduction in obese subjects treated for 2 years with orlistat: A randomized controlled trial. *JAMA* 281: 235-242.

Davis, A. 2000. Orchestra taken off list for school budget cuts. *Sentinel.* June 8.

Dhillo, W.S., and Bloom, S.R. 2001. Hypothalamic peptides as drug targets for obesity. *Curr. Opin. Pharmacol.* 1: 651-655.

Donnelly, J.E., Jacobsen, D.J., Heelan, K.S., Seip, R., and Smith, S. 2000. The effects of 18 months of intermittent vs. continuous exercise on aerobic capacity, body weight and composition, and metabolic fitness in previously sedentary, moderately obese females. *Int. J. Obes. Relat. Metab. Disord.* 24: 566-572.

Drenowski, A., and Popkin, B.M. 1997. The nutrition transition: New trends in the global diet. *Nutr. Rev.* 55: 31-43.

Dunn, A.L., Marcus, B.H., Kampert, J.B., Garcia, M.E., Kohl, H.W., and Blair, S.N. 1999. Comparison of lifestyle and structured interventions to increase physical activity and cardiorespiratory fitness: A randomized trial. *JAMA* 281: 327-334.

Durstine, J.L., and Haskell, W.L. 1994. Effects of exercise training on plasma lipids and lipoproteins. *Exerc. Sport Sci. Rev.* 22: 477-521.

Eaton, S.B., Konner, M., and Shostak, M. 1988. Stone agers in the fast land: Chronic degenerative diseases in evolutionary perspective. *Am. J. Med.* 84: 739-749.

Epstein, L.H., Paluch, R.A., Consalvi, A., Riordan, K., and Scholl, T. 2002. Effects of manipulating sedentary behavior on physical activity and food intake. *J. Pediatr.* 140: 334-339.

Epstein, L.H., and Roemmich, J.N. 2001. Reducing sedentary behavior: Role in modifying physical activity. *Exerc. Sport Sci. Rev.* 29: 103-108.

Erickson, J.C., Hollopeter, G., and Palmiter, R.D. 1996. Attenuation of the obesity syndrome of ob/ob mice by the loss of neuropeptide-y. *Science* 274: 1704-1707.

Esparza, J., Fox, C., Harper, I.T., Bennett, P.H., Schulz, L.O., Valencia, M.E., and Ravussin, E. 2000. Daily energy expenditure in Mexican and USA Pima Indians: Low physical activity as a possible cause of obesity. *Int. J. Obes. Relat. Metab. Disord.* 24: 55-59.

Farmer, M.E., Locke, B.Z., Moscicki, E.K. et al. 1988. Physical activity and depressive symptoms: The NHANES I epidemiologic follow-up study. *Am. J. Epidemiol.* 128: 1340-1351.

Finer, N., James, W.P.T., Kopelman, P.G., Lean, M.E.J., and Williams, G. 2000. One-year treatment of obesity: A randomized, double-blind, placebo-controlled, multicentre study of orlistat, a gastrointestinal lipase inhibitor. *Int. J. Obes. Relat. Metab. Disord.* 24: 306-313.

Flegal, K.M., Carroll, M.D., Kuczmarski, R.J. et al. 1998. Overweight and obesity in the United States: Prevalence and trends, 1960-1994. *Int. J. Obes. Relat. Metab. Disord.* 22: 39-47.

Flegal, K.M., Carroll, M.D., Ogden, C.L., and Johnson, C.L. 2002. Prevalence and trends in obesity among U.S. adults, 1999-2000. *JAMA* 288: 1723-1727.

Fontaine, K.R., and Bartlett, S.J. 2000. Access and use of medical care among obese persons. *Obes. Res.* 8: 403-406.

Foreyt, J.P. 1987. Issues in the assessment and treatment of obesity. *J. Consult. Clin. Psychol.* 55: 767-778.

Foreyt, J.P., and Goodrick, G.K. 1995. The ultimate triumph of obesity. *Lancet* 346: 134-135.

Foreyt J.P., and Pendleton V.R. 2000. Management of obesity. *Primary Care Reports* 6: 20-30.

Foreyt, J.P, Poston, W.S.C., and Goodrick, G.K. 1996. Future directions in obesity and eating disorders. *Addict. Behav.* 21: 767-778.

Foster, G.D., Wadden, T.A., Vogt, R.A., and Brewer, G. 1997. What is reasonable weight loss? Patient's expectations and evaluations of obesity treatment outcomes. *J. Consult. Clin. Psychol.* 65: 79-85.

Fox, C.S., Esparza, J., Nicolson, M., Bennett, P.H., Schulz, L.O., Valencia, M.E., and Ravussin, E. 1998.

Is low leptin concentration, a low resting metabolic rate, or both the expression of the "thrifty genotype"? *Am. J. Clin. Nutr.* 68: 1053-1057.

French, S.A., Story, M., and Jeffery, R.W. 2001. Environmental influences on eating and physical activity. *Annu Rev Public Health* 22: 309-335.

Fumento, M. 1997. *The fat of the land. The obesity epidemic and how overweight Americans can help themselves.* New York: Penguin Putnam.

Gauvin, L. and Spence, J.C. 1996. Physical activity and psychological well-being: Knowledge base, current issues, and caveats. *Nutr. Rev.* 54S: S53-S65.

Genuth, S. 2000. Implications of the United Kingdom Prospective Diabetes Study for patients with obesity and type 2 diabetes. *Obes. Res.* 8: 198-201.

Gill, T.P., and Carter, Y.H. 1999. Managing obesity in primary care: Do our patients deserve better? *Br. J. Gen. Pract.* 49: 515-516.

Giovannucci, E., Ascherio, A., Rimm, E.B., Colditz, G.A., Stampfer, M., and Willett, W.C. 1995. Physical activity, obesity, and risk for colon cancer and adenoma in men. *Ann. Intern. Med.* 122: 327-334.

Goran, M.I., and Weinsier, R.L. 2000. Role of environment vs. metabolic factors in the etiology of obesity: Time to focus on the environment. *Obes. Res.* 8: 407-409.

Gortmaker, S.L., Cheung, L.W.Y., Peterson, K.E. et al. 1999. Impact of a school-based interdisciplinary intervention on diet and physical activity among urban primary school children. *Arch. Ped. Adol. Med.* 153: 975-983.

Grady, K.L., Constanzo, M.R., Fisher, S., and Koch, D. 1996. Preoperative obesity is associated with decreased survival after heart transplantation. *J. Heart Lung Transplant* 15: 863-871.

Grilo, C.M. 1997. The role of physical activity in weight loss and weight loss maintenance. *Med. Exerc. Nutr. Health* 4: 60-76.

Gullo, K. 1999. Schools still serving plenty of fast food. *Seattle Times.* March 23.

Gwartney, D. 1998. Student dinning is like football: You Grab 'n' Go to score meal. *The Oregonian.* Nov 18.

Haddock, C.K., Poston, W.S., Dill, P.L., Foreyt, J.P., and Ericsson, M. 2002. Pharmacotherapy for obesity: A quantitative analysis of four decades of published randomized clinical trials. *Int. J. Obes. Relat. Metab. Disord.* 26 (2): 262-273.

Hägg, S., Joelsson, L., Mjörndal, T., Spigset, O., Oja, G., and Dahqvist, R. 1998. Prevalence of diabetes and impaired glucose tolerance in patients treated with clozapine compared with patients treated with conventional depot neuroleptic medications. *J. Clin. Psychiatry* 59: 294-299.

Haller, C.A., and Benowitz, N.L. 2000. Adverse cardiovascular and central nervous system events associated with dietary supplements containing ephedra alkaloids. *N. Engl. J. Med.* 343: 1833-1838.

Hanotin, C., Thomas, F., Jones, S.P. et al. 1998. Efficacy and tolerability of sibutramine in obese patients: A dose-ranging study. *Int. J. Obes. Relat. Metab. Disord.* 22: 32-38.

Helmrich, S.P., Ragland, D.R., Leung, R.W., and Paffenbarger, R.S. 1991. Physical activity and reduced occurrence of non-insulin-dependent diabetes mellitus. *N. Engl. J. Med.* 325: 147-152.

Hill, J.O., and Peters, J.C. 1998. Environmental contributions to the obesity epidemic. *Science* 280: 1371-1374.

Hollander, P.A., Elbein, S.C., Hirsch, I.B., Kelley, D., McGill, J., Taylor, T., Weiss, S.R., Crockett, S.E., Kaplan, R.A., Comstock, J., Lucas, C.P., Lodewick, P.A., Canovatchel, W., Chung, J., and Hauptman, J. 1998. Role of orlistat in the treatment of obese patients with type 2 diabetes. A 1-year randomized double-blind study. *Diabetes Care* 21: 1288-1294.

Iverson, D.C., Fieilding, J.E., Crow, R.S. et al. 1985. The promotion of physical activity in the United States population: The status of programs in medical, worksite, community, and school settings. *Pub. Health Rep.* 100: 212-224.

James, W.P., Avenell, A., Broom, J., and Whitehead, J. 1997. A one-year trial to assess the value of orlistat in the management of obesity. *Int. J. Obes. Relat. Metab. Disord.* 21 (Suppl. 3): S24-S30.

James, W.P.T., Astrup, A., Finer, N., Hilsted, J., Kopelman, P., Rössner, S., Saros, W.H.M., and Van Gaal, L.F. 2000. Effect of sibutramine on weight maintenance after weight loss: A randomized trial. *Lancet* 356: 2119-2125.

Jorenby, D.E., and Fiore, M.C. 1999. The Agency for Health Care Policy and Research smoking cessation practice guidelines: Basics and beyond. *Primary Care; Clinics in Office Practice* 26: 513-528.

Kaufman, J.S., Durazo-Arvizu, R.A., Rotimi, C.N. et al. 1996. Obesity and hypertension prevalence in populations of African origin. *Epidemiology* 7: 398-405.

Kopelman, P.G. 2000. Obesity as a medical problem. *Nature* 404: 635-643.

Kotz, K., and Story, M. 1994. Food advertisements during children's Saturday morning television programming. *J. Amer. Diet. Assoc.* 11: 1926-1929.

Lean, M.E.J. 1997. Sibutramine—A review of clinical efficacy. *Int. J. Obes. Relat. Metab. Disord.* 21: S30-S36.

Lee, A., and Morley, J.E. 1998. Metformin decreases food consumption and induces weight loss in subjects with obesity and type II non-insulin-dependent diabetes. *Obes. Res.* 6: 47-53.

Lenfant, C., and Ernst, N. 1994. Daily dietary fat and total food-energy intakes—Third national Health and Nutrition Examination Survey, Phase 1, 1988-91. *MMWR* 43(7): 116-125.

Lichtenstein, A.H., Kennedy, E., Barrier, P. et al. 1998. Dietary fat consumption and health. *Nutr. Rev.* 56: S3-S28.

Life Sciences Research Office, Federation of American Societies for Experimental Biology. 1995. *Third report on nutrition monitoring in the United States, Vol. 2.* Washington DC: U.S. Government Printing Office.

Lindsted, K.D., and Singh, P.N. 1998. Body mass and 26 year risk of mortality among men who never smoked: A re-analysis among men from the Adventist Mortality Study. *Int. J. Obes. Relat. Metab. Disord.* 22: 544-548.

Luke, A., Rotimi, C.N., Adeyemo, A.A., Durazo-Arvizu, R.A., Prewitt, T.E., Moragne-Kayser, L., Harders, R., and Cooper, R.S. 2000. Comparability of resting energy expenditure in Nigerians and U.S. Blacks. *Obes. Res.* 8: 351-359.

McGinnis, J.M., and Foege, W.H. 1993. Actual causes of death in the United States. *JAMA* 270 (18): 2207-2212.

McMahon, G.F., Fujioka, K., Singh, B.N., Mendel, C.M., Rowe, E., Rolston, K., Johnson, F., and Mooradian, A.D. 2000. Efficacy and safety of sibutramine in obese white and African American patients with hypertension: A 1-year, double-blind, placebo-controlled, multicenter trial. *Arch. Intern. Med.* 160: 2185-2191.

Meier-Kriesche, H.U., Vaghela, M., Thambuganipalle, R., Friedman, G., Jacobs, M., and Kaplan, B. 1999. The effect of body mass index on long-term renal allograft survival. *Transplantation* 68: 1294-1297.

Modlin, C.S., Flechner, S.M., Goormastic, M., Goldfarb, D.A., Papajcik, D., Mastroianni, B., and Novick, A.C. 1997. Should obese patients lose weight before receiving a kidney transplant? *Transplantation* 64: 599-604.

Morland, K., Wing, S., Diez Roux, A., and Poole, C. 2002. Neighborhood characteristics associated with the location of food stores and food service places. *Am J Prev Med* 22(1): 23-29.

Montague, C.T., Farooqui, I.S., Whitehead, J.P., Soos, M.A., Rau, H., Wareham, N.J. et al. 1997. Congenital leptin deficiency is associated with severe early-onset obesity in humans. *Nature* 387: 903-908.

National Health Service (NHS) 1997. Centre for Reviews and Dissemination. The prevention and treatment of obesity. *Effective Health Care* 3: 1-12.

National Institutes of Health (NIH). 1998. Clinical guidelines on the identification, evaluation, and treatment of overweight and obesity in adults—The evidence report. *Obes. Res.* 6: 51S.

National Institutes of Health Technology Assessment Conference Panel. 1993. Methods for voluntary weight loss and control. *Ann. Intern. Med.* 119: 764-770.

National Task Force on Prevention and Treatment of Obesity. 1994. Towards prevention of obesity: Research directions. *Obes. Res.* 2: 571-584.

Nestle, M. 2002. Food politics. How the food industry influences nutrition and health. Berkeley, CA: University of California Press.

Pavlou, K.I.N., Krey, S., and Steffee, W.P. 1989. Exercise as an adjunct to weight loss and maintenance in moderately overweight subjects. *Am. J. Clin. Nutr.* 49: 1115-1123.

Pearman, S.N., Thatcher, W.G., and Valois, R.F. 2000. Nutrition and weight management behaviors: Public and private high school adolescents. *Amer. J. Health Behav.* 23: 220-228.

Peturzzello, S.J., Landers, D.M., Hatfield, B.D. et al. 1991. A meta-analysis on the anxiety-reducing effects of acute and chronic exercise: Outcomes and mechanisms. *Sports Med.* 11: 143-182.

Pi-Sunyer, F.X. 2000. Obesity research and the new century. *Obes. Res.* 8: 1.

Poston, W.S.C., and Foreyt, J.P. 1999. Obesity is an environmental issue. *Atherosclerosis* 146: 201-209.

Poston, W.S.C., Foreyt, J.P., Borrell, L., and Haddock, C.K. 1998. Challenges in obesity management. *South. Med. J.* 1: 710-720.

Poston, W.S.C., Pavlik, V.N., Hyman, D.J., Ogbonnaya, K., Hanis, C.L., Haddock, C.K., Hyder, M.L., and Foreyt, J.P. 2001. Genetic bottlenecks, perceived racism, and hypertension risk among African Americans and first generation African immigrants. *J. Hum. Hypertens.* 15: 341-351.

Putnam, J.J., and Allshouse, J.E. 1999. *Food consumption, prices, and expenditures.* Washington DC.: U.S. Department of Agriculture, Economic Research Service, Statistical Bulletin No. 965.

Rejeski, W.J., Brawley, L.R., and Shumaker, S.A. 1996. Physical activity and health-related quality of life. *Exerc. Sport Sci. Rev.* 24: 71-108.

Richter, K.P., Haris, K.J., Paine-Andrew, A., Fawcett, S.B. et al. 2000. Measuring the health environment for physical activity and nutrition among youth: A review of the literature and applications for community initiatives. *Prev. Med.* 31: S98-111.

Robinson, T.N. 1999. Reducing children's television viewing to prevent obesity: A randomized controlled trial. *JAMA* 282: 1561-1567.

Ross, C.E., and Hayes, D. 1988. Exercise and psychological well being in the community. *Am. J. Epidemiol.* 127: 762-771.

Rössner, S., Sjöström, L., Noack, R., Meinders, E., and Noseda, G. 2000. Weight loss, weight maintenance, and improved cardiovascular risk factors after 2 years treatment with orlistat for obesity. *Obes. Res.* 8: 49-61.

Ryan, D.H., Kaiser, P., and Bray, G.A. 1995. Sibutramine: A novel new agent for obesity treatment. *Obes. Res.* 3 (Suppl. 4): 553S-559S.

Sandvik, L., Erikssen, J., Thaulow, E., Erikssen, G., Mundal, R., and Rodahl, K. 1993. Physical fitness as a predictor of mortality among healthy, middle-aged Norwegian men. *N. Engl. J. Med.* 328: 533-537.

School closings, budget cuts eyed to solve fiscal crisis. 1998. *Milwaukee J. Sentinel,* December 10.

Seagle, H.M., Bessesen, D.H., and Hill, J.O. 1998. Effects of sibutramine on resting metabolic rate and weight loss in overweight women. *Obes. Res.* 6: 115-121.

Seidell, J.C. 1999. Prevention of obesity: The role of the food industry. *Nutr. Metab. Cardiovasc. Dis.* 9: 45-50.

Shorter, N. 1997. Fast food gives area high school students choice. *In Depth: Restaurants & Food Service,* September 26.

Simkin-Silverman, L.R., and Wing, R.R. 1997. Management of obesity in primary care. *Obes. Res.* 5: 603-612.

Simons-Morton, D.G., Simon-Morton, B.G., Parcel, G.S., and Bunker, J.F. 1988. Influencing personal and environmental conditions for community health: A multilevel intervention model. *Fam. Commun. Health* 11: 25-35.

Sjöström, L. 1995. The natural history of massive obesity. *Obes. Res.* 3: 317.

Sjöström, L., Rissanen, A., Andersen, T., Boldrin, M., Golay, A., Koppeschaar, H.P.F., and Krempf, M. 1998. Randomised placebo-controlled trial of orlistat for weight loss and prevention of weight regain in obese patients. *Lancet* 352: 167-172.

Skender, M.L., Goodrick, K., Del Junco, D.J., Reeves, R.S., Darnell, L., Gotto, A.M., and Foreyt, J.P. 1996. Comparison of 2-year weight loss trends in behavioral treatments of obesity: Diet, exercise, and combination interventions. *J. Am. Diet. Assoc.* 96: 342-346.

Sooman, A., Macintyre, S., and Anderson, A. 1993. Scotland's health–a more difficult challenge for some? The price and availability of healthy foods in socially contrasting localities in the west of Scotland. *Health Bull (Edinb)* 51(5): 276-284.

South Carolina Department of Education. 1998. Physical Education Institute. Columbia, SC: South Carolina Department of Education, 1-5.

Stearns, P.N. 1997. *Fat history: Bodies and beauty in the modern West.* New York: NYU Press.

Stephen, A.M., and Wald, N.J. 1990. Trends in individual consumption of dietary fat in the United States, 1920-1984. *Am. J. Clin. Nutr.* 52: 457-469.

Stephens, T. 1988. Physical activity and mental health in the United States and Canada: Evidence from four population surveys. *Prev. Med.* 17: 35-47.

Stock, M.J. 1997. Sibutramine: A review of the pharmacology of a novel anti-obesity agent. *Int. J. Obes. Relat. Metab. Disord.* 21: S25-S29.

Stofan, J.R., DiPietro, L., Davis, D., Kohl, H.W. 3rd., and Blair, S.N. 1998. Physical activity patterns associated with cardiorespiratory fitness and reduced mortality: The Aerobics Center Longitudinal Study. *Am. J. Public Health* 88: 1807-1813.

Sturm, R. 2002. The effects of obesity, smoking and drinking on medical problems and costs. Obesity outranks both smoking and drinking in its deleterious effects on health and health costs. *Health Aff (Millwood),* Mar-Apr 21 (2): 245-253.

Swinburn, B., Egger, G., and Raza, F. 1999. Dissecting obesogenic environments: The development and application of a framework for identifying and prioritizing environmental interventions for obesity. *Prev. Med.* 29 (6 pt. 1): 563-570.

Thompson, D., Edelsberg, J., Colditz, G.A., Bird, A.P., and Oster, G. 1999. Lifetime health and economic consequences of obesity. *Arch. Intern. Med.* 159 (18): 2177-2183.

Tremblay, A., Doucet, E., Imbeault, P., Maurige, P., Depres, J.P., and Richard, D. 1999. Metabolic fitness in active reduced-obese individuals. *Obes. Res.* 7: 556-563.

U.S. Department of Agriculture Center for Nutrition Policy and Promotion. 1998. Is total fat consumption really decreasing? *Nutrition insights: A publication of the USDA Center for Nutrition Policy and Promotion* 5 (April): 1-2.

U.S. Department of Agriculture (USDA). Data tables: Results from USDA's 1994-1996 continuing survey of Food Intakes by Individuals and 1994-1996 Diet and Health Knowledge Survey, December 1997 (www.barc.usda.gov/bhnrc/foodsurvey/home.htm).

U.S. Department of Health and Human Services (USDHHS). 1996. *Physical activity and health: A report of the Surgeon General.* Atlanta, GA: U.S. Department of Health and Human Services, Centers for Disease Control and Prevention, National Center for Chronic Disease Prevention and Health Promotion.

Van Gaal, L.F., Wauters, M.A., and De Leeuw, I.H. 1998. Anti-obesity drugs: What does sibutramine offer? An analysis of its potential contribution to obesity treatment. *Exp. Clin. Endocrinol. Diabetes* 106 (Suppl. 2): 35-40.

Wadden, T.A., Berkowitz, R.I., Vogt, R.A., Steen, S.N., Stunkard, A.J., and Foster, G.D. 1997. Lifestyle modification in the pharmacologic treatment of obesity: A pilot investigation of a primary care approach. *Obes. Res.* 5: 218-226.

Wadden, T.A., Berkowitz, R.I., Womble, L.G., Sarwer, D.B., Arnold, M.E., and Steinberg, C.M. 2000. Effects of sibutramine plus orlistat in obese women following 1 year of treatment by sibutramine alone: A placebo-controlled trial. *Obes. Res.* 8: 431-437.

Wang, G.J., Volkow, N.D., Logan, J., Pappas, N.R., Wong, C.T., Zhu, W., Netusil, N., and Fowler, J.S. 2001. Brain dopamine and obesity. *Lancet* 357: 354-357.

Wannamethee, S.G., Shaper, A.G., and Walker, M. 1998. Changes in physical activity, mortality, and incidence of coronary heart disease in older men. *Lancet* 351: 1603-1608.

Wei, M., Kampert, J.B., Barlow, C.E., Nichaman, M.Z., Gibbons, L.W., Paffenbarger, R.S., and Blair, S.N. 1999. Relationship between low cardiorespiratory fitness and mortality in normal-weight, overweight, and obese men. *JAMA* 282: 1547-1553.

Wetterling, T., and Müßigbrodt, H.E. 1999. Weight gain: Side effect of atypical neuroleptics? *J. Clin. Psychopharmacol.* 19: 316-321.

Weyerer, S. 1992. Physical inactivity and depression in the community: Evidence from the Upper Bavarian field study. *Int. J. Sports Med.* 13: 492-496.

Wing, R.R. 1998. Behavioral approaches to the treatment of obesity. In *Handbook of obesity,* eds. G.A. Bray, C. Bouchard, and W.P.T. James, 855-873. New York: Marcel Dekker.

Wirshing, D.A., Spellberg, B.J., Erhart, S.M., Marder, S.R., and Wirshing, W.C. 1998. Novel antipsychotics and new onset diabetes. *Biol. Psychiatry* 44: 778-783.

Wirshing, D.A., Wirshing, W.C., Kysar, L., Berisford, M.A., Goldstein, D., Pashdag, J., Mintz, J., and Marder, S.R. 1999. Novel antipsychotics: Comparison of weight gain liabilities. *J. Clin. Psychiatry* 60: 358-363.

Wolf, A.M., and Colditz, G.A. 1998. Current estimates of the economic cost of obesity in the United States. *Obes. Res.* 6 (2): 97-106.

World Health Organization (WHO). 1990. *Diet, nutrition, and the prevention of chronic diseases.* WHO Technical Report Series nr, 129-130. Geneva, Switzerland: Author.

World Health Organization (WHO). 1998. *Obesity: Preventing and managing the global epidemic.* Report of a WHO consultation on obesity. Geneva, Switzerland: Author.

Young, L.R., and Nestle, M. 1995. Portion sizes in dietary assessment: Issues and policy implications. *Nutr. Rev.* 53: 149-158.

Zhang, Y., Proenca, R., Maffei, M., Barone, M., Leopold L., and Friedman, J.M. 1994. Positional cloning of the mouse obese gene and its human homologue. *Nature* 372: 425.

Index

Note: The italicized *f* and *t* following page numbers refer to figures and tables, respectively.

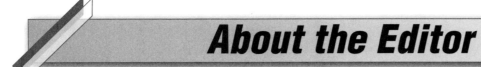

About the Editor

Ross Andersen, PhD, is associate director of fellowship training in the division of geriatric medicine at Johns Hopkins Medical Center. Since 1993, he has been conducting clinical trials examining the long-term effects of diet and exercise in helping people manage their weight. In addition, he has published several reports that have shaped current thinking about exercise for overweight individuals.

For 10 years Dr. Andersen operated community-based weight loss programs in health clubs, and he is the author of a book on how to implement weight loss programs in health club settings. He is a fellow of the American College of Sports Medicine (ACSM) and a member of the North American Association for the Study of Obesity (NAASO). He earned his PhD in exercise physiology at Temple University in 1992. He was a visiting scholar at the Cooper Institute in 1996.

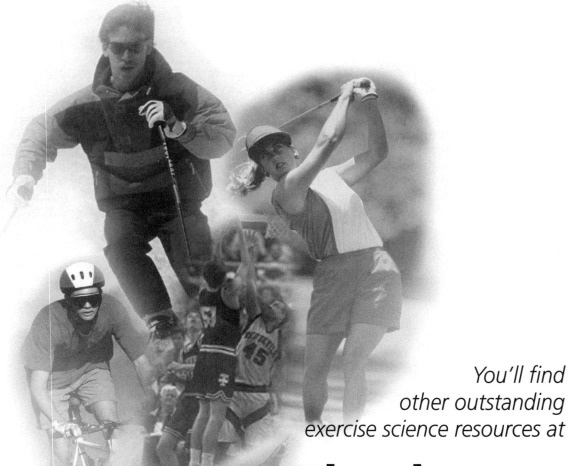

You'll find
other outstanding
exercise science resources at

www.HumanKinetics.com

In the U.S. call

1-800-747-4457

Australia... 08 8277 1555
Canada 1-800-465-7301
Europe...+44 (0) 113 255 5665
New Zealand..09-523-3462

 HUMAN KINETICS
The Information Leader in Physical Activity
P.O. Box 5076 • Champaign, IL 61825-5076 USA